Cracking the MRCS Part A

A unique revision guide aimed at candidates preparing for the MRCS examinations. The Part A exam tests knowledge of both basic science and the principles of surgery in general, and this textbook contains all the essential facts in one easy-to-read volume.

There is a focus on the most common questions asked pertaining to anatomy (representing 42% of the MRCS Part A paper 1) as well as other common areas frequently asked about in both the Part A and B examinations, although the focus of this book is the Part A examination. The Anatomy coverage includes line diagrams, short easy-to-recall text and bullet point lists to ensure that revision time is maximised for exam success. High-yield content in the areas of Physiology, Pathology, Pharmacology and Mathematics is also included.

The content has been designed specifically to help junior doctors memorise essential surgical facts, and further provides a convenient aide-memoire that will save hours of note taking. This will be particularly useful in the pressured run up to the MRCS examination.

T0138884

Cracking the MRCS Part A

A Revision Guide

Olivia A M Smith

MBBS (Hons), BSc (Hons), MSc (Dist),
PG cert, MRCS (Eng), MD
Plastic Surgery Registrar
South West Deanery, UK

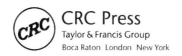

CRC Press is an imprint of the
Taylor & Francis Group, an **informa** business

First edition published 2024
by CRC Press
2385 NW Executive Center Drive, Suite 320, Boca Raton, FL 33431

and by CRC Press
4 Park Square, Milton Park, Abingdon, Oxon, OX14 4RN

CRC Press is an imprint of Taylor & Francis Group, LLC

ISBN: 9781032272627 (hbk)
ISBN: 9781032245126 (pbk)
ISBN: 9781003292005 (ebk)

DOI: 10.1201/9781003292005

Typeset in Palatino
by Apex CoVantage, LLC

In loving memory of my late father,
D.J.W. Smith.

To my mother—thank you for
supporting me every step of the way.

To those who have helped me over the years, you
know who you are, thank you.

Finally, to the surgical mentors who continue to inspire
me—with particular mention to the York Abdominal Wall Unit
(York Teaching Hospital) and the Department of Plastic, Reconstructive
& Burns Surgery, Southmead Hospital, Bristol.

Contents

Author

Olivia A M Smith MBBS (Hons) BSc Medical Sciences (Hons) MSc Human Anatomy (Dist) MD is a Plastic Surgery Registrar, South West Deanery, UK.

Acknowledgements

The author would like to thank the authors and publisher of *Bailey & Love's Essential Clinical Anatomy* (2019). Some line diagrams and clinical photographs originally published in *Bailey & Love's Essential Clinical Anatomy* have been used to illustrate much of the anatomy content, and the original contributions of John S P Lumley, John Craven, Peter Abrahams and Richard Tunstall are gratefully acknowledged.

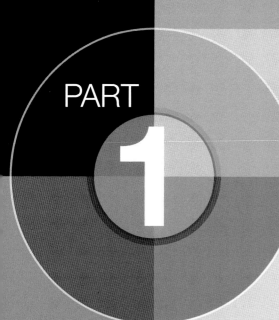

PART

1

ANATOMY

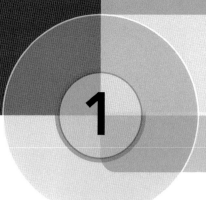

The Upper Limb and Breast

1

OSTEOLOGY OF THE CLAVICLE

The clavicle is a long, "s"-shaped bone that extends between the sternum and the scapula. The clavicle functions to transmit forces between the upper limb and axial skeleton. It is the first bone to ossify in the fetus (membranous ossification); a secondary ossification centre develops during the teenage years. It gains its name from the Latin *clavicula*, meaning "little key", which is what it looks like when rotated along its long axis. To identify which clavicle is the right or left clavicle, please note that the medial two-thirds are rounded and convex anteriorly whereas the lateral third is flat and convex posteriorly. The inferior surface of the clavicle is rough due to insertions of ligaments. The sternal end of the clavicle has a facet for the sternoclavicular joint. Laterally, the clavicle articulates with the acromion at the acromioclavicular joint. Six muscles are attached to the clavicle: medially, the clavicular head of the pectoralis major as well as a portion of the sternohyoid and the clavicular head of the sternocleidomastoid; laterally, the clavicular heads of the deltoid and trapezius insert. Within the clavicular groove inserts the subclavius. The subclavius protects the underlying subclavian vessels in the event of clavicular fractures (Figure 1.1).

CLINICAL POINTS

The clavicle is frequently fractured, typically between the middle and lateral third of the bone, i.e. always between the costoclavicular ligament and the coracoclavicular ligament (made up of the trapezoid and conoid ligament). When fractured, the trapezius cannot support the weight of the arm, leading to sagging. In addition to this, the pectoralis major abducts and medially rotates the upper limb. Therefore, the lateral fracture fragment is moved medially. The sternocleidomastoid elevates the medial fracture fragment.

OSTEOLOGY OF THE SCAPULA

This is a flat, triangular bone that lies on the postero-lateral surface of the thorax overlying ribs 2–7. The spine of the scapula unevenly divides the posterior surface of the scapula into the supraspinous fossa and the larger infraspinous fossa. The subscapular fossa is

DOI: 10.1201/9781003292005-2

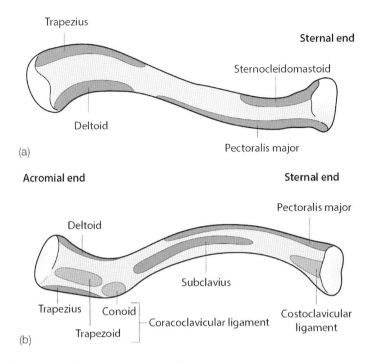

Figure 1.1 The clavicle: (a) superior surface; (b) inferior surface.

present on the anterior surface of the scapula. These fossae provide attachment for various muscles:

1. *Supraspinous fossa*—supraspinatus muscle
2. *Infraspinous fossa*—infraspinatus muscle
3. *Subscapular fossa*—subscapularis muscle

The spine of the scapula continues laterally as the acromion, articulating with the clavicle. The lateral border of the acromion has ridges formed by the attachment of the central portion of the deltoid muscle. The deltoid tubercle of the spine of the scapula is the medial point of attachment of the deltoid muscle.

The scapula has a glenoid cavity which articulates with the humeral head forming the glenohumeral joint. It is shallow, concave and oval. The socket accepts about 1/3 of the humeral head, thereby making the upper limb mobile but prone to dislocation. The glenoid labrum is a rim of fibrocartilage that serves to deepen the glenoid fossa. At its superior aspect is the supraglenoid tubercle which provides attachment for the long head of the biceps (within the capsule of the shoulder joint). Below the glenoid cavity is the infraglenoid tubercle, which provides the origin for the long head of the triceps.

The coracoid process is a beak-like process that provides attachment for three ligaments and three muscles listed here.

LIGAMENTS:

1. Coracoclavicular ligament
2. Coracoacromial ligament
3. Coracohumeral ligament

MUSCLES:

1. Pectoralis minor
2. Short head of the biceps
3. Coracobrachialis

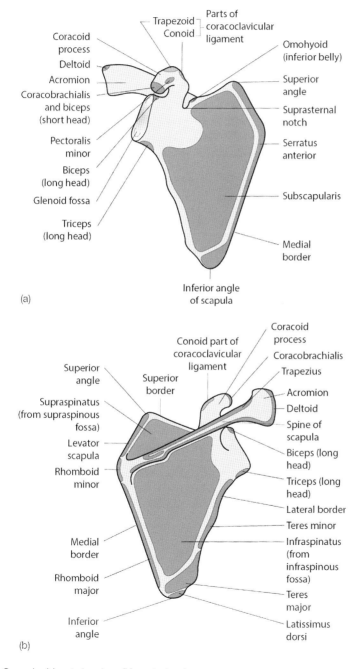

Figure 1.2 Scapula: (a) anterior view; (b) posterior view.

OSTEOLOGY OF THE HUMERUS

This is a long bone which articulates with the scapula at the glenohumeral joint and with the radius and ulna at the elbow joint.

The proximal end of the humerus has a distended head as well as two necks—an anatomical neck and a surgical neck. The anatomical neck indicates the line of attachment of the capsule of the shoulder joint (except medially where the capsule extends distally ~2 cm). The surgical neck is the narrow portion between the distended head and the shaft of the humerus. The axillary nerve and posterior circumflex humeral vessels lie against the surgical neck and may be injured here during fractures.

The greater (lateral) and lesser (projects anteriorly) tubercles form attachments for various muscles. The tubercles are separated by the bicipital groove. The tendon of the long head of the biceps muscle lies within this groove. The greater tubercle has three facets for the insertion of three of the following rotator cuff muscles—the supraspinatus, infraspinatus and teres minor. The lesser tubercle provides attachment for the remaining rotator cuff muscle, the subscapularis. The greater and lesser tubercles extend distally to form the lateral and medial lips of the bicipital groove. The lateral lip provides attachment for the pectoralis major, whereas the medial lip provides attachment for the teres major. The tendon of the latissimus dorsi inserts on the floor of the bicipital groove.

Important features of the shaft of the humerus include the radial (or spiral) groove and the deltoid tuberosity. The radial nerve and profunda brachii vessels lie in this groove and pass between the medial and lateral heads of the triceps. These structures may be injured in midshaft fractures of the humerus. The lateral head of the triceps originates from above the spiral groove, whereas the medial head originates below it. The deltoid tuberosity is "v"-shaped and is situated at the middle of the lateral side of the radial shaft. It provides attachment for the deltoid muscle.

Distally, the humerus widens to become the medial epicondyle and the less prominent lateral epicondyle. The epicondyles are extra-capsular and subcutaneous. The medial epicondyle has a groove in which runs the ulnar nerve. The medial epicondyle and lateral epicondyle provide the common origin of the flexors and the extensors of the forearm respectively. The capitulum of the humerus articulates with the radial head, whereas the trochlea (located medially) articulates with the trochlear notch of the ulna.

CLINICAL POINTS

There are three nerves that are related to the humerus that may be injured during fractures.

- *The axillary nerve*—fracture of the surgical neck of the humerus.
  The axillary nerve innervates the deltoid and teres minor muscles; therefore, injury causes weakness of shoulder abduction and external rotation.
- *The radial nerve*—fracture of the humeral shaft.
  The consequence of radial nerve paralysis is the inability to extend the wrist, i.e. "wrist drop", loss of extension of the fingers at the metacarpophalangeal joints and inability to extend and abduct the thumb. There may also be pain, numbness and/or paraesthesia affecting the dorsum of the hand/dorsum of the lateral three and a half digits i.e. in the distribution of the superficial branch of the radial nerve.
- *The ulnar nerve*—fractures involving the distal humerus.
  Consequences of ulnar nerve damage at this level may include paraesthesia and numbness in the ulnar nerve distribution, i.e. the little and ring fingers, hyperextension at the metacarpophalangeal joints and flexion at the proximal and distal interphalangeal joints with an inability to move the little and ring finger.

Note that the musculocutaneous nerve runs between the biceps and brachialis muscles and therefore is not in direct contact with the humerus and thus is not prone to injury during fractures of the humeral shaft.

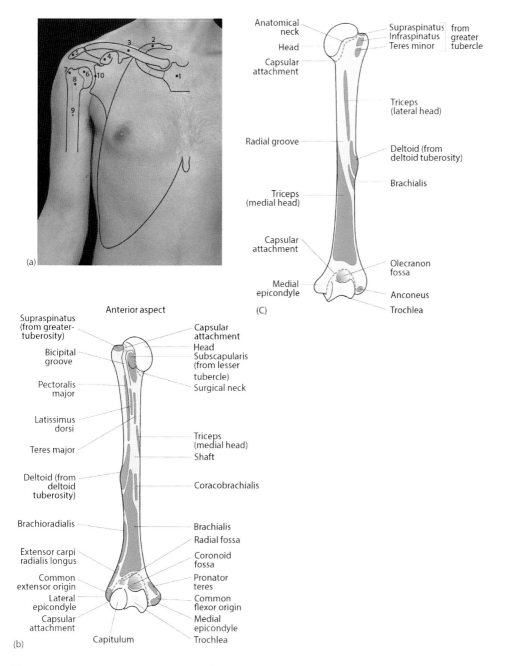

Figure 1.3 Bones of the shoulder joint. (a) Surface anatomy: 1, manubrium sterni; 2, first rib; 3, clavicle; 4, coracoid process; 5, acromion; 6, head of the humerus; 7, greater tuberosity; 8, intertubercular groove; 9, shaft of humerus; 10, glenoid fossa; (b) humerus anterior view and (c) humerus posterior view, each showing features, muscle attachments and capsular attachments.

OSTEOLOGY OF THE RADIUS AND ULNA

The ulna is larger at its proximal end, where it articulates with the humerus and the head of the radius. It has two prominent projections—the olecranon, which receives the triceps tendon, and the coronoid process, which provides insertion for the brachialis muscle. An olecranon bursa lies over the olecranon process and may become inflamed, causing "student's elbow". A small triangular muscle called the anconeus originates from the posterior surface of the lateral epicondyle and inserts into the lateral aspect of the olecranon. The medial aspect of the olecranon provides attachment for the flexor digitorum profundus. Proximal to this insertion is the attachment of the ulnar collateral ligament.

Just inferior to the coronoid process is the ulnar tuberosity where the brachialis attaches. The pronator teres is attached to the medial aspect of the coronoid process. There is a thin lip on the coronoid process that provides attachment for the articular capsule. Medially, this lip is more prominent and is called the sublime tubercle. The sublime tubercle provides another attachment for the flexor digitorum superficialis (in addition to the common flexor origin, i.e. the medial epicondyle of the humerus and the anterior oblique line of the radius).

The radial notch of the ulna articulates with the radial head. The margins of the notch receive attachments of the annular ligament. The quadrate ligament attaches inferior to this. Below this is the supinator fossa and an accompanying crest called the supinator crest. The pronator quadratus originates from the medial, anterior surface of the ulna and inserts into the lateral, anterior surface of the radius. Distally, the bone tapers into the ulnar head with a projection called the ulnar styloid process. There is a groove next to the styloid process which transmits the tendon of the extensor carpi ulnaris. The ulna is not part of the wrist joint, and the triangular fibrocartilage complex separates the radioulnar joint from the wrist joint.

The radius is the lateral and shorter of the two forearm bones. Its styloid process extends distally, and contributes to the wrist joint by articulating with the scaphoid and the lunate carpal bones. Proximally it has a radial head, neck and tuberosity. The head articulates with the capitulum of the humerus and with the radial notch of the ulna. The neck of the radius is distal to the head and there is an oval tuberosity projecting towards the ulna called the radial tuberosity. Here the biceps tendon inserts along the posterior lip of the radial tuberosity. The anterior oblique line is a ridge that extends from the radial tuberosity to the pronator tubercle. The posterior oblique line is found on the extensor surface of the radial shaft. Between these two lines is the insertion of supinator (this muscle has two heads—one from the lateral epicondyle and one from ulnar supinator crest and fossa). The deep branch of the radial nerve travels into the posterior forearm through the heads of the supinator muscle and emerges as the posterior interosseous nerve. The pronator teres inserts in an impression just distal to the insertion of the supinator muscle. This has clinical relevance in fractures of the radius. If the radius is fractured proximally to its attachment, then the proximal fragment is supinated due to the action of the biceps muscle and the distal fragment is pronated by the pronator teres.

Below the radial tuberosity, medially there is a sharp ridge for the insertion of the interosseous membrane. The fibres of the interosseous membrane pass inferiorly towards the ulna. The function of the interosseous membrane is to aid in the transmission of force from the hand. Distally, the radius is rectangular in appearance. There is a notch for articulation with the head of the ulna. Laterally the radial styloid process projects and here the lateral collateral ligament of the wrist joint attaches. The tendon of the brachioradialis inserts into the base of the radial styloid process. The posterior surface of the distal radius is characterised by a tubercle called Lister's tubercle. There are grooves on either side of this tubercle. The groove lateral to this tubercle houses the tendons of the extensor carpi radialis longus and brevis. Medially the groove is for the tendon of the extensor pollicis longus (for which the tubercle acts as a pulley).

CLINICAL POINTS

- Partial dislocation of the radial head through the annular ligament is also known as pulled elbow and can occur in children with a history of pulled arm.
- If the radius is fractured proximal to its attachment, then the proximal fragment is supinated due to the action of the biceps muscle and the distal fragment is pronated by the pronator teres.
- The radial styloid process always extends further distally (~1 cm) than the ulnar styloid process, and this relationship is disturbed in fractures and may be seen on radiographs.

OSTEOLOGY OF THE HAND

The hand is comprised of carpal bones, metacarpal bones and phalanges. There are eight carpal bones that are arranged in proximal and distal rows each containing four bones. Characteristics of these bones are outlined herein.

PROXIMAL ROW

- *Scaphoid*—boat shaped and forms part of the wrist joint. It has a prominent scaphoid tubercle which is palpable. It is the most frequently fractured carpal bone. The proximal bone has a poor blood supply and fractures may result in avascular necrosis.
- *Lunate*—moon shaped and articulates with the distal end of the radius at the wrist joint. It is the most frequently dislocated carpal bone (displacing anteriorly because it is broad anteriorly).
- *Triquetral*—pyramidal in shape. It articulates with the triangular fibrocartilage.
- *Pisiform*—pea-shaped bone which is within the tendon of the flexor carpi ulnaris.

DISTAL ROW

- *Trapezium*—table-shaped bone. Trapezium sits under the thumb. It has a saddle-shaped articular surface for the thumb metacarpal. It has a ridge and a groove on its palmar surface. The tendon of the flexor carpi radialis runs in this groove and then attaches to the base of the second metacarpal bone. The radial artery is related to the dorsal aspect of the trapezium and then passes between the two heads of the first dorsal interosseous muscle.
- *Trapezoid*—wedge-shaped bone.
- *Capitate*—largest of the carpal bones.
- *Hamate*—has a hook which extends anteriorly and is palpable. There is a groove on the distal surface of the base of the hamate hook where the deep branch of the ulnar nerve makes contact with the hamate. The ulnar nerve can be damaged here during hamate fractures or in handlebar neuropathy, where cyclists put pressure on the hook of the hamate when gripping handlebars with the hand in an extended position.

There are five metacarpal bones consisting of a base, shaft and head. The third metacarpal head is the most prominent and is characterised by a styloid process at the lateral aspect of its base. Fractures of the fifth metacarpal head are known as boxer's fractures. Each digit has three phalanges except for the thumb which has two.

Clinical Points

- The boundaries of the anatomical snuff box are the abductor pollicis longus and extensor pollicis brevis radially and the extensor pollicis longus on the ulnar side. The floor comprises the following bones from proximal to distal: the styloid process of the radius, the scaphoid, the trapezium and the base of the first metacarpal bone.

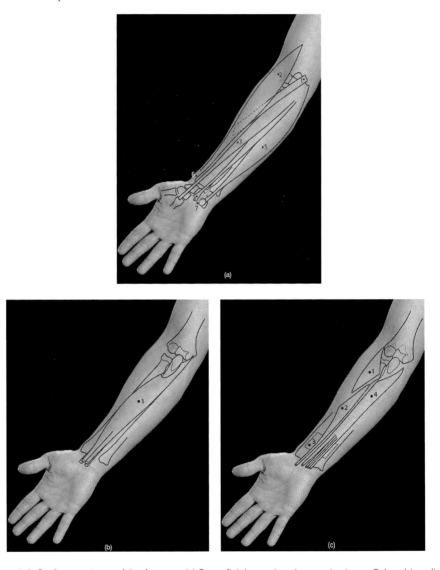

Figure 1.4 Surface anatomy of the forearm. (a) Superficial muscles: 1, pronator teres; 2, brachioradialis; 3, flexor carpi radialis; 4, palmaris longus; 5, flexor carpi ulnaris; 6, radial artery; 7, ulnar artery. (b) Intermediate muscles: 1, flexor digitorum superficialis. (c) Deep muscles: 1, supinator; 2, flexor pollicis longus; 3, pronator quadratus; 4, flexor digitorum profundus.

- The contents of the anatomical snuff box include the radial artery, the superficial branch of the radial nerve and the cephalic vein.
- Scaphoid bone avascular necrosis—this typically occurs at the proximal pole and is due to the relatively poor blood supply to this area. Typically, this bone is supplied from distal to proximal via branches of the radial artery. Fractures of the scaphoid disrupt this blood supply.
- The carpal bones are structured so that they form a curve, meaning that bones at the sides of the curve provide attachment for the flexor retinaculum.
- The flexor retinaculum attaches to:
  - The tubercle of the scaphoid and the lateral ridge of the trapezium on the radial aspect
  - The hook of the hamate and the pisiform on the ulnar aspect

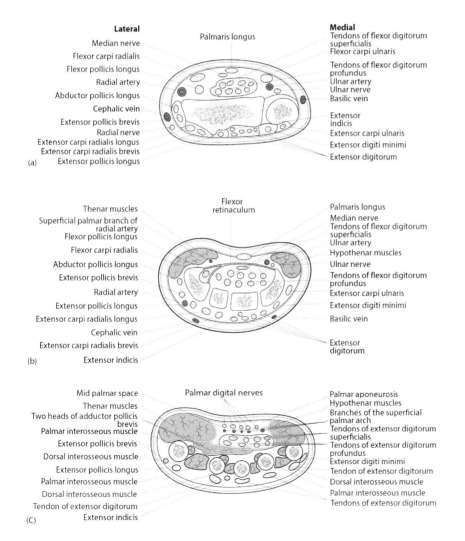

Figure 1.5 Transverse sections, viewed from below, through: (a) the right wrist; (b) the proximal carpus at the level of the flexor retinaculum; (c) the right palm at the mid-metacarpal level.

This results in the formation of a tunnel called the carpal tunnel
- The carpal tunnel contains 10 structures:
  - The median nerve—which may be compressed resulting in carpal tunnel syndrome
  - Tendons of the:
    - Flexor pollicis longus (1)
    - Flexor digitorum superficialis (4)
    - Flexor digitorum profundus (4)

MUSCLES OF THE PECTORAL GIRDLE

Summary of the Muscles of the Shoulder (Excluding the Rotator Cuff Muscles)

Muscle	Proximal attachment	Distal attachment	Innervation	Action
Pectoralis major	Clavicular head—medial aspect of the clavicle Sternal head—sternum, superior six costal cartilages and the external oblique aponeurosis	Lateral lip of the bicipital groove of the humerus	Medial and lateral pectoral nerves	Adducts humerus, flexes humerus and medially rotates humerus Draws scapula anteriorly
Pectoralis minor	Ribs 3–5	Coracoid process	Medial pectoral nerve	Stabilises scapula Assists serratus anterior in protraction of the scapula
Serratus anterior	Ribs 1–8	Medial border of the scapula	Long thoracic nerve	Protracts and rotates scapula
Subclavius	Costochondral junction of first rib	Subclavian groove	Nerve to subclavius	Stabilises clavicle
Trapezius	Superior nuchal line, nuchal ligament, external occipital protuberance, C7-T12 spinous processes	Lateral 1/3 of clavicle, acromion, spine of scapula	Spinal accessory nerve	Elevation, depression and retraction of scapula Superior rotation of the glenoid fossa
Latissimus dorsi	Spinous processes of T6–12, thoracolumbar fascia, iliac crest, ribs 9–12	Floor of the bicipital groove	Thoracodorsal nerve	It is the climber's muscle, so it adducts, extends and medially rotates the humerus

Muscle	Proximal attachment	Distal attachment	Innervation	Action
Levator scapulae	Transverse processes of C1–4	Medial border and superior angle of scapula	Dorsal scapular nerve	Elevates the scapula
Rhomboid major	Spinous processes of T2–5	Medial border of scapula	Dorsal scapular nerve	Retracts and rotates scapula
Rhomboid minor	Spinous process of C7–T11 and the nuchal ligament	Spine of the scapula	Dorsal scapular nerve	Retracts and rotates scapula
Deltoid	Clavicle, acromion and spine of scapula	Deltoid tuberosity	Axillary nerve	Anterior portion— flexes and medially rotates humerus Middle portion— arm abduction Posterior portion—extends and laterally rotates humerus
Teres major	Inferior angle of scapula	Medial lip of the bicipital groove	Lower subscapular nerve	Adducts and medially rotates humerus

CLINICAL POINTS

- The lower medial aspect of the pectoralis major is thinner and therefore more prone to rupture. The perforating branches of the internal thoracic artery are prone to damage during subpectoral dissection.
- The pectoralis minor muscle is largely functionally unimportant, but it is a very important landmark muscle for the levels of the axillary lymph nodes and the branches of the axillary artery.
- The levels of the axillary lymph nodes are:
  - *Level 1*—nodes inferior to pectoralis minor
  - *Level 2*—nodes behind/posterior to pectoralis minor
  - *Level 3*—nodes above/medial to pectoralis minor
- The axillary artery is split into three parts based on its relationship to the pectoralis minor muscle:
  - *First part*—superior to the pectoralis minor
  - *Second part*—posterior to the pectoralis minor
  - *Third part*—inferior to the pectoralis minor
- The branches of the axillary artery are frequently examined and may be remembered by the mnemonic "Screw The Lawyer Save A Patient":
  - *First part (1 branch)*—superior thoracic artery
  - *Second part (2 branches)*—thoraco-acromial artery, lateral thoracic artery
  - *Third part (3 branches)*—subscapular artery, anterior circumflex humeral artery, posterior circumflex humeral artery

- The axillary artery continues as the brachial artery at the inferior border of the teres major muscle.
- The subclavius muscle serves to protect the subclavian vein when the clavicle is fractured.
- When the long thoracic nerve (C5–7) is damaged, the serratus anterior muscle is paralysed, and this results in winging of the scapula.
- The axillary nerve tends to be damaged in fractures of the surgical neck of the humerus and in inferior dislocation of the glenohumeral joint. This causes atrophy of the deltoid muscle and loss of sensation in the regimental patch distribution.
- The clavipectoral fascia is an important structure that lies between the pectoralis minor and the subclavius muscle and serves to protect the axillary artery, vein and nerve. This fascia is pierced by four things that can be remembered as two inwards and two outwards.
  - *Two inwards*—lymphatics from the infraclavicular nodes (drain to the apical nodes) and the cephalic vein
  - *Two outwards*—the lateral pectoral nerve and the thoraco-acromial artery

THE ROTATOR CUFF

Four muscles comprise the rotator cuff, and they may be remembered by the mnemonic "**SITS**". Their attachments, innervation and actions are summarised in the table below.

Rotator Cuff Muscles

Muscle	Proximal attachment	Distal attachment	Innervation	Action
Supraspinatus	Supraspinous fossa	Greater tubercle of the humerus	Suprascapular nerve	Initiates arm abduction
Infraspinatus	Infraspinous fossa	Greater tubercle of the humerus	Suprascapular nerve	Laterally rotates arm
Teres minor	Lateral border of scapular	Greater tubercle of the humerus	Axillary nerve	Laterally rotates arm
Subscapularis	Subscapular fossa	Lesser tubercle of humerus	Upper and lower subscapular nerves	Medially rotates arm Adducts arm

CLINICAL POINTS

- Rotator cuff injuries and how they present are common in the MRCS examination; therefore, it is important that you familiarise yourself with the mechanism of action of each muscle and how loss of its action would present clinically.

POSTERIOR SHOULDER SPACES

Posterior shoulder spaces are also frequently asked about in Multiple Choice Questions (MCQs). They will now be discussed. Familiarise yourself with their boundaries and contents.

Posterior Shoulder Spaces

Shoulder space	Boundaries	Contents
Quadrangular space	*Superiorly*—teres minor *Inferiorly*—teres major *Laterally*—surgical neck of the humerus *Medially*—long head of the triceps	Axillary nerve Posterior circumflex humeral artery
Upper triangular space	*Superiorly*—teres minor *Inferiorly*—teres major *Laterally*—long head of the triceps	Circumflex scapular artery (branch of the scapular artery)
Lower triangular space (also called the triangular interval)	*Superiorly*—teres major *Laterally*—medial head of the triceps *Medially*—long head of the triceps	Radial nerve Deep brachial artery

MUSCLES OF THE ARM

Summary of Muscles of the Arm

Muscle	Proximal attachment	Distal attachment	Innervation	Action
Coracobrachialis	Coracoid process	Humerus	Musculocutaneous nerve	Flexes and adducts arm
Biceps brachii	Long head—supraglenoid tubercle Short head—coracoid process	Radial tuberosity	Musculocutaneous nerve	Flexes arm Flexes forearm Supinates
Brachialis	Distal humerus, medial supracondylar ridge	Ulnar tuberosity	Musculocutaneous nerve	Flexes forearm
Triceps brachii	Long head—infraglenoid tubercle Lateral head—lateral to radial groove Medial head—medial to radial groove	Olecranon process	Radial nerve	Extends forearm
Anconeus	Lateral epicondyle	Olecranon process	Radial nerve	Extends forearm

MUSCLES OF THE FOREARM

Summary of Muscles of the Forearm

Muscle	Proximal attachment	Distal attachment	Innervation	Action
Pronator teres	Medial epicondyle of the humerus and the coronoid process of the ulna	Middle of the radius	Median nerve	Pronates elbow Flexes elbow
Flexor carpi radialis	Medial epicondyle of the humerus	Second metacarpal	Median nerve	Flexes wrist Abducts hand
Palmaris longus (absent in up to 10% population)	Medial epicondyle of the humerus	Flexor retinaculum and palmar aponeurosis	Median nerve	Flexes wrist
Flexor carpi ulnaris	Medial epicondyle of the humerus, olecranon process and posterior ulna	Pisiform (sesamoid bone), hook of hamate, fifth metacarpal	Ulnar nerve	Flexes wrist Adducts hand
Flexor digitorum superficialis	Medial epicondyle of the humerus, ulnar coronoid process and anterior radius	Middle phalanges of medial four digits	Median nerve	Flexes proximal interphalangeal joints of the medial four digits, flexes metacarpophalangeal joints and flexes wrist
Flexor digitorum profundus	Ulna and interosseous membrane, deep fascia of the forearm	Base of the distal phalanges of medial four digits	Medial portion— ulnar nerve Lateral portion— median nerve (anterior interosseous nerve)	Flexes distal interphalangeal joints of the medial four digits, flexes wrist
Flexor pollicis longus	Radius and interosseous membrane	Distal phalanx of thumb	Median nerve (anterior interosseous nerve)	Flexes thumb
Pronator quadratus	Distal ulna	Distal radius	Median nerve (anterior interosseous nerve)	Pronates forearm

Muscle	Proximal attachment	Distal attachment	Innervation	Action
Brachioradialis	Lateral supracondylar ridge of the humerus	Styloid process of the radius	Radial nerve	Flexes forearm at the elbow joint
Extensor carpi radialis longus	Lateral supracondylar ridge of the humerus	Second metacarpal	Radial nerve	Extends hand at the wrist joint Abducts wrist
Extensor carpi radialis brevis	Lateral epicondyle of the humerus	Third metacarpal	Radial nerve (deep)	Extends hand at the wrist joint Abducts hand at the wrist joint
Extensor digitorum	Lateral epicondyle of the humerus	Extensor expansion of the medial four digits	Radial nerve (posterior interosseous)	Extends medial four digits
Extensor digiti minimi	Lateral epicondyle of the humerus	Extensor expansion of the fifth digit	Radial nerve (posterior interosseous)	Extends fifth digit
Extensor carpi ulnaris	Lateral epicondyle of the humerus and ulna	Fifth metacarpal	Radial nerve (posterior interosseous)	Extends hand at the wrist joint Adducts hand at the wrist joint
Supinator	Lateral epicondyle of the humerus, radial collateral ligament, supinator crest and supinator fossa of the ulna	Proximal radius	Radial nerve (deep)	Supinates forearm
Abductor pollicis longus	Ulna, radius and interosseous membrane	First metacarpal	Radial nerve (posterior interosseous)	Abducts thumb
Extensor pollicis longus	Ulna and interosseous membrane	Distal phalanx of thumb	Radial nerve (posterior interosseous)	Extends thumb
Extensor pollicis brevis	Radius and interosseous membrane	Proximal phalanx of thumb	Radial nerve (posterior interosseous)	Extends thumb
Extensor indicis	Ulna and interosseous membrane	Extensor expansion of the second digit	Radial nerve (posterior interosseous)	Extends second digit

CLINICAL POINTS

- The extensor tendons at the level of the wrist are divided into six extensor compartments which are described from lateral to medial as:
  - I—abductor pollicis longus (APL), extensor pollicis brevis (EPB)
  - II—extensor carpi radialis longus (ECRL), extensor carpi radialis brevis (ECRB)
  - III—extensor pollicis longus (EPL)
  - IV—extensor digitorum (ED), extensor indicis (EI)
  - V—extensor digiti minimi (EDM)
  - VI—extensor carpi ulnaris (ECU)
- Note that compartments II and III are divided by Lister's tubercle
- The ECU runs in the groove of the ulnar head.
- The radial nerve innervates the BEST muscles—brachioradialis, the extensors, supinator muscles and the triceps muscles.
- The cubital fossa is another space which is frequently asked about in MRCS examinations. Its boundaries are as follows:
  - *Superiorly*—a line drawn between the medial and lateral epicondyles
  - *Medially*—pronator teres
  - *Laterally*—brachioradialis
  - *Floor*—brachialis and supinator muscles
  - *Roof*—bicipital aponeurosis and the deep fascia of the forearm and skin
- The contents of the cubital fossa from lateral to medial are:
  - The biceps tendon
  - The brachial artery (with its venae comitantes)
  - The median nerve
- The cubital tunnel transmits the ulnar nerve, and this nerve may be compressed here (amongst other areas which will be discussed later in the chapter). The roof of this tunnel is formed from an aponeurotic expansion between the two heads of the flexor carpi ulnaris. The floor is formed by the medial collateral ligament of the elbow.

Tests for Ulnar Nerve Motor Function

Muscle innervated by ulnar nerve	Test	Sign if positive result
FCU	Flex wrist in ulnar direction against resistance	Weakness
FDP (ulnar portion)	Flexion at the distal interphalangeal joint (DIPJ) of the fifth finger against resistance	Weakness
Abductor digiti minimi	Abduction of the little finger against resistance	Weakness
First dorsal interosseous	Index finger abduction against resistance	Weakness
Adductor pollicis	Pinch a piece of paper between the thumb and index finger	Froment's sign—the thumb interphalangeal joint will flex if the adductor pollicis muscle is weak
Third palmar interosseous and small finger lumbricals	Adduct all fingers	Wartenberg's sign—small finger begins to abduct relative to other digits

MUSCLES OF THE HAND

Summary of Muscles of the Hand

Muscle	Proximal attachment	Distal attachment	Innervation	Action
Opponens pollicis	Flexor retinaculum and trapezium	First metacarpal	Recurrent branch of the median nerve	Rotates and pulls first metacarpal medially
Abductor pollicis	Flexor retinaculum, trapezium and scaphoid	Proximal phalanx of the thumb	Recurrent branch of the median nerve	Abducts thumb Aids opposition
Flexor pollicis brevis	Flexor retinaculum and trapezium	Proximal phalanx of the thumb	Superficial head—recurrent branch of the median nerve Deep head—deep branch of ulnar nerve	Flexes thumb
Adductor pollicis	Oblique head—second and third metacarpals, capitate and adjacent carpal bones Transverse head—third metacarpal	Proximal phalanx of the thumb	Deep branch of the ulnar nerve	Adducts thumb
Abductor digiti minimi	Pisiform	Proximal phalanx of fifth digit	Deep branch of the ulnar nerve	Abducts fifth digit
Flexor digiti minimi	Flexor retinaculum and hamate	Proximal phalanx of fifth digit	Deep branch of the ulnar nerve	Flexes fifth digit
Opponens digiti minimi	Flexor retinaculum and hamate	Fifth metacarpal	Deep branch of the ulnar nerve	Opposes fifth digit
First and second lumbricals	Tendons of the flexor digitorum profundus	Extensor expansion of the second to fifth digits	Median nerve	Flexes digits at the metacarpophalangeal joints and extends at the interphalangeal joints
Third and fourth lumbricals	Tendons of the flexor digitorum profundus	Extensor expansion of the second to fifth digits	Deep branch of the ulnar nerve	Flexes digits at the metacarpophalangeal joints and extends at the interphalangeal joints

(Continued)

Summary of Muscles of the Hand (Continued)

Muscle	Proximal attachment	Distal attachment	Innervation	Action
Palmar interossei	Second, fourth and fifth metacarpals (none insert at the third)	Proximal phalanges and extensor expansions of second, fourth and fifth digits	Deep branch of the ulnar nerve	Adducts second, fourth and fifth digits Flexes digits at the metacarpophalangeal joints and extends at the interphalangeal joints *Remember PAD and DAB—palmar interossei adduct and dorsal interossei abduct*
Dorsal interossei	Metacarpals	Proximal phalanges and extensor expansions of second, third and fourth digits	Deep branch of ulnar nerve	Abducts second, third and fourth digits Flexes digits at the metacarpophalangeal joints and extends at the interphalangeal joints

KEY POINTS CONCERNING ARTERIES OF THE UPPER LIMB

THE AXILLARY ARTERY

The axillary artery is a continuation of the subclavian artery and starts at the lateral border of the first rib.

It becomes the brachial artery at the inferior border of the teres major muscle.

It is divided into three parts by the pectoralis minor muscle. Each part of the axillary artery gives off one, two and three branches respectively.

The branches of the axillary artery are the superior thoracic artery, the thoraco-acromial artery, the lateral thoracic artery, the subscapular artery, the anterior circumflex humeral artery and the posterior circumflex humeral artery.

THE BRACHIAL ARTERY

The brachial artery the continuation of the axillary artery. It splits into its terminal branches, the radial and the ulnar artery at the level of the radial neck. Its branches are:

- The deep brachial artery (profunda). This artery accompanies the radial nerve in the spiral groove.
- The superior and inferior ulnar collateral arteries.
- The nutrient branch.

THE RADIAL ARTERY

- Starts at the radial neck.
- It lies on the biceps tendon.
- In the forearm it lies between the brachioradialis and flexor carpi radialis.
- In the wrist it may be palpated between the tendon of the brachioradialis and the flexor carpi radialis.
- It provides a branch which contributes to the superficial palmar arch and also contributes to the deep palmar arch.
- It may be palpated in the anatomical snuff box.
- It pierces the first dorsal interosseous muscle and the adductor pollicis.

THE ULNAR ARTERY

- Passes deep to the muscles of the common flexor origin and lies on the flexor digitorum profundus.
- The median nerve superficially crosses this artery.
- In the forearm, it passes between the tendons of flexor carpi ulnaris and flexor digitorum superificialis, passing over the flexor retinaculum through Guyon's canal and then contributing to the superficial palmar arch.
- Distally, the ulnar nerve is always medial to the artery.

VEINS OF THE UPPER LIMB

The basilic and cephalic veins are the main venous drainage for both the arm and hand.

The basilic vein commences on the medial aspect of the dorsal venous network of the hand. It is superficial for much of its course and joins the cephalic vein at the cubital fossa. The cephalic vein drains the dorsal venous network that crosses the anatomical snuff box.

The cephalic vein drains to the axillary vein and the median cubital vein.

Halfway up the humerus the basilic vein passes deep to the muscles, and at the inferior aspect of the teres major muscles the anterior and posterior circumflex humeral veins drain into it. The basilic vein and the venae comitantes of the brachial artery join to form the axillary vein. The axillary vein continues as the subclavian vein from the outer border of the first rib to the medial border of the anterior scalene muscle.

Path of the Cephalic v Basilic Vein

Vein	Path
Cephalic vein	Through snuff box to ascend lateral aspect of arm
	Communicates with median cubital vein
	Runs along deltopectoral groove
	Enters clavipectoral triangle
	Pierces clavipectoral fascia to drain to the axillary vein
Basilic vein	Medial aspect of arm
	Deep when piercing brachial fascia but runs parallel and superior to brachial artery

THE BRACHIAL PLEXUS

The brachial plexus extends from the neck to the axilla. It has contributions from C5–T1. The plexus may be pre-fixed or post-fixed if it receives contributions from C4 or T2 respectively. The sections of the brachial plexus are the roots, trunks, divisions, cords and branches, which may be remembered by the mnemonic: "Reach To Drink Cold Beer". The roots are located posterior to scalenus anterior, the trunks traverse the lower part of the posterior triangle, the divisions lie posterior to the clavicle and the cords embrace the axillary artery posterior to the pectoralis minor. There are three terminal cords: the lateral cord (musculocutaneous nerve and a contribution to the median nerve), the medial cord (ulnar nerve and a contribution to the median nerve) and the posterior cord (axillary nerve and radial nerve).

The following image and table provide an illustration of the plexus as well as the muscles innervated.

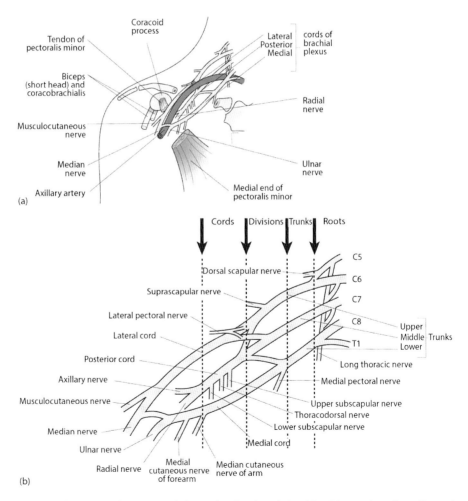

Figure 1.6 (a) Diagram of the brachial plexus showing the relationship of the cords to the axillary artery with a segment of clavicle and pectoralis minor removed. (b) Brachial plexus—diagram showing its roots, trunks, divisions, cords and branches.

Summary of Nerves of the Brachial Plexus*

Nerve	Origin	Muscle innervated
Dorsal scapular nerve	C5	Rhomboids major and minor Levator scapulae
Long thoracic nerve	C5,6,7	Serratus anterior
Suprascapular nerve	C5,6	Supraspinatus Infraspinatus
Nerve to subclavius	C5,6	Subclavius
Lateral pectoral nerve	Lateral cord C5,6,7	Pectoralis major
Musculocutaneous nerve	Lateral cord C5,6,7	Anterior compartment of the arm
Upper subscapular nerve	Posterior cord C5,6	Subscapularis
Thoracodorsal nerve	Posterior cord C6,7,8	Latissimus dorsi
Lower subscapular nerve	Posterior cord C5,6	Subscapularis Teres major
Axillary nerve	Posterior cord C5,6	Deltoid Teres minor
Radial nerve	Posterior cord** C5,6,7,8,T1	Posterior compartment of the arm Posterior compartment of the forearm
Median nerve	Contribution from lateral and medial cord C5,6,7,8,T1	Flexor muscles in the forearm, (except flexor the carpi ulnaris the ulnar head of the flexor digitorum profundus, which are supplied by the ulnar nerve) Thenar muscles Radial two lumbricals Mnemonic: The median nerve supplies the "**LOAF**" muscles in the hand: **L**—lateral two **L**umbricals **O**—**O**pponens pollicis **A**—**A**bductor pollicis brevis **F**—superficial head of the **F**lexor pollicis brevis
Medial pectoral nerve	Medial cord C8/T1	Pectoralis major Pectoralis minor
Medial cutaneous nerve of arm	T1	Cutaneous supply of arm
Medial cutaneous nerve of forearm	C8	Cutaneous supply of forearm
Ulnar	C8/T1	Flexor carpi ulnaris Ulnar head of the flexor digitorum profundus Intrinsic muscles of the hand including the palmaris brevis, lumbricals, hypothenar and interossei muscles

The composition of the plexus includes the ventral rami and the roots of the plexus, which lie between the scalenus medius and anterior. Entering the posterior triangle, the upper two (C5,6) and lower two (C8, T1) roots of the plexus unite, forming the upper and lower trunks of the plexus respectively. C7 continues as the middle trunk. The lower trunk may groove the superior surface of the first rib posterior to the subclavian artery, and the root from the first ventral ramus is always in contact with it. Each trunk divides into ventral and dorsal divisions which supply the anterior (flexor) and posterior (extensor) portions of the upper limb.

** Branches of the posterior cord of the brachial plexus can be remembered as "**STAR**": **S**ubscapular (upper and lower), **T**horacodorsal, **A**xillary and **R**adial.

Summary of the Cutaneous Supply of the Terminal Branches of the Brachial Plexus

Nerve	Area supplied
Musculocutaneous nerve	Skin of lateral forearm since it continues as the lateral cutaneous nerve of the forearm
Median nerve	Palmar cutaneous branch—innervates the lateral aspect of the palm
	Digital cutaneous branch—innervates the lateral three and a half fingers on the palmar surface of the hand including the fingertips
Ulnar nerve	Medial one and half fingers and the associated palm area
Radial nerve	Innervates most of the skin of the posterior forearm, the lateral aspect of the dorsum of the hand and the dorsal surface of the lateral three and a half digits.
Axillary nerve	Regimental patch area

CLINICAL POINTS

Compression of the brachial plexus and its terminal branches may occur at many points which will now be explored.

At the neck the nerves pass through the posterior triangle, which is bounded inferiorly by the clavicle, anteriorly by sternocleidomastoid and posteriorly by trapezius. Triangles of the neck and the full contents of the posterior triangle will be explored later in the Anatomy section. The brachial plexus passes between the scalenus anterior and medius* (these are prevertebral muscles and are invested in prevertebral fascia). They then enter the apex of the axilla and run to the arm.

Areas of compression in the neck may occur:

- If the scalenus anterior and medius are joined together.
- Due to cervical ribs or bands. About 95% are asymptomatic; they are more common in females and up to 50% are bilateral. Usually patients have T1 symptoms, but patients may also present with changes in their pulse since the subclavian artery is also compressed.
- At Sibson's suprapleural membrane, which is tensed by the scalenus minimus**. The scalenus minimus may also be multiple and can be interwoven in the plexus, causing compression.
- A Pancoast tumour in the apex of the lung may compress or infiltrate the plexus.

* The scalene muscles are three paired muscles— the scalenus anterior and medius, which serve to elevate the first rib and laterally flex the neck to same side, and the scalenus posterior, which elevates the second rib and tilts the cervical spine they originate from the transverse processes of C2–7 and insert onto the first and second ribs. They are innervated by spinal nerves C4–6. The subclavian vein and the phrenic nerve pass anteriorly to the scalenus anterior as it crosses over the first rib.

** Scalenus minimus—this is also known as Sibson's muscle, and it is an inconsistently present fourth scalene muscle that may be found behind the lower portion of the anterior scalene. When present, it originates from the anterior tubercle of transverse process C6 or C7 and inserts onto the first rib and Sibson's fascia. It functions to support the suprapleural membrane and to elevate the first rib.

Summary of the Compression Sites of the Five Main Terminal Branches of the Brachial Plexus

Nerve	Origin	Location of compression	Symptoms
Musculocutaneous	Lateral cord	Compressions uncommon Supplies the powerful flexors of the arm and ends as the lateral cutaneous nerve of the forearm	Injury to musculocutaneous nerve may present with: • Weakness of elbow flexion and forearm supination • Sensory loss over the lateral and volar aspects of the forearm • Weak or absent biceps tendon reflex
Median	Medial and lateral cords	Proximal group: 1. *Struther's ligament*—this is a fibrous condensation at the medial aspect of the distal humerus 2. *Bicipital aponeurosis*—blends into the deep fascia of the forearm, which probably confers a greater mechanical advantage, but it can form a sharp edge that can compress the median nerve at the cubital fossa 3. *Pronator teres (commonest of the proximal group)*—the median nerve enters between the two heads of this muscle and may be compressed 4. *Lische of vessels*—part of the anastomosis around the elbow that may cross the nerve, compressing it Distal group: 1. *Carpal tunnel*—commonest overall	In pronator syndrome (proximal group): • Pain in the proximal volar forearm that increases with activity and with resisted forearm pronation • Decreased sensation in median nerve distribution • Loss of precision pinch • Palmar cutaneous branch of median nerve is affected • No Tinel's sign at the wrist • Fewer nocturnal symptoms With AION syndrome: Anterior interosseous nerve syndrome is rare. The AION is a branch of the median nerve that arises approximately 4–6 cm below the elbow. It supplies: 1. The flexor pollicis longus 2. Flexor digitorum profundus to the index and middle digit 3. The pronator quadratus The condition presents with forearm pain and weakness of pinch grip (can't perform the OK sign) In carpal tunnel syndrome: • Weakness and decrease in fine motor skills • Hyperaesthesia/paraesthesia in the median nerve distribution (palm spared due to palmar cutaneous branch) • Sensory disturbance, particularly at night • Thenar muscle wasting • Phalen's and Tinel's test positive

(Continued)

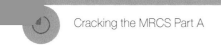

Summary of the Compression Sites of the Five Main Terminal Branches of the Brachial Plexus   (Continued)

Nerve	Origin	Location of compression	Symptoms
Ulnar nerve	Medial cord	Proximal group: 1. Compressed when piercing the intermuscular septum when the nerve moves from the flexor compartment to the extensor compartment 2. *Triceps*—especially when the medial head is hypertrophied over a short period of time 3. *Cubital tunnel**—this is the commonest site of compression 4. Flexor carpi ulnaris arch Distal group: 1. *Guyon's canal***—second commonest 2. *Opponens digiti minimi*—has a sharp arch 3. *Hook of hamate*—runs along its ulnar side and can be compromised in arthritis or fractures here 4. Pisotriquetral arthritis	Cubital tunnel syndrome (proximal): • Pain in forearm • Paraesthesia in the ulnar nerve distribution • Pain with elbow flexion • Weakness of pinch grip (due to affected innervation to adductor pollicis) • Wasting of the first dorsal interosseous, intrinsic muscles of the hand and the hypothenar muscles • *Ulnar claw*—if palsy occurs above the branch to the ulnar aspect of flexor digitorum profundus then no clawing. If more distal to this, then the long flexors cause interphalangeal flexion but in the absence of lumbrical action (i.e. extension at the interphalangeal joints and flexion at the metacarpophalangeal joints). The rhyme to remember this *"the nearer the injury is to the paw the worse the claw"* • Specific signs, e.g. Wartenberg's sign—abducted little finger and claw or Froment's sign—holding a piece of paper between the radial border of the index finger and the thumb; patients compensate by flexing the thumb/finger due to lack of functioning adductor pollicis Ulnar tunnel syndrome (distal compression at Guyon's canal): • Nerve signs as above • Dysaesthesia in the ulnar distribution • Weakness of the intrinsic muscles of the hand • Weakness of thumb adduction

Nerve	Origin	Location of compression	Symptoms
Radial nerve	Posterior cord Largest branch of the brachial plexus	1. Radial tunnel/arcade of Fröhse 2. Wartenburg syndrome 3. *Trauma/iatrogenic injury*—midshaft fractures of the humerus (radial nerve runs in the spiral groove), post orthopaedic repair of fractures, fractures of the radial neck (the radial nerve motor branch wraps around it), external compression, e.g. Saturday night palsy	Pain in the radial tunnel Tenderness over the supinator bulk Sensory disturbance in the distribution of the superficial radial nerve (not present in compression of the posterior interosseous nerve) In posterior interosseous nerve (PIN) syndrome the main features are weakness of the wrist and finger extension (here the BR, ERCB and ECRL are spared)
Axillary nerve	Posterior cord	Fractures of the surgical neck of the humerus and shoulder dislocations	Innervates the deltoid and the teres minor muscles and also has a cutaneous branch Wasting of the deltoid, weakness of arm abduction, weakness of arm external rotation and reduced sensation in the regimental patch distribution

* *Boundaries of the cubital tunnel:* the roof of the cubital tunnel is formed by the fascia of the FCU and the cubital tunnel retinaculum (or the arcuate ligament of Osbourne). The floor is formed by the elbow capsule and the medial collateral ligament.

** *The ulnar nerve and artery run through Guyon's canal, which is on top of the flexor retinaculum but under the palmar carpal ligament of this canal. It is about 4 cm long.*

THE AXILLA AND THE BREAST

The axilla is an area of great clinical importance.

It contains the axillary artery, axillary vein, the brachial plexus and between 35–50 lymph nodes that are divided into surgical groups I, II and III lying lateral, posterior and medial to the pectoralis minor muscle.

THE BOUNDARIES OF THE AXILLA ARE AS FOLLOWS

- *Floor*—axillary fascia
- *Anteriorly*—pectoralis major and minor, subclavius and clavipectoral fascia
- *Posteriorly*—subscapularis, teres major and tendon of the latissimus dorsi
- *Medially*—serratus anterior
- *Laterally*—bicipital groove (or the intertubercular groove) of the humerus
- *Apex*—outlet/inlet which is bounded medially by the edge of the first rib, anteriorly by the clavicle and posteriorly by the scapula

CLINICAL POINTS

The axilla contains a variety of important structures that may be seen and potentially damaged during breast surgeries like axillary node clearances. These structures and some important information about them are described in the following table.

Summary of Important Structures within the Axilla

Structures	Comment
Long thoracic nerve	Derived from C5–7
	Passes posterior to the brachial plexus to enter the axilla
	Innervates the serratus anterior
	Damage results in winging of the scapula
Thoracodorsal nerve	C6–8
	Innervates and supplies the latissimus dorsi muscle
Intercostobrachial nerve	Lateral cutaneous branch of the second intercostal nerve (occasionally the third intercostal)
	Provides cutaneous sensation to the medial aspect of the upper arm
	Most commonly injured during sentinel lymph node biopsies/axillary node dissections
Lateral pectoral nerve	C6–8
	Arises from the lateral cord
	Crosses the axillary vein to enter the deep surface of the pectoralis minor, then through to pectoralis major
Axillary vein	Lies on the medial side of the axillary artery
	Not invested within the axillary sheath; able to expand
	Formed by the union of the venae comitantes of the brachial artery and the basilic vein
	Receives the cephalic vein in its first part
	Becomes continuous with the subclavian vein at the lateral border of the first rib
Axillary artery	Continuation of the subclavian artery after it passes the inferior border of the first rib
	Continues as the brachial artery at the inferior border of teres major
	Divided into three parts relative to the pectoralis minor muscle, as previously discussed
	The cords of the brachial plexus are related to this artery:
	• **First part** of the axillary artery—the lateral and posterior cords lie superolateral, whereas the medial cord lies posteriorly; a loop connecting the medial and lateral pectoral nerves also lies anterior to the axillary artery.
	• **Second part** of the axillary artery—the posterior, lateral and medial cords are related to the artery as per their names.
	• **Third part** of the axillary artery—the cords branch into their respective terminal branches.

THE BREAST

The breast spans the second to sixth ribs and lies superficially over the pectoralis and serratus anterior muscles. It consists of a circular body and the axillary tail of Spence. It comprises 15–20 lobules. Each lobule has many alveoli drained by a single lactiferous duct. The fibrous connective stroma supports the mammary glands and condenses to form the suspensory ligaments of Cooper, which separate the lobules and secure the breast to the dermis and pectoral fascia.

ARTERIAL SUPPLY

1. *Medially*—internal mammary artery (a branch of the subclavian artery), anterior intercostal arteries (from internal mammary artery)
2. *Laterally*—lateral thoracic artery (from the axillary artery), thoraco-acromial artery (from the axillary artery) via pectoral branches, posterior intercostal arteries (from the thoracic aorta) via lateral mammary branches

Venous drainage is to the axillary and internal thoracic veins.

The breast is innervated by the anterior and lateral cutaneous branches of the fourth to sixth intercostal nerves. Lymphatic drainage is to the axillary lymph nodes (75%), parasternal nodes (20%) and posterior intercostal lymph nodes (5%). The levels of the axillary lymph nodes and their relationship to the pectoralis minor muscle has been discussed earlier in this chapter.

The Lower Limb

2

The lower limb holds important functions in terms of locomotion and supporting the weight of the body. The lower limb is attached to the axial skeleton via the pelvis (the ischium, ilium and pubis). It is divided into the gluteal region, the thigh, the knee, the leg, the ankle and the foot. These regions will be considered in turn throughout this chapter. First, we will consider the transition points of the lower limb.

TRANSITION POINTS OF THE LOWER LIMB

The transition points of the lower limb are the femoral triangle, the popliteal fossa and the tarsal tunnel. Important structures run through these regions, and it is not uncommon to be asked questions about these areas, their contents and their boundaries in the MRCS examination.

THE FEMORAL TRIANGLE:

- Boundaries
  - *Superiorly*—the inguinal ligament, which runs from the anterior superior iliac spine to the pubic tubercle
  - *Medial*—medial border of the adductor longus
  - *Lateral*—medial border of sartorius
  - *Roof*—skin, superficial fascia and deep fascia lata
  - *Floor*—pectineus, iliopsoas and adductor longus
- Contents (from lateral to medial)
  - Lateral cutaneous nerve of the thigh.
  - Femoral nerve.
  - The femoral sheath containing the femoral branch of the genitofemoral nerve, the femoral artery (present at the mid-inguinal point, i.e. the midpoint between the anterior superior iliac spine and the pubic symphysis), the femoral vein and the femoral canal containing Cloquet's node. Cloquet's node receives lymphatics from the glans penis/clitoris, as well as from the superficial inguinal lymph nodes and the deep lymphatics of the lower limb.

The **femoral sheath** is a conical structure contained within the femoral triangle. It is variable in length but generally runs about 4 cm below the inguinal ligament and facilitates smooth movement of the femoral vessels during movement of the hip.

DOI: 10.1201/9781003292005-3

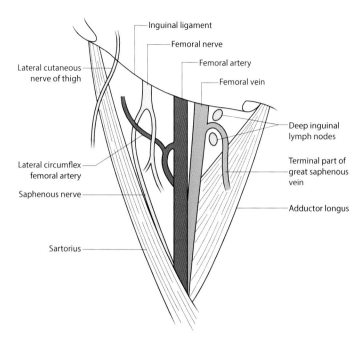

Inguinal ligament

Femoral nerve

Femoral artery

Lateral cutaneous
nerve of thigh

Femoral vein

Deep inguinal
lymph nodes

Lateral circumflex
femoral artery

Terminal part of
great saphenous
vein

Saphenous nerve

Adductor longus

Sartorius

Figure 2.1 The femoral triangle and relationship of structures within the femoral triangle.

The femoral sheath is split into three compartments by two septae, each with its own contents:

- The lateral compartment contains the femoral artery and femoral branch of the genitofemoral nerve.
- The intermediate compartment contains the femoral vein.
- The medial compartment is the femoral canal containing Cloquet's node.

Please do not become confused re: the boundaries of the femoral triangle and the boundaries of the femoral canal. The femoral canal is the medial compartment of the femoral sheath. Its purpose is to allow expansion of the femoral vein and it also houses important lymphatics.

The boundaries regarding the **femoral ring** (the opening of the femoral canal), are as follows:

- *Anteriorly*—the inguinal ligament
- *Posteriorly*—the pectineal ligament
- *Medially*—the lacunar ligament
- *Laterally*—the femoral vein

CLINICAL POINT

The clinical importance here is that femoral hernia occur through the femoral ring, and since three of the boundaries are ligamentous, the risk of hernia incarceration is high.

THE POPLITEAL FOSSA:

This is a diamond-shaped structure at the posterior aspect of the knee.

- Boundaries:
  - *Superomedial*—the semimembranosus muscle and the semitendinosus muscle
  - *Superolateral*—the biceps femoris

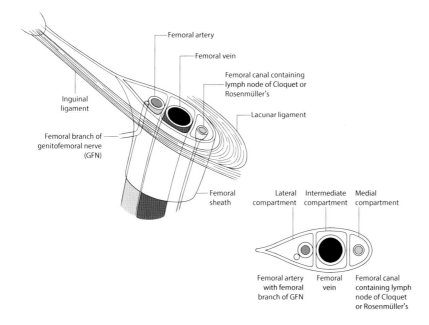

Figure 2.2 Cross-section of the femoral sheath showing the different compartments and their contents.

- *Inferomedial*—the medial head of gastrocnemius
- *Inferolateral*—the lateral head of gastrocnemius and plantaris
- *Roof*—skin, superficial fascia and the popliteal fascia
- *Floor*—popliteal surface of the femur, oblique popliteal ligament and fascia over the popliteus muscle
- Contents (from superficial to deep)
  - Tibial nerve
  - Common peroneal nerve
  - Popliteal vein
  - Popliteal artery
  - Small saphenous vein
  - Popliteal vessels and lymph nodes

THE TARSAL TUNNEL:

This is a tunnel found at the posterior medial aspect of the ankle. The boundaries of this tunnel are as follows:

- *Roof*—flexor retinaculum of the foot
- *Floor*—medial malleolus and calcaneus

Contents from anterior to posterior (mnemonic = "**T**om **D**ick **A**nd **V**ery **N**aughty **H**arry"):

- *Tom*—**T**ibialis posterior tendon
- *Dick*—flexor **D**igitorum longus tendon
- *And*—posterior tibial **A**rtery
- *Very*—posterior tibial **V**ein
- *Naughty*—tibial **N**erve
- *Harry*—flexor **H**allucis longus tendon

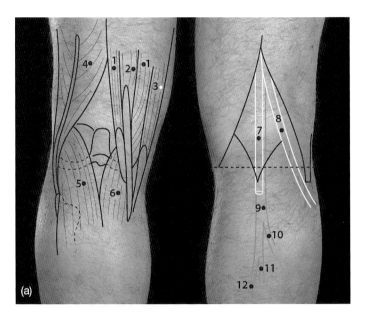

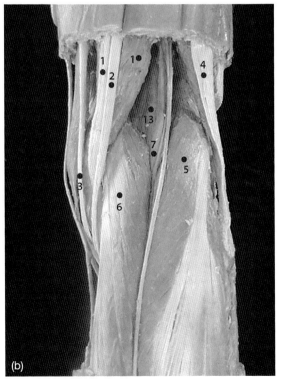

Figure 2.3 (a) Surface anatomy of the popliteal fossa: 1, semimembranosus; 2, semitendinosus; 3, gracilis; 4, biceps femoris; 5, lateral and 6, medial head of gastrocnemius; 7, tibial nerve; 8, common peroneal (fibular) nerve; 9, popliteal artery; 10, anterior tibial artery; 11, peroneal (fibular) artery; 12, posterior tibial artery (the popliteal vein, 13, between the artery and main nerves has been omitted in the diagram) (b) Dissection of the right popliteal fossa with numbers corresponding to (a).

THE FEMORAL HEAD AND NECK

The femur is the largest bone in the body. It has a head, neck and shaft, and the distal end has two prominent condyles separated by the intercondylar notch. The normal neck-shaft angle is 130 +/− 7 degrees, with 10 +/− 7 degrees of neck anteversion. The head of the femur has a smooth surface that articulates with the acetabulum of the pelvis, but it also has a pit (fovea). This pit is the attachment point for the ligamentum teres. The other end of the ligamentum teres attaches to the transverse acetabular ligament. The transverse acetabular ligament bridges the acetabular notch.

The hip joint and most of the neck of the femur are enclosed by a fibrous capsule. It attaches proximally to the edge of the acetabulum and the transverse acetabular ligament. Distally and anteriorly the capsule is attached to the intertrochanteric line. Distally and posteriorly the capsule is attached midway down the neck of the femur, i.e. proximal to the intertrochanteric crest. Some fibres of the capsule are reflected backwards along the neck of the femur to form retinacular fibres. These fibres house the nutrient arteries derived from the trochanteric anastomosis, which provide the femoral head with a rich blood supply. Three ligaments reinforce the capsule; the iliofemoral ligament ("Y"-shaped and the strongest), the pubofemoral ligament and the ischiofemoral ligament.

Knowledge concerning the trochanteric anastomosis and blood supply to the femoral head is vital for the MRCS exam. The blood supply to the femoral head comes from:

1. The trochanteric anastomosis. This consists of:
   a. Ascending branches (retinacular arteries) from the **medial and lateral circumflex arteries** (which are branches of the profunda femoris). These are the major contributors to the femoral head blood supply.
   b. Descending branch from the superior and inferior gluteal arteries.
2. A branch of the obturator artery (which runs in the ligamentum teres).

CLINICAL POINTS

Fracture of the neck of the femur usually occurs following high-energy trauma in the young or in the elderly/osteoporotic following a fall from standing height.

In an AP radiograph, Shenton's line is disrupted. Typically, the affected leg is shortened and externally rotated. The external rotation is caused by the short muscles of the gluteal region, including the piriformis, the superior and inferior gemelli, the obturator internus and the quadratus femoris aided by the gluteus maximus. Shortening (as measured from the ASIS to the medial malleolus) is due to the action of the gluteal muscles, the hamstrings, the iliopsoas and the adductors as well as some action from the rectus femoris and sartorius.

Hip fractures may be classified as intra-capsular or extra-capsular. Fractures of the femoral neck involving the capsule, i.e. intra-capsular fractures, rupture the retinacular fibres and adversely affect the blood supply via the nutrient arteries. The result is avascular necrosis of the femoral head. These fractures are classified using the Garden classification.

The Garden Classification of Femoral Neck fractures is as follows:

I: Incomplete and minimally displaced
II: Complete and non-displaced
III: Complete fracture and partially displaced
IV: Complete fracture with full displacement

Management of these fractures depends on several factors such as whether the fracture is intra-capsular or extra-capsular and whether the patient is young or elderly, amongst others, but decisions are made by the orthopaedic team on a case-by-case basis. The following diagrams provide an idea regarding operative management for exam MCQ purposes, but please refer to the most up-to-date BOAST and NICE guidelines.

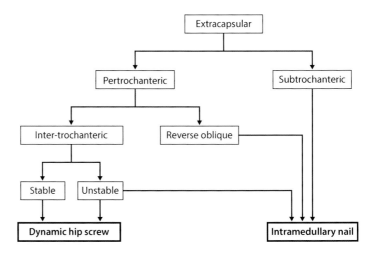

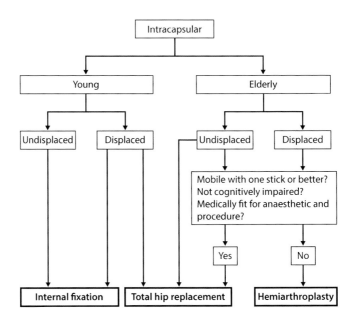

Figure 2.4 Algorithm for the operative management of intracapsular and extracapsular hip fractures (refer to latest published guidelines).

THE KNEE

The knee joint is a synovial hinge joint. It is formed by articulations between the femur and the tibia as well as the femur and the patella. Movements primarily are flexion and extension; however, rotation is permitted when the knee is in flexion.

Stability of the joint is due to several structures outlined below.

MUSCLES:

- *Quadriceps*—these muscles are strong extensors of the knee and they attach to the patella by way of the patella tendon. Here, the patella acts as a sesamoid bone and inserts into the tibial tuberosity through the ligamentum patellae.
- The gluteus maximus and tensor fascia lata also confer some stability through their action on the iliotibial tract.

LIGAMENTS:

- External ligaments (outside the joint capsule)
  - *Collateral ligaments*—the medial collateral ligament attaches to the medial epicondyle of the femur and inserts into the medial condyle of the tibia. It is also attached to the medial meniscus. The lateral collateral ligament runs from the lateral epicondyle of the femur and inserts into the head of the fibula. It is cord-like in structure and is separated from the lateral meniscus.
  - *Oblique popliteal ligament*—this is an extension of the semitendinosus muscle.
  - *Arcuate popliteal ligament*—this is a thickening of the knee joint where the tendon of popliteus passes through the capsule.
- Internal ligaments
  - *Cruciate ligaments (anterior and posterior)*—the anterior cruciate ligament is the weaker of the two and attaches to the anterior intercondylar area, and then its fibres extend upwards and laterally to insert at the lateral condyle of the femur. It serves to prevent backwards displacement of the femur on the tibia. Conversely, the posterior cruciate ligament runs from the posterior intercondylar area of the tibia and attaches to the medial condyle of the femur. It prevents forwards displacement of the femur on the tibia.

CARTILAGE:

- *Menisci*—these are plates of fibrocartilage that are semi-lunar in shape, with the medial meniscus being "C"-shaped and larger than the more rounded lateral meniscus. They are thicker and increasingly wedged shaped at their peripheral margins, where they are attached to the tibial plateau via the coronary ligaments. The menisci are attached to each other via the transverse ligament. The lateral meniscus is also attached to the femur via the meniscofemoral ligament. The menisci serve as shock absorbers and deepen the articular surface of the joint.

CLINICAL POINT

Meniscus tears represent the most common intra-articular knee injury. The meniscus has variable blood supply to different regions, with more blood supply being associated with higher potential for recovery. Blood supply is from the medial and lateral genicular arteries. The meniscus is broken into three zones based on its vascularity.

- *Red zone*—the outer perimeter of the meniscus which receives adequate blood supply
- *Red–white zone*—the mid-zone of the meniscus where blood supply is decreased
- *White zone*—the innermost portion of the meniscus which has almost zero vascularity

The medial meniscus is more frequently torn than the lateral meniscus for the following reasons:

- The lateral meniscus is not attached to the lateral collateral ligament.
- The lateral meniscus is also attached to fibres from the popliteus and to the meniscofemoral ligament, meaning that it will be moved out of the way of potential injury during sudden destabilising movements of the knee.

The medial collateral ligament is more likely to be injured due to trauma to the lateral aspect of the knee.

The combination of a medial collateral ligament rupture, ACL injury and a torn medial meniscus is known as O'Donoghue's unhappy triad of the knee.

MUSCLES OF THE GLUTEAL REGION

The muscles of the gluteal region consist of extensors (gluteus maximus), abductors (gluteus medius and minimus) as well as rotators (piriformis, obturator internus, gemelli and quadratus femoris) of the hip joint.

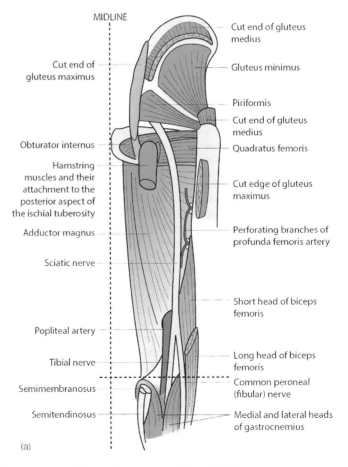

Figure 2.5a Deep muscles of the posterior aspect of the right thigh.

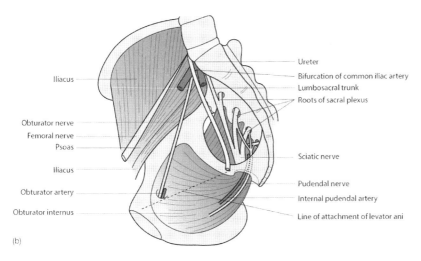

Ureter
Bifurcation of common iliac artery
Lumbosacral trunk
Roots of sacral plexus

Iliacus

Obturator nerve
Femoral nerve
Psoas

Iliacus

Sciatic nerve

Obturator artery

Pudendal nerve
Internal pudendal artery

Obturator internus

Line of attachment of levator ani

(b)

Figure 2.5b Muscles and nerves of the lateral pelvic wall.

Summary of Muscles of the Gluteal Region

Muscle	Proximal attachment	Distal attachment	Innervation	Action
Gluteus maximus	Ilium, posterior to the posterior gluteal line, the sacrum, the coccyx and the sacrotuberous ligament	The gluteal tuberosity and the iliotibial tract	Inferior gluteal nerve	Laterally rotates and extends thigh
Gluteus medius	Ilium between the anterior and posterior gluteal lines	Greater trochanter of the femur	Superior gluteal nerve	Hip abduction Medially rotates thigh Helps to level pelvis when the contralateral leg is not supported*
Gluteus minimus	Ilium between the anterior and inferior gluteal lines	Greater trochanter of the femur	Superior gluteal nerve	Hip abduction Medially rotates thigh Helps to level pelvis when the contralateral leg is not supported
Tensor fascia lata	Anterior superior iliac spine	Via the iliotibial tract into the lateral condyle of the tibia	Superior gluteal nerve	Hip abduction Medially rotates thigh Helps to level pelvis when the contralateral leg is not supported

(*Continued*)

Summary of Muscles of the Gluteal Region   (Continued)

Muscle	Proximal attachment	Distal attachment	Innervation	Action
Piriformis	Sacrum and the sacrotuberous ligament	Greater trochanter of the femur	S1 and S2	Lateral rotator of the hip** Helps to hold femoral head in the acetabulum
Obturator internus	Obturator foramen and the obturator membrane	Greater trochanter of the femur	Nerve to obturator internus	Lateral rotator of hip Helps to hold femoral head in the acetabulum
Superior gemellus	Ischial spine	Greater trochanter of the femur	Nerve to obturator internus	Lateral rotator of hip Helps to hold femoral head in the acetabulum
Inferior gemellus	Ischial tuberosity	Greater trochanter of the femur	Nerve to quadratus femoris	Lateral rotator of hip Helps to hold femoral head in the acetabulum
Quadratus femoris	Ischial tuberosity	Intertrochanteric crest	Nerve to quadratus femoris	Lateral rotator of hip Helps to hold femoral head in the acetabulum

* Damage to the hip abductors results in a Trendelenburg gait.

** The lateral rotators of the hip are also known as the POGO-Q muscles, i.e. piriformis, obturator internus, gemelli, obturator externus and quadratus femoris.

CLINICAL POINTS

- *Trendelenburg test*—the Trendelenburg test assesses the stability of the hip and the ability of the hip abductors (gluteus medius and gluteus minimus) to stabilise the pelvis on the femur. If these hip abductors are paralysed in any way, e.g. injury to the superior gluteal nerve via a stab injury, hip dislocation or infections (polio), then when the patient stands on one leg, the pelvis will tilt down on the contralateral side.
- *Dislocation of the hip*—dislocations of the hip can be classified as congenital or acquired. Congenital dislocations result from the position of the fetus against the maternal abdominal wall, with a posterior force acting against a dysplastic hip joint in flexion.

Acquired dislocation of the hip is generally rare but when it does occur, it is frequently associated with high-velocity, significant mechanisms of injury, e.g. road traffic accidents. Since the anterior ligaments of the hip are stronger, trauma to the hip commonly presents as a posterior dislocation when discovered (90% of cases).

Hip dislocations are time-sensitive emergencies that require prompt treatment. No more than 6 hours should elapse between presentation and reduction. Please see BOAST guidelines for up-to-date management. Some closed reduction techniques for posterior dislocations include the Allis manoeuvre, the Bigelow manoeuvre, the Lefkowitz manoeuvre and the Captain Morgan technique.

MUSCLES OF THE THIGH

The muscles of the thigh are separated into three compartments.

1. *The anterior compartment*—the extensors (quadriceps)
2. *The medial compartment*—the adductors (pectineus; adductor longus, brevis and magnus; gracilis; obturator externus)
3. *The posterior compartment*—the flexors (hamstrings)

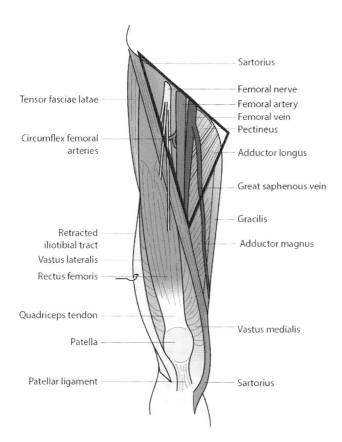

Figure 2.6a Anterior aspect of the thigh and femoral triangle (outlined in bold).

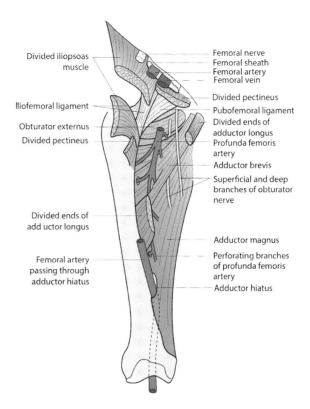

Figure 2.6b Deep aspect of the medial thigh and relations of the profunda femoris artery.

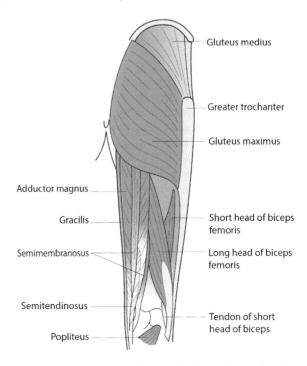

Figure 2.6c Anatomy of the muscles of the right gluteal region and posterior thigh.

Summary of Muscles of the Thigh

Muscle	Proximal attachment	Distal attachment	Innervation	Action
Anterior compartment = hip flexors and knee extensors				
Pectineus	Pubis	Pectineal line	Femoral nerve or obturator nerve	Adducts, flexes and medially rotates thigh
Psoas major	T12 and lumbar vertebrae	Lesser trochanter	L1–L3	Flexes thigh Stabilises hip joint
Psoas minor	T12–L1	Pectineal line	L1–L3	Flexes thigh Stabilises hip joint
Iliacus	Iliac fossa	Lesser trochanter	Femoral nerve	Flexes thigh Stabilises hip joint
Sartorius	Anterior superior iliac spine	Via the pes anserinus ("the goose's foot") into the medial condyle of the tibia	Femoral nerve	Abducts, flexes and laterally rotates thigh Flexes leg
Rectus femoris	Anterior superior iliac spine	Tibial tuberosity via the patellar tendon/ligamentum patellae	Femoral nerve	Extensor of the leg Flexes thigh
Vastus lateralis	Greater trochanter Linea aspera of femur	Tibial tuberosity via patellar tendon/ligamentum patellae	Femoral nerve	Extensor of leg
Vastus intermedius	Femoral shaft	Tibial tuberosity via patellar tendon/ligamentum patellae	Femoral nerve	Extensor of leg
Vastus medialis	Intertrochanteric line Linea aspera of femur	Tibial tuberosity via patellar tendon/ligamentum patellae	Femoral nerve	Extensor of leg
Medial compartment = thigh adductors				
Adductor longus	Pubis	Linea aspera	Obturator nerve	Adducts thigh
Adductor brevis	Pubis	Linea aspera	Obturator nerve	Adducts thigh
Adductor magnus	Adductor part—pubis Hamstring part—ischial tuberosity	Adductor part—gluteal tuberosity and linea aspera Hamstring part—adductor tubercle	Adductor part—obturator nerve Hamstring part—tibial nerve	Adductor part—adducts thigh Hamstring part—extends thigh

(Continued)

Summary of Muscles of the Thigh   (Continued)

Muscle	Proximal attachment	Distal attachment	Innervation	Action
Gracilis	Pubis	Via the pes anserinus ("the goose's foot") into the medial condyle of the tibia	Obturator nerve	Adducts thigh Flexes and medially rotates leg
Obturator externus	Obturator foramen and external aspect of obturator membrane	Trochanteric fossa	Obturator nerve	Laterally rotates thigh
Posterior compartment = knee flexors and hip extensors				
Semitendinosus	Ischial tuberosity	Via the pes anserinus ("the goose's foot") into the medial condyle of the tibia	Tibial division of the sciatic nerve	Extends thigh Flexes and medially rotates leg
Semimembranosus	Ischial tuberosity	Medial condyle of the tibia	Tibial division of the sciatic nerve	Extends thigh Flexes and medially rotates leg
Biceps femoris	Long head—ischial tuberosity Short head—linea aspera	Head of fibula	Long head—tibial division of the sciatic nerve Short head—common peroneal nerve	Flexes and laterally rotates leg Extends thigh at the hip joint (long head only)

THE ADDUCTOR CANAL

There is an important canal to consider in the thigh which is high-yield for MRCS questions—the adductor canal, also known as Hunter's canal.

The adductor canal extends from the femoral triangle to the adductor hiatus.

- Boundaries
  - *Anteromedially*—sartorius
  - *Anterolaterally*—vastus medialis
  - *Posteriorly*—adductor longus and adductor magnus

- Contents
  - Superficial femoral artery
  - Superficial femoral vein
  - Saphenous nerve
  - Nerve to the vastus medialis

The femoral artery and vein exit the canal through the adductor hiatus, which is situated between the oblique and medial heads of adductor magnus.

CLINICAL POINT

The saphenous nerve may be compressed in the adductor canal.

THE PES ANSERINUS

The pes anserinus, also known as the goose's foot, refers to three tendons that conjoin and insert into the proximal anteromedial tibial surface. From superficial to deep, these are the sartorius tendon, the gracilis tendon and the semitendinosus tendon.

CLINICAL POINT

The submuscular anserine bursa may become inflamed causing painful pes anserine bursitis. This is typically painful when climbing stairs.

MUSCLES OF THE LEG

The leg is divided into four fascial compartments by the interosseous membrane of the leg, the transverse intermuscular septum and the anterior intermuscular (crural) septum.

Compartments of the Leg and Their Contents

Compartment	Muscles	Vessels	Nerve
Anterior	Tibialis anterior Extensor hallucis longus Extensor digitorum longus Peroneus tertius	Anterior tibial vessels	Deep peroneal
Lateral	Peroneus longus Peroneus brevis	—	Superficial peroneal
Superficial posterior	Gastrocnemius Plantaris Soleus	—	Sural
Deep posterior	Tibialis posterior Flexor hallucis longus Flexor digitorum longus Popliteus	Posterior tibial vessels	Tibial

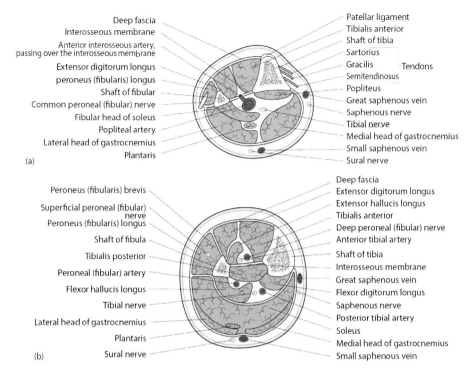

Figure 2.7 Transverse section: (a) through the right lower leg at the level of the lower popliteal fossa and (b) through the mid-calf.

Summary of Muscles of the Leg

Muscle	Proximal attachment	Distal attachment	Innervation	Action
Anterior compartment				
Tibialis anterior	Tibia and interosseous membrane	Base of the first metatarsal Medial cuneiform	Deep peroneal (fibular) nerve	Dorsiflexes ankle Inverts the foot
Extensor digitorum longus	Tibia and interosseous membrane	Middle and distal phalanges of digits 2–5	Deep peroneal (fibular) nerve	Dorsiflexes ankle Extends digits 2–5
Extensor hallucis longus	Fibula and interosseous membrane	Distal phalanx of digit 1 (the great toe)	Deep peroneal (fibular) nerve	Dorsiflexes ankle Extends digit 1
Peroneus tertius	Fibula and interosseous membrane	Dorsum of fifth metatarsal	Deep peroneal (fibular) nerve	Dorsiflexes ankle Everts the foot
Lateral compartment				
Peroneus longus	Fibula	First metatarsal Medial cuneiform	Superficial peroneal nerve	Plantarflexes ankle Everts the foot

Muscle	Proximal attachment	Distal attachment	Innervation	Action
Peroneus brevis	Fibula	Tuberosity of fifth metatarsal	Superficial peroneal nerve	Plantarflexes ankle Everts the foot
Posterior compartment				
Gastrocnemius*	Medial and lateral femoral condyles	Via the calcaneal tendon into the calcaneus	Tibial nerve	Plantarflexes the ankle Flexes the leg
Soleus	Soleal line	Via the calcaneal tendon into the calcaneus	Tibial nerve	Plantarflexes the ankle
Plantaris	Oblique popliteal ligament Lateral supracondylar ridge of femur	Via the calcaneal tendon into the calcaneus	Tibial nerve	Plantarflexes the ankle
Popliteus	Lateral femoral condyle Lateral meniscus	Tibia	Tibial nerve	Unlocks the knee
Tibialis posterior	Fibula and interosseous membrane	Navicular tuberosity	Tibial nerve	Plantarflexes ankle Inverts the foot
Flexor hallucis longus	Fibula and interosseous membrane	Distal phalanx of digit 1	Tibial nerve	Plantarflexes ankle Flexes digit 1 Supports longitudinal foot arches
Flexor digitorum longus	Tibia and fibula	Distal phalanges digits 2–5	Tibial nerve	Plantarflexes ankle Flexes digits 2–5 Supports longitudinal foot arches

* The triceps surae = the gastrocnemius, soleus and plantaris.

CLINICAL POINTS

Compartment syndrome:

This is a limb threatening emergency which occurs when tissue pressure within a closed osteofascial compartment is greater than tissue perfusion pressure, thereby resulting in muscle ischaemia.

Compartment syndrome may occur in many regions of the body including the abdomen, upper limb and the lower limb. Here, the focus will be on the lower limb which is the most frequently tested area for compartment syndrome in the MRCS examination. The anterior compartment of the lower is the most affected by compartment syndrome followed by the deep posterior compartment.

Compartment syndrome may be caused by:

1. Things that increase volume within the compartment e.g. trauma—fractures/dislocation, haemorrhage, vessel injury—ischaemic/reperfusion injury, burns (oedema) and
2. Things that restrict volume within the compartment e.g. tight bandages/casts, circumferential full thickness burns.

These factors result in an increase in the intracompartment pressure to the point at which it overwhelms capillary perfusion pressure and the capillaries collapse. Eventually, tissue perfusion pressure drops to a level where no oxygen is available for cellular metabolism. Cells switch to anaerobic respiration resulting in a build up of lactic acid, dysfunction of the ATP Na^+/K^+ pump, more oedema and more ischaemia.

Symptoms may be remembered as "The Six P's": pain, pulselessness, paraesthesia, paralysis, poikilothermia and pallor. Supporting investigations include Hb (haemorrhage), U&Es (increase K^+, creatinine and CK) and myoglobin in the urine. Compartment pressures may be measured (ICP is greater than or equal to 30 mmHg).

Two incision four-compartment fasciotomy of the leg is the surgery of choice. The aim of which is to completely open and decompress all tight fascial envelopes of the lower limb.

LOWER LIMB TRAUMA

The Gustilo Anderson system is often used to classify any open fracture. The following table outlines the grading system.

Gustilo Anderson Grading System

Grade I—open fracture, wound <1 cm
Grade II—open fracture, wound >1 cm without extensive soft tissue damage
Grade IIIA—open fracture with extensive soft tissue injury
Grade IIIB—open fracture with extensive soft tissue injury, bone damage, periosteal stripping, massive contamination, often needs soft tissue coverage
Grade IIIC—open fracture with extensive soft tissue injury and arterial injury requiring vascular repair

With respect to tibial plateau fractures specifically, one classification system used is the Schatzker classification system, outlined in the following table.

Type	Anatomical description	Features
1	Vertical split of lateral condyle	Fracture through dense bone. It may be undisplaced, or the condylar fragment may be pushed inferiorly and tilted.
2	Vertical split of the lateral condyle combined with an adjacent load-bearing part of the condyle	The wedge fragment (which may be of variable size) is displaced laterally. The joint is widened. Untreated, a valgus deformity may develop.
3	Depression of the articular surface with intact condylar rim	Split does not extend to the edge of the plateau. Depressed fragments may be embedded in subchondral bone; the joint is stable.
4	Fragment of the medial tibial condyle	Two injuries are seen in this category: (1) a depressed fracture of osteoporotic bone in the elderly, (2) a high-energy fracture resulting in a condylar split that runs from the intercondylar eminence to the medial cortex. Associated ligamentous injury may be severe.

Type	Anatomical description	Features
5	Fracture of both condyles	Both condyles fractured but the column of the metaphysis remains in continuity with the tibial shaft.
6	Combined condylar and subcondylar fractures	High-energy fracture with marked comminution.

MUSCLES OF THE FOOT

Summary of Muscles of the Foot

Muscle	Proximal attachment	Distal attachment	Innervation	Action
Dorsum				
Extensor digitorum brevis	Calcaneus	Tendons of the extensor digitorum longus	Deep peroneal nerve	Extends digits 2–5
Extensor hallucis brevis	Calcaneus	Proximal phalanx of digit 1	Deep peroneal nerve	Extends digit 1
Plantar surface (layer 1)				
Abductor hallucis	Calcaneus	Proximal phalanx of digit 1	Medial plantar nerve	Abducts digit 1
Flexor digitorum brevis	Calcaneus	Middle phalanges of digits 2–5	Medial plantar nerve	Flexes phalanges of digits 2–5
Abductor digiti minimi	Calcaneus	Proximal phalanx of digit 5	Lateral plantar nerve	Abducts digit 5
Plantar surface (layer 2)				
Quadratus plantae	Calcaneus	Tendons of the flexor digitorum longus	Lateral plantar nerve	Flexes toes
Lumbricals	Tendons of flexor digitorum longus	Extensor expansion	First lumbrical = medial plantar nerve All others via the lateral plantar nerve	Flexes metatarsophalangeal joints Extends interphalangeal joints
Plantar surface (layer 3)				
Flexor hallucis brevis	Cuboid and third cuneiform	Proximal phalanx of digit 1	Medial plantar nerve	Flexes digit 1
Adductor hallucis	Oblique head— metatarsals 1–4 Transverse head— metatarsophalangeal joints	Proximal phalanx of digit 1	Lateral plantar nerve	Adducts hallux Maintains transverse arch
Flexor digiti minimi brevis	Fifth metatarsal	Proximal phalanx of the little toe	Lateral plantar nerve	Flexes little toe
Plantar surface (layer 4)				
Plantar interossei (3)	Metatarsals 3–5	Proximal phalanges 3–5	Lateral plantar nerve	Flexion of metatarsophalangeal joints Adduction of digits 2–4
Dorsal interossei (4)	Metatarsals 1–5	Proximal phalanges 2–5	Lateral plantar nerve	Flexion of metatarsophalangeal joints Adduction of digits 2–4

CLINICAL POINTS

Arches of the foot—the arches of the foot are maintained by the shape of the interlocking bones, ligaments and muscles. The arches to consider here are the longitudinal arches (medial and lateral) and the transverse arches (proximal and distal).

- *The longitudinal arches*
  The longitudinal arches are higher medially than laterally. The posterior part of the calcaneum forms a posterior pillar to support the arch. The lateral part of this structure passes via the cuboid bone and the lateral two metatarsal bones. The medial part of this structure is the more important part. The head of the talus marks the summit of this arch, located between the sustentaculum tali and the navicular bone. The anterior pillar of the medial arch is composed of the navicular bone, the three cuneiforms and the medial three metatarsal bones.

- *The transverse arches*
  These are located on the anterior part of the tarsus and the posterior part of the metatarsus. The inferior narrowing of the cuneiforms and metatarsals contribute to the shape of the arch.

The ligaments involved in maintaining the arches are supported by the plantar aponeurosis. These ligaments are:

- *The spring ligament*—runs from the sustentaculum tali to the tuberosity of the navicular.
- *The plantar, dorsal and interosseous ligaments*—between the small bones of the foot.
- *The long plantar ligament*—runs from the posterior tuberosity of the calcaneus to the bases of the second, third and fourth metatarsals.
- *The short plantar ligament*—from the plantar surface of the calcaneus to the cuboid.

KEY POINTS CONCERNING ARTERIES OF THE LOWER LIMB

THE FEMORAL ARTERY

This is a continuation of the external iliac artery after it crosses the inguinal ligament, and it supplies the anterior compartment of the thigh. The femoral artery may be found in the femoral triangle enclosed in the lateral compartment of the femoral sheath. It then passes through Hunter's canal within adductor magnus and becomes the popliteal artery when it passes through the adductor hiatus. It is accompanied by the femoral vein, which lies medial to the artery. The anatomical surface marking of the femoral artery is the mid-inguinal point.

The femoral artery has many branches, including:

- *The superficial circumflex iliac artery*—this is a small branch in the region of the anterior superior iliac spine.
- *The superficial epigastric artery*—this branch crosses the inguinal ligament.
- *The superficial external pudendal artery*—this branch supplies the skin of the scrotum or labia majora.
- *The deep external pudendal artery*—this branch supplies the skin of the scrotum or labia majora.
- *The profunda femoris artery*—this is a very important branch that arises from the lateral side of the femoral artery about 4 cm inferior to the inguinal ligament. It passes medially and posteriorly to the femoral vessels and enters the medial fascial compartment of the thigh. It gives off the medial and lateral femoral circumflex arteries which are important in supplying the femoral neck. It terminates at the fourth perforating artery.

- *The descending genicular artery*—this is a small branch from the femoral artery near its termination within the adductor canal. It is one of many genicular arteries that supply the knee.

THE POPLITEAL ARTERY

This is a continuation of the femoral artery once it has passed through the adductor hiatus. It traverses the popliteal fossa, where it is the deepest structure. It terminates as the anterior and posterior tibial arteries after crossing the inferior border of popliteus.

The branches of the popliteal artery are:

- The anterior tibial artery
- The posterior tibial artery
- The sural artery
- The medial superior genicular artery
- The lateral superior genicular artery
- The middle genicular artery
- The lateral inferior genicular artery
- The medial inferior genicular artery

The relationships of structures to the popliteal artery are sometimes questioned in the MRCS exam, and they are as follows:

- *Anteriorly*—the popliteal surface of the femur, the knee joint, and the popliteus muscle
- *Posteriorly*—the popliteal vein, the tibial nerve, fascia and skin
- *Laterally*—the biceps femoris, the lateral condyle of femur, plantaris and the lateral head of gastrocnemius
- *Medially*—the semimembranosus and the medial condyle of the femur, the tibial nerve, the popliteal vein and the medial head of the gastrocnemius

THE ANTERIOR TIBIAL ARTERY

This is a branch of the popliteal artery. It passes medially to the fibular neck, where it is vulnerable to damage. It then descends between the tibialis anterior and extensor digitorum longus muscles via an opening in the interosseous membrane.

The branches of the anterior tibial artery are:

- The posterior tibial recurrent artery
- The anterior tibial recurrent artery
- Muscular branches
- The anterior medial malleolar artery
- The anterior lateral malleolar artery
- The dorsalis pedis artery—palpated easily laterally to the extensor hallucis longus tendon

THE POSTERIOR TIBIAL ARTERY

This is another branch of the popliteal artery and supplies the posterior compartment of the leg. Of significance is that it may be palpated posterior to the medial malleolus, and it runs through the tarsal tunnel as previously described.

The branches of the posterior tibial artery are:

- The medial plantar artery
- The lateral plantar artery

- The peroneal artery (from the bifurcation of the tibio-fibular trunk and the posterior tibio-fibular artery)
- The calcaneal branch which supplies the medial aspect of calcaneus

KEY POINTS CONCERNING VEINS OF THE LOWER LIMB

There are deep and superficial venous systems in the lower limb. The deep veins follow their respective arteries as previously described. The superficial system consists of the great saphenous vein and the small saphenous vein as well as their tributaries.

THE GREAT SAPHENOUS VEIN

This vein originates at the great toe where the dorsal vein merges with the dorsal venous arch of the foot. It ascends anteriorly to the medial malleolus, advancing up the medial side of the leg. The vein traverses the posterior border of the medial epicondyle of the femur at the knee and runs on the anterior surface of the thigh. It passes through the saphenous opening whereupon it drains into the femoral vein at the saphenofemoral junction.

Tributaries of the great saphenous vein include:

- The medial marginal vein
- The superficial epigastric vein
- The superficial circumflex iliac vein
- The superficial external pudendal veins

CLINICAL POINTS

The great saphenous vein may be harvested for bypass surgery or removed as treatment for varicose veins with saphenofemoral junction incompetence.

THE SHORT SAPHENOUS VEIN

This vein originates at the little toe where the dorsal vein merges with the dorsal venous arch of the foot. It passes inferiorly and posteriorly to the lateral malleolus and then ascends the posterior aspect of the leg with the sural nerve. It runs between the heads of the gastrocnemius muscle and drains into the popliteal vein at the level of the knee joint.

CLINICAL POINTS

The sural nerve may be damaged during stripping of the short saphenous vein. The sural nerve is purely sensory, providing innervation to the skin of the lateral foot and lateral lower ankle.

KEY POINTS CONCERNING NERVES OF THE LOWER LIMB

THE LUMBAR PLEXUS

The lumbar plexus originates from the anterior rami of L1–4. The trunks appear at the lateral border of the psoas major, except for the genitofemoral nerve (anterior to muscle) and the obturator nerve (at medial border of psoas major). The nerves of the lumbar plexus and their branches and innervations are summarised in the following table.

Summary of the Nerves of the Lumbar Plexus

Nerve	Segment of lumbar plexus	Cutaneous branches	Muscles innervated
Iliohypogastric	T12–L1	Anterior cutaneous ramus Lateral cutaneous ramus	Transversus abdominus Internal oblique
Ilioinguinal	L1	Anterior scrotal/labial nerves	Transversus abdominus Internal oblique
Genitofemoral	L1–L2	Femoral branch Genital branch	Cremaster
Lateral femoral cutaneous	L2–L3	Lateral femoral cutaneous	—
Obturator	L2–4	Cutaneous branch to medial aspect of thigh	Obturator externus Adductor longus and brevis Adductor magnus Gracilis Pectineus
Femoral	L2–4	Anterior cutaneous branches Long saphenous nerve	Quadriceps femoris Sartorius Pectineus Iliacus
Short branches	L1–3	—	Psoas major
Short branches	T12–L4	—	Quadratus lumborum Intertransversarii

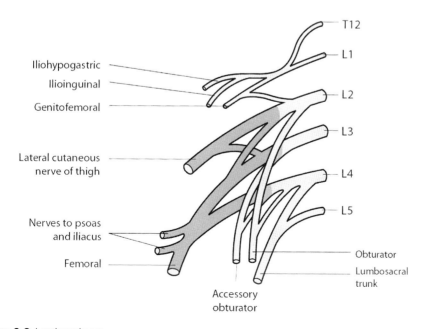

Figure 2.8 Lumbar plexus.

THE SACRAL PLEXUS

The sacral plexus is a web of nerves that supply motor and cutaneous supply to the posterior thigh and the lower leg. It is formed from the anterior primary rami of L4–5 and S1–S4. The nerves of the sacral plexus and their branches and innervations are summarised in the following table. Some of the nerves will then be considered in greater detail.

Summary of the Nerves of the Sacral Plexus

Nerve	Segment of sacral plexus	Cutaneous branches	Muscles innervated
Superior gluteal	L4–S1	–	Gluteus medius and minimus Tensor fasciae latae
Inferior gluteal	L5–S2	–	Gluteus maximus
Posterior cutaneous femoral	S1–3	–	–
Perforating cutaneous	S2–3	–	–
Nerve to piriformis	S1–2	–	Piriformis
Nerve to obturator internus	L5, S1–2	–	Obturator internus Superior gemellus
Nerve to quadratus femoris	L4–5, S1	–	Quadratus femoris Inferior gemellus
Sciatic	L4–S3	–	Semitendinosus Semimembranosus Biceps femoris (long head—tibial division of sciatic nerve; short head—common peroneal division of sciatic nerve) Adductor magnus (hamstring portion)
Common peroneal	L4–S2	Superficial peroneal—medial dorsal cutaneous Intermediate dorsal cutaneous Deep peroneal—medial branch goes on to provide cutaneous innervation to the webbing between the first and second toe	Superficial peroneal—lateral compartment of the leg, i.e. peroneus longus and brevis Deep peroneal—anterior compartment of the leg, i.e. tibialis anterior, extensor digitorum longus, extensor digitorum brevis, extensor hallucis longus, extensor hallucis brevis, peroneus tertius

Nerve	Segment of sacral plexus	Cutaneous branches	Muscles innervated
Tibial	L4–S3	Medial sural cutaneous Medial calcaneal Lateral dorsal cutaneous Medial plantar—proper digital plantar Lateral plantar—proper digital plantar	Triceps surae Plantaris Tibialis posterior Flexor digitorum longus Flexor hallucis longus Medial plantar—abductor hallucis Flexor digitorum brevis Flexor hallucis brevis (medial head) Lumbrical (first and second) Lateral plantar—flexor hallucis brevis (lateral head) Quadratus plantae Abductor digiti minimi Flexor digiti minimi Lumbrical (third and fourth) Plantar interossei (first to third) Dorsal interossei (first to fifth) Adductor hallucis
Pudendal	S2–4	Inferior rectal Perineal region, e.g. posterior scrotal/labial Dorsal penis/clitoris Prostatic urethra	*Muscles of the pelvic floor:* Levator ani (the pubococcygeus, the iliococcygeus and the puborectalis) Ischiococcygeus Superficial transverse perineal Deep transverse perineal Bulbospongiosus Ischiocavernosus Sphincter anus externus Urethral sphincter
Coccygeal	S4,5–Co1	Anococcygeal Dorsal branches	Ischiococcygeus

THE PUDENDAL NERVE

Originates from S2–4. It is responsible for innervating the perineum. It runs through the greater and lesser sciatic foramen.

The boundaries of the greater sciatic foramen are:

- *Anterolaterally*—greater sciatic notch of the ilium
- *Posteromedially*—the sacrotuberous ligament
- *Inferiorly*—sacrospinous ligament and the ischial spine
- *Superiorly*—anterior sacroiliac ligament

The contents of the greater sciatic foramen may be summarised in the following table:

Summary of the Structures Passing through the Greater Sciatic Foramen

Nerves	Vessels
Sciatic nerve	Superior gluteal artery and vein
Superior and inferior gluteal nerves	Inferior gluteal artery and vein
Pudendal nerve	Internal pudendal artery and vein
Posterior femoral cutaneous nerve	
Nerve to quadratus femoris	
Nerve to obturator internus	

Note: The piriformis is the landmark muscle for structures passing out of the sciatic notch. *Superior* to this muscle pass the *superior* gluteal vessels, *inferior* to it pass the *inferior* gluteal vessels and the sciatic nerve.

The boundaries of the lesser sciatic foramen are:

- *Anteriorly*—the tuberosity of the ischium
- *Superiorly*—the spine of the ischium and sacrospinous ligament
- *Posteriorly*—the sacrotuberous ligament

The structures passing through the lesser sciatic foramen are:

- Tendon of the obturator internus
- *Nerves*—the pudendal nerve and the nerve to obturator internus
- *Vessels*—the internal pudendal artery and vein

Structures that pass through both the greater and lesser sciatic foramina from medial to lateral may be remembered by the mnemonic "**PIN**":

- **P—P**udendal nerve
- **I—I**nternal pudendal artery
- **N—N**erve to obturator internus

The sciatic, tibial and common peroneal nerves:

The sciatic nerve is the largest nerve in the body and arises from the ventral rami of L4–S3. Typically, it passes through the greater sciatic notch and then emerges beneath piriformis but there are some anatomical variations. It lies beneath the gluteus maximus muscle and is supplied by the inferior gluteal artery. The nerve has multiple muscular and cutaneous branches which will be summarised below. It terminates into the tibial nerve and common peroneal nerve approximately halfway down the posterior thigh. The tibial nerve innervates the flexor muscles and all muscles of the foot except the extensor digitorum brevis (which is innervated by the common peroneal nerve). The common peroneal nerve supplies the extensor muscles and the evertor muscles of the foot.

Summary of the Branches of the Sciatic Nerve

Branches	Comment
Muscular branches	Hamstring portion of adductor magnus
	The hamstring muscles
Articular branches	To the hip joint
	To the knee joint
Terminal branches	Tibial nerve
	Common peroneal nerve

CLINICAL POINTS

The clinical presentations for lower limb nerve injuries are frequently asked about in the MRCS. It is important to know what muscles each nerve innervates and what would happen if that nerve were to be injured during trauma; e.g. the common peroneal nerve is intimately related to the fibular neck and therefore is frequently damaged in fractures of the fibular neck. The following table outlines what happens when the nerves of the leg are injured. The illustrations outline the cutaneous supply of nerves of the lower limb.

Summary of Leg Nerve Injury Sequalae

Nerve	Outcome
Common peroneal nerve	Damaged before bifurcation, therefore loss of function of both superficial and deep peroneal nerves (outlined below)
	Results in talipes equinovarus, which is defined as fixation of the foot in adduction, in supination and in varus
Superficial peroneal nerve	Supplies the peroneal muscles, therefore loss of ankle eversion
	Supplies cutaneous sensation to the distal two-thirds of the lateral aspect of the leg and the dorsum of the foot (except the first dorsal webspace); therefore, when injured, sensation to this region is lost
Deep peroneal nerve	Supplies the anterior compartment of the leg therefore loss of ability to dorsiflex the foot
	Also, loss of sensation to the first dorsal web space

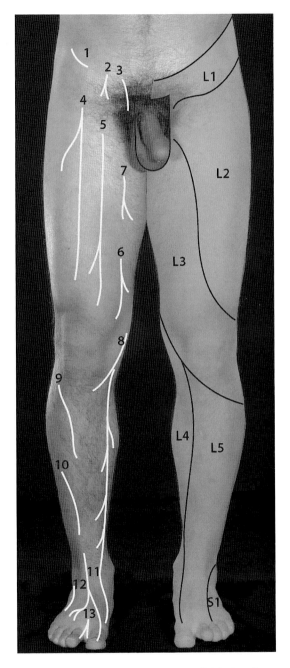

Figure 2.9a Surface anatomy showing lower leg dermatomes (left leg) and cutaneous nerves (right leg), anterior aspect: 1, subcostal; 2, femoral branch of genitofemoral; 3, ilioinguinal; 4, lateral cutaneous of thigh; 5, intermediate cutaneous of thigh; 6, medial cutaneous of thigh; 7, obturator; 8, saphenous; 9, lateral cutaneous of calf; 10 and 11, superficial peroneal (fibular); 12, sural; 13, deep peroneal (fibular).

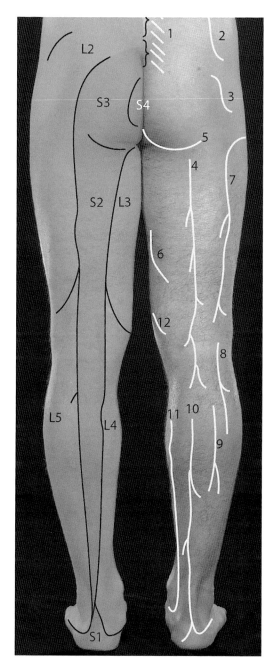

Figure 2.9b Surface anatomy of lower limb dermatomes (left leg) and cutaneous nerves (right leg), posterior aspect: 1, dorsal rami; 2, subcostal; 3, posterior lumbar rami; 4, posterior cutaneous nerve of thigh; 5, gluteal and perineal branch; 6, obturator; 7, lateral cutaneous nerve of thigh; 8, lateral cutaneous nerve of calf; 9, sural communicating; 10, sural; 11, saphenous; 12, medial cutaneous nerve of thigh.

(Continued)

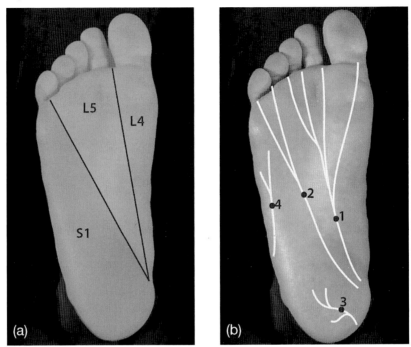

Figure 2.9c Surface anatomy of the sole. (a) Dermatomes. (b) Cutaneous nerves: 1, medial plantar; 2, lateral plantar; 3, medial calcaneal branch of the tibial nerve; 4, sural. L = lumbar, S = sacral.

The Abdomen and Pelvis

3

MUSCLES OF THE ANTERIOR ABDOMINAL WALL

The abdominal wall comprises muscles and fascial layers that enclose the abdominal cavity. These muscles serve to maintain the correct anatomical position of intra-abdominal viscera, protect internal organs from injury, assist in coughing/vomiting by increasing intra-abdominal pressure, assist in expiration by pushing organs towards the diaphragm and stabilise the vertebral column as well the trunk in rotation, bending and walking.

The anterolateral abdominal wall consists of symmetrically paired muscles and, typically, the anatomical layers are described from superficial to deep as skin, subcutaneous tissue, Scarpa's and Camper's fascia, external oblique muscle, internal oblique muscle, transversus abdominis muscle, transversalis fascia and parietal peritoneum. The table provided herein summarises their origin, insertion, innervation and function.

The "flat muscles" of the abdominal wall are the external oblique, the internal oblique and the transversus abdominus. They serve to flex and rotate the trunk and, due to the orientation of their muscular fibres, they aim to strengthen the abdominal wall and lower the risk of hernia development. The external oblique muscle has fibres running in an infero-medial direction. Deep to this is the thinner internal oblique muscle with fibres running supero-medially. The deepest muscle is the transversus abdominus with transverse fibres.

The "vertical muscles" are the rectus abdominus and the pyramidalis muscle. The rectus abdominus is a long, paired muscle that runs either side of the linea alba. The linea semilunaris forms its lateral border, and at multiple loci, the muscle is intersected by fibrous bands which form the "six-pack". The pyramidalis muscle is a small, triangular muscle which is inconsistently present in humans. An intimate understanding of abdominal wall anatomy is crucial for a surgeon. It allows surgeons to make the most appropriate abdominal incision and is essential for an appreciation of abdominal wall pathologies, with hernia being the commonest.

Summary of Muscles of the Anterior Abdominal Wall

Muscle	Proximal attachment	Distal attachment	Innervation	Action
External oblique	Ribs 5–12	Linea alba, pubic crest and pubic tubercle, anterior iliac crest	T5–12	Protects and supports abdominal contents Flexes and rotates trunk

(Continued)

DOI: 10.1201/9781003292005-4

Summary of Muscles of the Anterior Abdominal Wall   (Continued)

Muscle	Proximal attachment	Distal attachment	Innervation	Action
Internal oblique	Thoracolumbar fascia, anterior iliac crest, inguinal ligament	Ribs 10–12, linea alba, pectin pubis (via the conjoint tendon)	T6–12 and L1	Protects and supports abdominal contents
Transversus abdominus	Thoracolumbar fascia, costal cartilages 7–12, iliac crest, inguinal ligament	Pubic crest, linea alba, pectin pubis (via the conjoint tendon)	T6–12 and L1	Protects and supports abdominal contents
Rectus abdominus	Pubic symphysis, pubic crest	Xiphoid process, costal cartilage 5–7	T6–12	Protects and supports abdominal contents Flexes trunk
Pyramidalis (inconsistently present)	Pubis	Linea alba	T12	Tenses linea alba

Below the level of the arcuate line of Douglas there is no posterior rectus sheath. The rectus lies on the transversalis fascia. This is demonstrated by the following diagram.

The contents of the rectus sheath are frequently asked about and include:

- The recti
- The pyramidalis
- Segmental nerves
- Segmental vessels
- Superior and inferior epigastric arteries

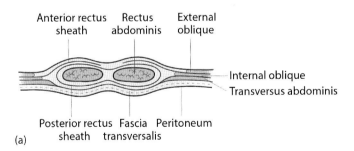

(a)

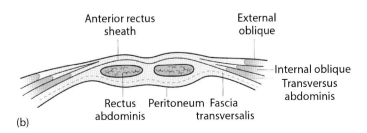

(b)

Figure 3.1 Anatomy of anterior abdominal wall. (a) Transverse section at the supraumbilical level. (b) Transverse section below the level of the arcuate line.

Summary of Muscles of the Posterior Abdominal Wall

Muscle	Proximal attachment	Distal attachment	Innervation	Action
Psoas minor (inconsistently present)	T12–L1 vertebrae and intervertebral discs	Pectineal line Iliopubic eminence	L1	Weak trunk flexor
Psoas major	T12–L5 vertebrae and intervertebral discs	Lesser trochanter of femur	L2–4	With the iliacus forms the iliopsoas which flexes the thigh
Iliacus	Iliac fossa	Lesser trochanter of femur	L2–4	With the psoas major forms the iliopsoas which flexes the thigh
Quadratus lumborum	Twelfth rib	Iliolumbar ligament and iliac crest	T12–L4	Extends and laterally rotates the vertebral column

THE INGUINAL CANAL

The inguinal canal is an incredibly high-yield topic for surgical exams, and it is imperative that you know this thoroughly. The inguinal canal is a passage, usually around 4–6 cm in length, that extends from the external/superficial ring, and then travels medially and inferiorly to the internal/deep ring.

The inguinal canal may be thought of as a box with each wall representing a different structure.

- *The anterior wall*—the aponeurosis of the external oblique muscle, reinforced laterally by the internal oblique muscle. The ring contributes to the medial third.
- *The posterior wall or floor*—the transversalis fascia and conjoint tendon.
- *The superior wall or roof*—the medial crus of the aponeurosis of the external oblique, the musculoaponeurotic arches of the internal oblique and transverse abdominal muscles and the transversalis fascia.
- *The inferior wall*—the inguinal ligament, which is reinforced medially by the lacunar ligament and reinforced laterally by the iliopubic tract. The inguinal ligament is a thickened inferior portion of the external oblique aponeurosis.

In males, the inguinal canal transmits the spermatic cord as well as the gonadal vessels and lymphatics. In females, it transmits the round ligament of the uterus (which can be ligated and divided so that the external/superficial ring may be completely closed). The contents of the spermatic cord include three fascia, three arteries, three veins, three nerves and three other structures.

THREE FASCIA:

1. External spermatic fascia (from the external oblique aponeurosis)
2. Cremasteric fascia (from the internal oblique aponeurosis)
3. Internal spermatic fascia (from the transversalis fascia)

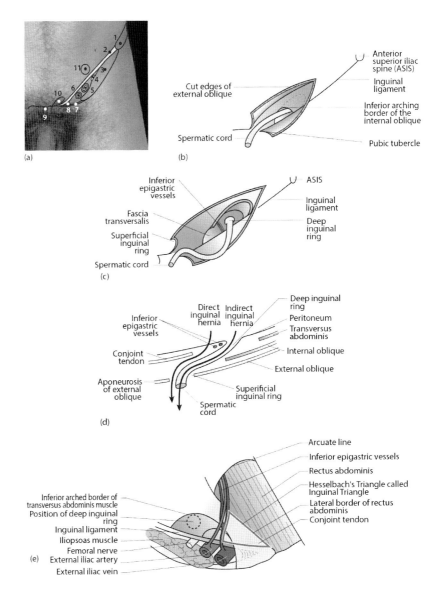

Figure 3.2 Inguinal canal. (a) Surface anatomy: 1, anterior superior iliac spine; 2, inguinal ligament; 3, iliopsoas muscle; 4, femoral nerve; 5, femoral artery passing beneath mid-inguinal point; 6, femoral vein; 7, origin of pectineus muscle; 8, reflected part of the inguinal ligament (pectineal [lacunar] ligament); 9, symphysis pubis; 10, superficial inguinal ring; 11, position of deep inguinal ring above midpoint of the inguinal ligament. (b) Anatomy of the inguinal region, external oblique being divided to demonstrate the course of the inguinal canal. (c) Deeper dissection through the internal oblique. (d) Diagram of horizontal section through the inguinal canal (e) Posterior aspect, as viewed laparoscopically, of the inguinal region showing the inguinal (Hesselbach's) triangle (thick lines).

THREE ARTERIES:

1. Testicular artery (from the abdominal aorta L2)
2. Cremasteric artery (from the inferior epigastric artery)
3. Artery to vas (from the inferior vesical artery)

THREE VEINS:

1. Pampiniform plexus (right side drains to the inferior vena cava, left side drains to the left renal vein).
2. Cremasteric vein (follows artery).
3. Vein of vas (follows artery).

THREE NERVES:

1. Nerve to cremaster (from the genitofemoral nerve)
2. Sympathetic fibres T10–11
3. Genital branch of the genitofemoral nerve

THREE OTHER STRUCTURES:

1. Vas deferens
2. Lymphatics which drain to the para-aortic lymph nodes
3. Processus vaginalis (if patent results in indirect hernia)

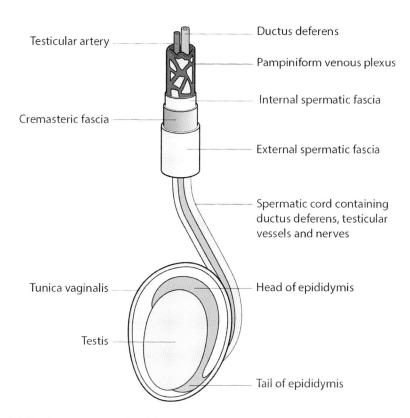

Figure 3.3 Testis, spermatic cord and their coverings.

CLINICAL POINTS

The significance of the inguinal canal comes into play when considering hernias. Hernias are the commonest cause of small-bowel obstruction worldwide (second is adhesions). A hernia is defined as the protrusion of a viscus or part of a viscus through the wall of its containing cavity into an anatomically abnormal position. There are many different types of hernias, but here we shall consider groin hernias.

Inguinal hernias are defined as direct or indirect. A direct hernia is caused by a weakness in the posterior wall of the inguinal canal, whereas in the case of an indirect hernia, abdominal contents pass through the deep inguinal, then the inguinal canal and exit via the superficial ring. The deep ring is located at the midpoint of the inguinal ligament, i.e. halfway between the anterior superior iliac spine and the pubic tubercle. This is not to be confused with the mid-inguinal point, which is the surface landmark for the femoral artery, i.e. halfway between the anterior superior iliac spine and the pubic symphysis.

Anatomically speaking, direct hernias are said to protrude through Hesselbach's triangle. The boundaries of this triangle are:

- *Medially*—lateral margin of the rectus sheath
- *Superolaterally*—inferior epigastric vessels
- *Inferiorly*—inguinal ligament

Direct hernias are found medial to the inferior epigastric vessels, whereas indirect hernias are found lateral to these vessels. Hernia tend to be acquired and are associated with risk factors such as chronic cough, obesity, smoking, poor nutrition, ascites or anything that will increase intra-abdominal pressure. Indirect hernias are usually the result of a patent processus vaginalis. Femoral hernias are more common in females, although women are still more likely to have inguinal hernias overall. They are classically found below and lateral to the pubic tubercle within the femoral canal. The anatomy of the femoral canal has been described earlier in this book.

Hernia repair can be performed as an elective or emergency procedure.

Strangulated hernias warrant emergency repairs; worrisome symptoms include obstructive symptoms, a non-reducible lump, skin changes over the lump and intractable pain.

In the elective setting, repairs can be done open or laparoscopically. Laparoscopic repairs are recommended for bilateral or recurrent hernias. Repairs should be tension-free, normally using a mesh. Inguinodynia (chronic pain) is common following this procedure, and can be related to intra-operative injury or complications relating to the mesh.

The principle of hernia repair (in general) is one which is tension-free, and the cause of a recurrent hernia is often related to wound infection. In an open repair the ilioinguinal nerve is the most commonly injured nerve. It is found after opening of the external oblique fascia. In a laparoscopic repair the lateral femoral cutaneous is the most commonly injured, usually by an improperly placed tack lateral to the cord.

The "corona mortis" may be encountered during laparoscopic inguinal hernia repair when the mesh is tacked to Cooper's ligament. This is an anatomical variant (an aberrant obturator), an anastomosis between the obturator and the external iliac or inferior epigastric arteries. It is located behind the superior pubic ramus at a variable distance from the symphysis pubis.

EPONYMOUS HERNIAS:

- *Amyand's hernia*—when the appendix is found within an inguinal hernia.
- *Littre's hernia*—Meckle's diverticulum within an inguinal hernia.
- *Canal of Nuck hernia*—ovary within the inguinal hernia.
- *Richter's hernia*—a herniation of only a portion of the circumference of the bowel wall through the fascial defect. Usually, it is the anti-mesenteric portion of the bowel. This may result in strangulation without obstructive symptoms.
- *Pantaloon hernia*—co-existing direct and indirect hernias.

IMPORTANT EMBRYOLOGICAL STRUCTURES TO CONSIDER AT THE UMBILICUS:

- *The medial umbilical ligaments*—obliterated portion of the umbilical arteries (×2)
- *The median umbilical ligament*—obliterated urachus
- *The round ligament of the liver*—obliterated umbilical vein

THE LESSER SAC

This is a sac that lies posterior to the lesser omentum and stomach. It projects downwards between the layers of the greater omentum. The greater omentum is supplied by:

1. The right gastro-omental artery (from the gastroduodenal artery)
2. The left gastro-omental artery (the largest branch of the splenic artery)

Left wall—the spleen which is attached by the gastrosplenic ligament and the splenorenal ligament.

The gastrosplenic ligament contains the short gastric vessels and the left gastro-epiploic vessels. The splenorenal ligament contains the splenic vessels and the tail of the pancreas.

Right wall—the foramen of Winslow.

The boundaries of the foramen of Winslow are:

- *Anteriorly*—free edge of the lesser omentum, which contains the common bile duct (right), the hepatic artery (left) and the portal vein (posteriorly)
- *Posteriorly*—the inferior vena cava
- *Interiorly*—the first part of the duodenum
- *Superiorly*—the caudate lobe of the liver

CLINICAL POINT

The Pringle manoeuvre compresses the hepatic artery here to control bleeding.

THE COELIAC AXIS

- The coeliac axis is located at T12.
- Branches are: the common hepatic artery, the splenic artery and the left gastric artery.
- It supplies blood to the abdominal viscera of the foregut.

- It is affected by a wide range of pathologic conditions, including mesenteric isch-aemia due to intrinsic occlusion (secondary to causes such as atherosclerosis or thromboembolic events) and extrinsic compression from masses or the median arcuate ligament.
- Symptoms of mesenteric ischaemia are non-specific and include postprandial abdomi-nal pain and weight loss.
- More unusual pathologic conditions include dissection, aneurysm, and vascular malformations.

THE STOMACH

This is a "J"-shaped organ that has anterior and posterior surfaces as well as lesser and greater curvatures and two orifices (the cardia and the pylorus).

The relationships of the stomach are as follows:

- *Anteriorly*—the abdominal wall, the left costal margin, the diaphragm and the liver
- *Posteriorly*—the lesser sac, the splenic artery, the transverse colon, the left kidney, the left adrenal gland, the spleen and the pancreas
- *Superiorly*—the diaphragm

ARTERIAL SUPPLY:

- *Left gastric artery*—from the coeliac axis (T12)
- *Right gastric artery*—from the hepatic artery
- *Right gastro-epiploic artery*—from the gastroduodenal branch of the hepatic artery
- *Left gastro-epiploic artery*—from the splenic artery (largest branch)
- *Short gastric artery*—from the splenic artery

The correspondingly named veins drain into the portal system.

The lymphatic drainage follows the blood supply. The regions are as follows:

- *I*—to the aortic nodes
- *II*—to the subpyloric lymph nodes and then the aortic nodes
- *III*—to the suprapancreatic lymph nodes and the aortic lymph nodes

NERVE SUPPLY (WHICH PASSES THROUGH THE OESOPHAGEAL HIATUS AT T10):

- *The anterior vagus*—anterior branch is close to the stomach and supplies the cardia and lesser curvature.
- *The posterior vagus*—the posterior branch is larger and supplies the anterior and posterior part of the stomach forming the coeliac branch and runs along the left gastric artery.

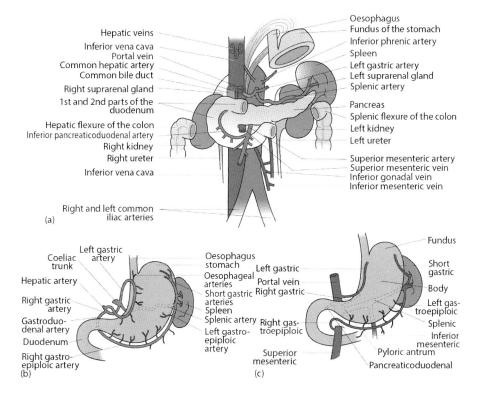

Figure 3.4 (a) Posterior relations of the stomach (shown with the major part of the stomach removed). (b) Arterial blood supply of the stomach. (c) Venous drainage of the stomach to the portal vein.

THE DUODENUM

This is the first part of the small intestine. At its origin it is completely covered by the peritoneum for one inch, and then it is retroperitoneal. Classically, it is described in four parts.

BLOOD SUPPLY:

- Superior pancreaticoduodenal artery (from the gastroduodenal artery)
- Inferior pancreaticoduodenal artery (from the first branch of the superior mesenteric artery)

CLINICAL POINTS

- The differences between the jejunum and the ileum are important to be aware of. The jejunum lies in the umbilical region and has:
  - A thicker wall (valvulae conniventes are larger and thicker more proximally)
  - A greater diameter
  - A mesentery that is less fat laden
  - One or two arterial arcades with a long, infrequent terminal branches
- The ileum is shorter with more numerous arterial arcades (3–5 usually).

Parts of the Duodenum

Part of duodenum	Length	Anatomical points	Clinical points
D1	5 cm	Overlapped by liver and gallbladder Posterior—portal veins, common bile duct and gastroduodenal artery	Duodenal ulcers— massive bleeding Gallstone ileus
D2	8 cm	Curves around head of pancreas Crossed by transverse colon and right kidney/ureter Halfway posteromedially is the pancreatic duct of Wirsung on an eminence (duodenal papilla) Accessory duct of Santorini opens a little above this papilla	May be damaged in right hemicolectomy and right nephrectomy
D3	10 cm	Crossed by superior mesenteric vessels	
D4	2.5 cm	Ends at the ligament of Treitz, which is a well demarcated peritoneal fold descending from the right crus of the diaphragm	

THE LARGE BOWEL

The large bowel may anatomically be divided into eight parts: the caecum, appendix, ascending colon, transverse colon, descending colon, sigmoid colon, rectum and anal canal.

The colon (not the appendix, rectum or caecum) has appendices epiploicae over its surface. Furthermore, the colon and caecum have taenia coli, which are three flattened bands of longitudinal muscle. The taenia coli are responsible for the saccular shape of the large bowel. The ascending and descending colon attached directly to the posterior abdominal wall. They do not have a mesocolon. The sigmoid colon and the transverse colon are peritonealised.

The bowel is divided into foregut, midgut and hindgut structures which each have a dominant blood supply. The foregut is from the oral cavity to the ligament of Treitz. The midgut runs from the ligament of Treitz to the initial two-thirds of the transverse colon. The hindgut is from the latter one-third of the transverse colon to the upper third of the anus. Foregut structures receive their blood supply from the coeliac axis (located at T12), midgut structures from the superior mesenteric artery (SMA, located at L1) and hindgut structures from the inferior mesenteric artery (IMA, at L3). The following diagram highlights this blood supply as well as the relevant branches.

CLINICAL POINTS

- Please be aware of Griffith and Sudeck's points, which are the watershed areas of the bowel. These are the areas in the colon between two major arteries that supply the colon and are therefore more prone to ischaemia.
- Note that the SMA has five branches—diagram below.

- Branches of the SMA (LI):
  - Jejunal branches

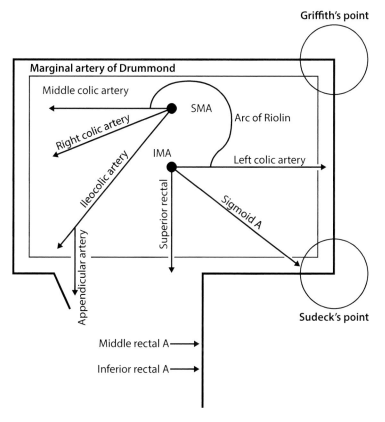

Figure 3.5 Blood supply to the large bowel.

- Ileal branches
- Ileocolic artery
- Right colic artery
- Middle colic artery

THE RECTUM AND ANAL CANAL

The rectum starts anterior to the third segment of the sacrum and finishes at the level of the prostate in men or the intrapelvic vagina in women. Here it passes through the levator to become the anal canal. The rectum is fully extraperitoneal in its lower third, extraperitoneal posteriorly and laterally in the middle third and extraperitoneal only posteriorly in its upper third.

Anterior structures are separated from the rectum by Denonvilliers' fascia, and posterior structures by Waldeyer's fascia. Laterally, structures are supported by the levator ani. The levator ani is a broad muscular sheet that, together with the coccygeus muscle and their associated fascias, forms the pelvic diaphragm. The levator ani is a collection of three muscles: the puborectalis, pubococcygeus and iliococcygeus.

The anal canal is 4 cm long and is directed downwards and backwards. The middle part of the anal canal represents the embryological junction between endoderm (hindgut) and ectoderm (proctodaeum). The lower half of the anal canal is composed of the squamous epithelium and the upper half is the columnar epithelium. Anteriorly the anal canal is related to the perineal body, posteriorly to the anococcygeal body and laterally to the ischioanal fossa.

The anal sphincter is made up of two parts—internal and external. The internal sphincter is involuntary and is continuous superiorly with the smooth coat of the rectum. The external sphincter is voluntary and some of its fibres fuse with the levator ani.

Clinically they can be differentiated, as smooth muscle is white and skeletal is red. This is relevant when doing a lateral sphincterotomy (you only want to cut the internal sphincter).

BLOOD SUPPLY

FROM THREE ARTERIES:

1. The superior rectal artery (from the IMA)
2. The middle rectal artery (from the IIA)
3. The inferior rectal artery (from the pudendal artery, which is a branch of the IIA)

VENOUS DRAINAGE:

- Superior rectal vein to the inferior mesenteric vein (portal system)
- Middle rectal vein to the internal iliac vein (systemic system)
- Inferior rectal vein to the pudendal vein and then to the internal iliac vein (systemic system)

LYMPHATIC DRAINAGE:

- *Above the dentate line*—drains to the lumbar nodes/mesorectal nodes
- *Below the dentate line*—drains to the inguinal lymph nodes

NERVE SUPPLY:

- *Upper*—autonomic plexus
- *Lower*—somatic inferior rectal nerve (terminal branch of the pudendal nerve)

CLINICAL POINTS

Haemorrhoids are dilatations of the superior rectal veins. They are classified in the following way:

- *Grade I*—first-degree or primary haemorrhoids
  Normal or near normal. Prominent vasculature with engorgement but no prolapse.
- *Grade II*—second-degree or secondary haemorrhoids
  Some symptoms. Haemorrhoidal tissue prolapses only with straining but spontaneously reduces.
- *Grade III*—third-degree or tertiary haemorrhoids
  Haemorrhoidal tissue prolapses beyond the dentate line with straining and can only be reduced manually. Itching, staining from mucous discharge, soilage and swelling may occur.

- *Grade IV*—fourth-degree or quaternary haemorrhoids
  Prolapsed tissues are evident and they cannot be reduced manually. Chronic inflammatory changes with maceration, mucosal atrophy, friability and ulceration are commonly observed.

Cancers associated with the lower half of the anal cancer include SCC (due to the squamous epithelium); the upper half is columnar and therefore associated with adenocarcinomas. These are managed differently.

An intimate understanding of the anal canal and the sphincter mechanism is vital in the management of perianal abscesses and fistulae.

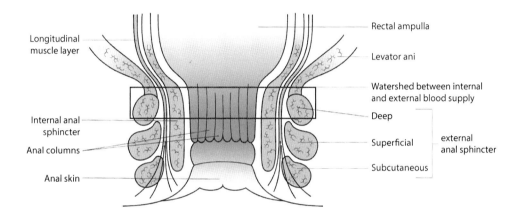

Figure 3.6 Anal sphincter—coronal section.

THE PORTAL VENOUS SYSTEM

The portal venous system drains blood from the gallbladder, spleen, pancreas, stomach and small and large intestines.

Key points to remember are:

- The portal vein is a confluence of the superior mesenteric vein, inferior mesenteric vein and splenic vein (with other tributaries).
- The portal vein enters the liver within the hepatoduodenal ligament.
- The portal vein runs posterior to the proper hepatic artery and the common bile duct within the hepatoduodenal ligament.

CLINICAL POINTS

- Portal hypertension arises when blood flow through the liver is compromised and blood pressure in the portal vein rises. Complications of portal hypertension include oesophageal varices, ascites and hepatorenal syndrome.

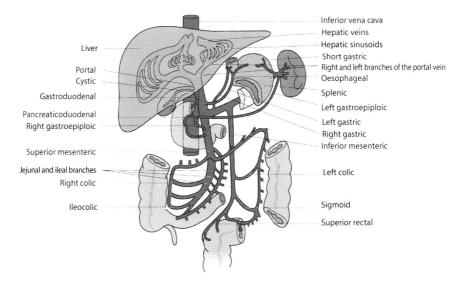

Figure 3.7 Portal venous system showing the portal vein and its branches.

Sites of Porto-Systemic Anastomoses Include

Lower oesophagus	Left gastric veins (portal system)—lower branches of oesophageal veins (systemic veins)
Upper part of the anal canal	Superior rectal veins (portal)—inferior and middle rectal veins (systemic)
Umbilicus	Paraumbilical veins (portal)—epigastric veins (systemic)
Area of the liver	Intraparenchymal branches of right division of portal vein (portal)—retroperitoneal veins (systemic)
Hepatic and splenic flexures	Omental and colonic veins (portal)—retroperitoneal veins (systemic)

- Anatomical variants of the portal vein occur in up to 35% of individuals. Some examples of these variations include trifurcation of the main portal vein, the right posterior branch arising from the main portal vein or the right anterior branch originating from the left portal vein.

THE LIVER

The liver is the largest organ in the body. It has a variety of functions, including metabolism, immunity, detoxification and vitamin storage amongst others. It is unique in its dual blood supply from the portal vein (75%) and the hepatic artery (25%). There are three hepatic veins (left, middle and right) which drain into the IVC.

The functional unit of the liver is the lobule. Each lobule is hexagonal, and a portal triad (portal vein, hepatic artery, bile duct) sits at each corner of the hexagon. Lobules comprise hepatocytes, and depending on the degree of perfusion and function, these organised hepatocytes are classified into three distinct zones, as follows:

1. *Zone I*—the periportal region of hepatocytes. These are the best perfused and the first to regenerate due to closeness to oxygenated blood and nutrients. This zone plays an

important role in oxidative metabolism, gluconeogenesis, bile formation and cholesterol formation as well as amino acid catabolism.

2. *Zone II*—the pericentral region of the hepatocytes.
3. *Zone III*—hepatocytes situated the furthest from the portal triad. This zone is important in detoxification, biotransformation, ketogenesis, glycolysis, lipogenesis and glycogen synthesis.

Macroscopically the liver is divided into a right lobe and a left lobe by the falciform ligament. The right lobe is the larger of the two. The base of the liver is divided into an "H"-shaped arrangement of fossae. Within the H is the porta hepatis. Details about the porta hepatis and its importance are listed in the next section.

THE PORTA HEPATIS

- *Location*—postero-inferior surface of the liver
- Separates the caudate lobe (posterior) from the quadrate lobe (anterior)
- Transmits the:
  - Common hepatic duct
  - Hepatic artery
  - Portal vein (most posterior structure)
  - Sympathetic and parasympathetic nerves
  - Lymphatic drainage and nodes

CLINICAL POINTS

- The hepatocystic triangle (aka Calot's triangle) is a triangular space at the porta hepatis. It is of surgical importance as it is dissected during cholecystectomy. Its boundaries are as follows:

  - *Superiorly*—the inferior surface of the liver
  - *Right*—the cystic duct
  - *Left*—common hepatic duct
  - *Contents*—the cystic artery and the cystic lymph node of Lund

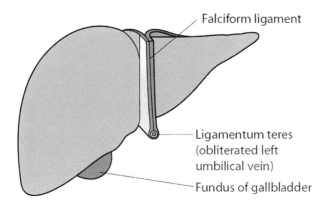

Falciform ligament

Ligamentum teres (obliterated left umbilical vein)

Fundus of gallbladder

Figure 3.8a Liver, anterior surface.

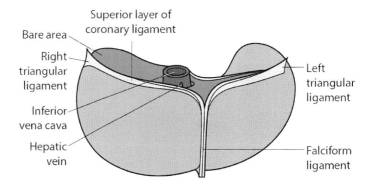

Figure 3.8b Liver, superior surface.

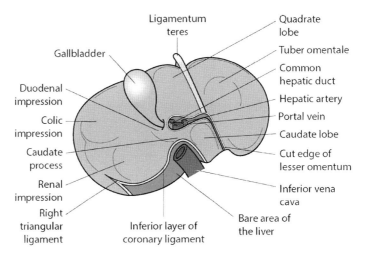

Figure 3.8c Liver, inferior (visceral) surface.

The falciform ligament is a useful anatomical division, but a more useful physiologic separation is Cantlie's line. This is a line drawn from the gallbladder fossa to the IVC. This separates the lobes into divisions which have their own arterial and portal blood supply.

The Couinaud classification of liver anatomy divides the liver into eight functionally independent segments. An intimate understanding of these divisions is not required for the MRCS Part A. The caudate lobe or segment I is located posteriorly and is anatomically different from other lobes since it often has direct connections to the IVC through hepatic veins which are separate from the main hepatic veins.

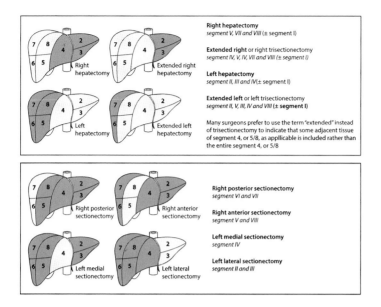

Figure 3.9 Liver resections with respect to the Couinaud classification of liver anatomy.

CLINICAL POINTS

- An awareness of the lobes of the liver is important for liver resections.
- The middle hepatic vein is located at the level of Cantlie's line and may complicate hepatic resection.
- The ligamentum teres is the obliterated left umbilical vein.
- The ligamentum venosum was the ductus venosus which shunted oxygenated blood from the left umbilical vein to the IVC in the fetus.

THE GALLBLADDER

The gallbladder is a small, hollow organ that serves to store and concentrate bile. It lies beneath the liver in the gallbladder fossa and inferiorly is related to both the duodenum and the transverse colon. It comprises a fundus, body and neck.

BLOOD SUPPLY

ARTERIAL SUPPLY:

- Cystic artery, which is a branch of the right hepatic artery.
- Small vessels from the hepatic bed supply the gallbladder.

VENOUS DRAINAGE:

- There is no cystic vein. Small veins drain the gallbladder bed into the tributaries of the right portal vein.

LYMPHATIC DRAINAGE:

- Via the cystic node/Lund's node of the gallbladder. All the lymph finally drains into coeliac lymph nodes.

CLINICAL POINTS

- Pringle's manoeuvre may be used to controlled bleeding during cholecystectomy.
- Anatomic variants of gallbladder duplication are differentiated according to Boyden's classification:
  - *Type I*—split primordium group
    Septate, "V"-shaped (bilobed) and "Y"-shaped
  - *Type 2*—accessory gallbladder group
    "H"-shaped (ductular and trabecular)

THE SPLEEN

The spleen is the largest reticuloendothelial organ in the body. During week 6 of gestation, the spleen develops from the cephalic aspect of the dorsal mesogastrium as irregular hillocks. It comprises two types of pulp:

1. *Red pulp*—filters damaged/old red blood cells
2. *White pulp*—immunologic function

There are four ligaments of the spleen: the gastrosplenic ligament, the colicosplenic ligament, the phrenocolic ligament and the splenorenal ligament. The gastrosplenic ligament contains the short gastric artery and the left gastro-epiploic artery. The splenorenal ligament contains the splenic artery and the tail of the pancreas.

ARTERIAL SUPPLY:

- Splenic artery (from the coeliac axis)

VENOUS DRAINAGE:

- Splenic vein, which is joined by the SMV to drain to the portal vein.

CLINICAL POINTS

- Functions of the spleen:
  - Platelet storage
  - Culls damaged or old red blood cells
  - Pitting—this is the removal of intracellular products
  - Immune function
  - Generates proteins, e.g. tuftsin—important for opsonisation
- Indications for splenectomy:
  - Major trauma
  - Haemorrhage
  - Haemolytic anaemia

The severity of a splenic injury can objectively be described with a grading system developed by the American Association for the Surgery of Trauma (AAST).

The AAST Splenic Injury Scale*

Grade	Definition
I	Subcapsular haematoma <10% of surface area
	Parenchymal laceration <1 cm depth
	Capsular tear
II	Subcapsular haematoma 10–50% of surface area
	Intraparenchymal haematoma <5 cm
	Parenchymal laceration 1–3 cm in depth
III	Subcapsular haematoma >50% of surface area
	Ruptured subcapsular or intraparenchymal haematoma ≥5 cm
	Parenchymal laceration >3 cm in depth
IV	Any injury in the presence of a splenic vascular injury or active bleeding confined within splenic capsule
	Parenchymal laceration involving segmental or hilar vessels producing >25% devascularisation
V	Shattered spleen
	Any injury in the presence of splenic vascular injury with active bleeding extending beyond the spleen into the peritoneum

* Low-grade injuries I–III may be managed conservatively, IV and V may be amenable to interventional radiology and angio-embolisation or may proceed to laparotomy and splenectomy.

Splenectomy patients are at increased risk of infections, particularly those caused by encapsulated bacteria (Streptococcus pneumoniae, Haemophilus influenzae and Neisseria meningitidis). On some occasions, infection may result in a severe case of sepsis known as overwhelming post-splenectomy infection (OPSI). OPSI has a high mortality rate and is considered a medical emergency that requires prompt treatment. OPSI is usually caused by the aforementioned encapsulated bacteria.

THE PANCREAS

The pancreas is a retroperitoneal structure that is descriptively divided into a head, neck, tail, body and uncinate process.

ARTERIAL SUPPLY:

- Splenic artery—supplies pancreatic branches, the largest of which is called the greater pancreatic artery.
- Superior and inferior pancreaticoduodenal arteries from the gastroduodenal artery (coeliac axis) and SMA.

VENOUS DRAINAGE:

- Splenic vein
- Pancreaticoduodenal veins

LYMPHATIC DRAINAGE:

- Splenic lymph nodes
- Coeliac lymph nodes
- Superior mesenteric lymph nodes

- The pancreas appears at 5 weeks of gestation as two outpouchings of the endodermal lining of the duodenum. These are the ventral and dorsal pancreas. The dorsal pancreas grows more rapidly than the ventral pancreas. Eventually the ventral and dorsal pancreas join, and their ductal systems combine so that secretions from the ventral pancreas enter the shared ductal system of the ventral pancreas and common bile duct. The dorsal pancreas becomes the body and tail of the pancreas. The ventral pancreas becomes the uncinate process. The dorsal and ventral pancreas both contribute to the head of the pancreas.
- Cancers at the head of the pancreas may compress the common bile duct, resulting in obstructive jaundice.

THE ADRENAL GLANDS

These are exocrine glands found above the kidneys. They are in the retroperitoneum.

The adrenal gland is made up of two distinct parts, the medulla and the cortex. Each part is responsible for producing different hormones.

ARTERIAL SUPPLY:

- Superior adrenal arteries (from the inferior phrenic arteries)
- Middle adrenal arteries (from the aorta)
- Inferior adrenal arteries (from the renal arteries)

VENOUS DRAINAGE:

- Right adrenal gland directly to inferior vena cava
- Left adrenal gland to left renal vein to inferior vena cava

LYMPHATIC DRAINAGE:

- Lumbar lymph nodes

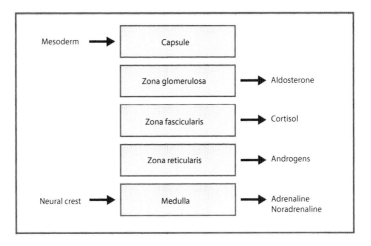

Figure 3.10 Anatomy of the adrenal cortex and adrenal medulla.

THE KIDNEYS

The kidneys are retroperitoneal structures which are approximately 11 cm long, 6 cm wide and 4 cm thick. The right kidney lies slightly lower than the left due to the presence of the liver in the right upper quadrant. The hilum of the left kidney is at the level of L1. The adrenal glands are related to the kidneys at their superior pole. The relationship of structures at the renal hilum anterior to posterior is as follows: the renal vein, the renal artery and the pelvis of the ureter.

The kidney has three capsules:

1. The renal fascia
2. Perinephric fat
3. The true fibrous capsule

ARTERIAL SUPPLY:

- Renal artery (from the abdominal aorta, L1)

VENOUS DRAINAGE:

- Renal vein

LYMPHATIC DRAINAGE:

- Para-aortic lymph nodes

CLINICAL POINTS

The American Association for the Surgery of Trauma (AAST) renal injury scale is the most widely used grading system for renal trauma. It classifies renal injury as follows.

Grade	Description
I	• Subcapsular haematoma or contusion, without laceration
II	• Superficial laceration ≤1 cm depth not involving the collecting system (no evidence of urine extravasation)
	• Perirenal haematoma confined within the perirenal fascia
III	• Laceration >1 cm not involving the collecting system (no evidence of urine extravasation)
	• Vascular injury or active bleeding confined within the perirenal fascia
IV	• Laceration involving the collecting system with urinary extravasation
	• Laceration of the renal pelvis and/or complete ureteropelvic disruption
	• Vascular injury to segmental renal artery or vein
	• Segmental infarctions without associated active bleeding (i.e. due to vessel thrombosis)
	• Active bleeding extending beyond the perirenal fascia (i.e. into the retroperitoneum or peritoneum)
V	• Shattered kidney
	• Avulsion of renal hilum or laceration of the main renal artery or vein; devascularisation of a kidney due to hilar injury
	• Devascularised kidney with active bleeding

THE URETER

The ureters are approximately 25 cm long and connect the kidneys to the bladder. Anatomically they may be split into an abdominal portion, a pelvic portion and an intravesical portion.

ABDOMINAL PORTION:

- Lies on the medial edge of the psoas major muscle.
- At the bifurcation of the common iliac artery, it enters the pelvis.

PELVIC PORTION:

- Runs anterior to the internal iliac artery and in front of the iliac spine.
- In men it runs above the seminal vesicle and is crossed by the vas deferens.
- In women it passes above and lateral to the vaginal fornix.

INTRAVESICAL PORTION:

- Passes through the wall of the bladder obliquely.

The ureters are supplied by arterial branches from the aorta, the renal arteries, the testicular/ovarian arteries and the internal iliac and inferior vesical arteries.

CLINICAL POINTS

The ureter is narrowed at three anatomical points:

1. The junction of the pelvis of the ureter with the abdominal portion of the ureter
2. The pelvic brim
3. The ureteric orifice

THE BLADDER

The bladder is a temporary capacitance organ that, in an average adult, stores about 300 mL of urine. It has an internal lining with folds (known as rugae) and it assists in the expulsion of urine. Anteriorly the bladder is related to the pubic symphysis, posteriorly to the rectum/seminal vesicles in males and the vagina/supravaginal part of the cervix in females. Laterally, the bladder is related to the levator ani and the obturator internus. Superiorly it is covered by peritoneum.

BLOOD SUPPLY:

Its blood supply is conferred from the superior and inferior vesical branches of the internal iliac artery. The plexus of vesical veins drains to the internal iliac vein.

LYMPHATIC DRAINAGE:

Lymphatics drain to the iliac and para-aortic lymph nodes.

NERVE SUPPLY:

The nerve supply to the bladder is both parasympathetic and sympathetic:

1. *Parasympathetic*—efferent, from S2–4. Conveys motor fibres to stimulate the bladder wall muscles. Inhibitory to the internal sphincter.
2. *Sympathetic*—efferent. Stimulates the internal sphincter and inhibit the detrusor.

The striated muscle of the external sphincter is under control of the pudendal nerve.

THE URETHRA

The male urethra is divided anatomically into the prostatic, membranous and spongy portions. The female urethra is significantly shorter, and it lies immediately anterior to the vagina.

Blood supply to the urethra is via the inferior vesical artery, middle rectal artery and internal pudendal artery. Venous drainage is via the inferior vesical vein, middle rectal vein and internal pudendal vein.

The nerve supply to the urethra comes from the pudendal nerve, the pelvic splanchnic nerves and the inferior hypogastric plexus.

Lymphatics drain via the internal iliac and the deep inguinal lymph nodes.

CLINICAL POINTS

- The narrowest part of the urethra is the external orifice.
- The ureter and bladder are lined by the transitional epithelium (uroepithelium).
- The urethra is lined by the transitional epithelium as far as the entry of the ejaculatory ducts in the prostatic urethra, whereupon the urethra is then lined by the squamous epithelium.

THE PROSTATE

The prostate is a chestnut-sized fibromuscular and glandular structure. It is anatomically split into the fibromuscular zone, the peripheral zone, the transitional zone and the central zone. It has two capsules: the true capsule, which is a fibrous, thin sheath which surrounds the gland, and the false capsule, which is a condensed extraperitoneal fascia. Between these capsules is the prostatic venous plexus. The prostatic plexus drains to the internal iliac vein. Some venous blood drains to the valveless vertebral veins of Batson. The prostate receives its arterial supply from a branch of the internal iliac artery, the inferior vesical artery.

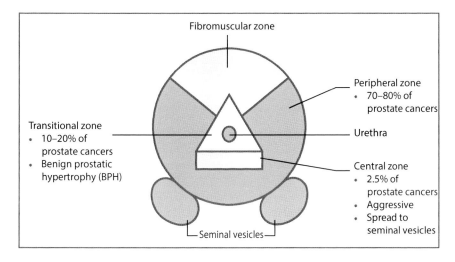

Figure 3.11 Zones of the prostate gland.

- The Batson venous plexus drains the vertebrae and skull. It forms anastomoses with veins draining the thoracic, abdominal and pelvic organs. Since this venous system is valveless, it acts as a pathway to transmit metastatic cells to the spinal column.

THE SCROTUM, TESTES AND EPIDIDYMIS

The scrotum is a pouch of skin in which overlies the testes and their surrounding coverings. The subcutaneous tissue contains the dartos muscle. The dartos muscle is the thin, rugate fascial muscle of the scrotum made of smooth muscle. This muscle is innervated by the genital branch of the genitofemoral nerve. The scrotum protects the testes and is important in thermoregulation. Arteriovenous anastomoses and subcutaneous plexuses provide blood supply to the scrotum. The external pudendal branches and the scrotal branches of the internal pudendal arteries play a role in supplying blood to the scrotum. The wall of the scrotum drains into the superficial inguinal lymph nodes. The contents of the scrotum drain to the lumbar lymph nodes.

The layers of the scrotum may be remembered with the following mnemonic.

"SOME DAMN ENGLISHMAN CALLED IT THE TESTES"

S—Skin
D—Dartos fascia and muscle
E—External spermatic fascia
C—Cremaster muscle
I—Internal spermatic fascia
T—Tunica vaginalis
T—Tunica albuginea

The testicle itself is supplied by the testicular artery (from the abdominal aorta) as well as an anastomosis with the artery to the vas (from the inferior vesical branch of the internal iliac artery). The testicles are drained by the pampiniform plexus of veins becoming a singular testicular vein. The right testicular vein drains into the inferior vena cava whereas the left testicular vein drains into the left renal vein. Testicular lymphatics drain to the para-aortic lymph nodes. The testes receive their nerve supply from T10 and T11 sympathetic fibres via the renal and aortic plexus.

THE PERINEUM

The perineum is a diamond-shaped structure that is split into two triangles: the urogenital triangle and the anal triangle. The triangles are divided by a line drawn between the two ischial tuberosities. The neurovascular supply to the perineum is the pudendal nerve and the internal pudendal artery/vein.

The boundaries of the perineum are as follows:

- *Anteriorly*—the pubic symphysis
- *Posteriorly*—tip of the coccyx
- *Laterally*—the inferior pubic rami, the inferior ischial rami and the sacrotuberous ligament

- *Roof*—formed by the pelvic floor
- *Base*—formed by skin and fascia

The urogenital triangle is bounded by a line drawn between the ischial tuberosities, the ischio-pubic rami and the pubic symphysis.

The layers of the urogenital triangle (deep to superficial) are as follows:

1. *Deep perineal pouch*—a potential space between the deep fascia of the pelvic floor and the perineal membrane.
   In females, it contains the urethra, external urethral sphincter and vagina.
   In males, it contains the urethra, external urethral sphincter, bulbourethral glands and deep transverse perineal muscles.
2. *Perineal membrane*—this is tough fascia which is pierced by the urethra in men and by the urethra and the vagina in women. It provides attachment for external genital muscles.
3. *Superficial perineal pouch*—this contains (a) the erectile tissues of the penis and clitoris, (b) three muscles (ischiocavernosus, bulbospongiosus and superficial transverse perineal muscles) and (c) the Bartholin's glands.
4. *Fascia of the perineum*—this is the fascia which covers the muscles of the superficial perineal pouch. The muscles surrounded by the deep perineal fascia are the bulbospongiosus, ischiocavernosus and superficial transverse perineal muscles. The lateral attachment of the fascia is to the ischiopubic ramus, and anteriorly it is attached to the suspensory ligament of the clitoris/penis.
5. Skin.

The anal triangle is the posterior half of this diamond-shaped structure. It is bounded by the theoretical line between the ischial tuberosities, the coccyx and the sacrotuberous ligaments. The anal triangle contains the following structures: the anal aperture, the external anal sphinc-ter muscle, the ischioanal fossae and the pudendal nerve (S2, 3, 4), which runs through Alcock's canal. Alcock's canal is formed by a thickening of the obturator fascia. This canal transmits three structures: the pudendal nerve, the internal pudendal artery and the internal pudendal veins. These structures cross the pelvic surface of the obturator internus muscle. Clinically, the pudendal nerve can be compressed in this region, causing Alcock canal syndrome.

The perineal body is located at the junction between the anterior and posterior triangles. It provides attachment for the following structures:

- Levator ani (part of the pelvic floor)
- Bulbospongiosus muscle
- Superficial and deep transverse perineal muscles
- External anal sphincter muscle
- External urethral sphincter muscle fibres

THE VAGINA

The posterior fornix of the vagina is the only part which is intraperitoneal.

BLOOD SUPPLY:

- The vaginal artery
- The uterine artery

- The pudendal artery
- The middle rectal artery

(* All the above are branches of the internal iliac artery.)

VENOUS DRAINAGE:

- Venous plexus → vaginal vein → internal iliac vein

LYMPHATIC DRAINAGE:

- *Upper third*—external and internal iliac lymph nodes
- *Middle third*—internal iliac lymph nodes
- *Lower third*—superficial inguinal lymph nodes

*N.B. BRANCHES OF THE INTERNAL ILIAC ARTERY:

"**I** Love **G**oing **P**laces **I**n **M**y **V**ery **O**wn **U**nderwear":

- **I**liolumbar A
- **L**ateral sacral A
- **G**luteal A (superior + inferior)
- **P**udendal A (internal)
- **I**nferior vesicle A
- **M**iddle rectal A
- **V**aginal A
- **O**bturator A
- **U**terine A

THE UTERUS

ARTERIAL SUPPLY:

- Its blood supply is from the uterine artery (which originates from the internal iliac artery and runs in the base of the broad ligament).
- It forms an anastomosis with the ovarian artery and gives off a branch to the upper vagina and cervix.

VENOUS DRAINAGE:

- Drains to the internal iliac vein and communicates via the pelvic plexus with the vagina and bladder.

LYMPHATIC DRAINAGE:

- *Fundus*—para-aortic lymph nodes (some pass along the round ligament to the superficial inguinal lymph nodes).
- *Body*—via the broad ligament to the external iliac lymph nodes.
- *Cervix*—laterally via the broad ligament to the external iliac lymph nodes, postero-laterally with the uterine vessels to the internal iliac lymph nodes and posteriorly to the sacral lymph nodes.

THE OVARIES

The ovaries are attached to the broad ligament by the mesovarium and to the cornu of the uterus by the ovarian ligament.

They receive blood via the ovarian arteries, which are branches from the aorta. Drainage is via the ovarian veins. The right ovarian vein drains to the inferior vena cava directly; the left ovarian vein drains to the left renal vein and then to the inferior vena cava. The ovarian vessels run in the infundibulopelvic ligament. Lymphatic drainage is to the para-aortic lymph nodes. There are two sources of sympathetic innervation of the ovary; one is through the ovarian plexus, and the other is via the superior ovarian nerve (which is carried within the ovarian ligament). Parasympathetic innervation is via the pelvic plexus (which arises from the pelvic splanchnic nerves).

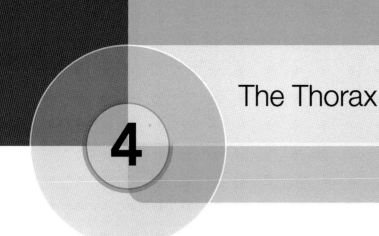

The Thorax

4

SURFACE MARKINGS

C6—cricoid cartilage
T2—superior angle of the scapula
T2/3—suprasternal notch
T3—spine of the scapula
T4/5—angle of Louis
T8—inferior angle of the scapula
T9—xiphisternal joint

THE RIBS

There are 12 pairs of ribs. There are seven "true" ribs that are attached via costal cartilages to the sternum. The "false" ribs are ribs 8, 9 and 10, and they are so called because their cartilages articulate with the cartilage of the rib above. Ribs 11 and 12 are "floating" ribs.

The atypical ribs are frequently asked about in the MRCS examination. These are the first rib, the second rib, the tenth rib and the floating ribs. Each will be addressed in turn.

THE FIRST RIB

This rib is the flattest and the shortest rib. It is the most curvaceous of all the ribs and has a prominent scalene tubercle. The anterior scalene muscle inserts here. There are a number of grooves present on the first rib, and it is important to know how these grooves relate to surrounding structures. Anterior to the tubercle for the anterior scalene muscle is the groove for the subclavian vein, behind it the groove for the subclavian artery. The inner border of the first rib provides attachment for Sibson's fascia.

From medial to lateral, the following structures cross the neck of the first rib: the sympathetic trunk, the superior intercostal artery and a branch of the first thoracic nerve.

CLINICAL POINTS

The first rib plays an important role in thoracic outlet syndrome. The lower trunk of the brachial plexus and the subclavian artery may be compressed between the first rib and the clavicle, causing neurovascular symptoms.

DOI: 10.1201/9781003292005-5

THE SECOND RIB

Is twice as long as the first rib and it has a small subcostal groove. It articulates with the sternum at the angle of Louis.

THE 10TH RIB

Only has one articular facet rather than two.

THE 11TH AND 12TH RIBS

These are floating ribs. They have one articular facet and do not have tubercles.

THE INTERCOSTAL SPACES

This space contains three inter-related muscles and a neurovascular bundle. From superior to inferior, the neurovascular bundle contains "**VAN**"—the intercostal **V**ein, **A**rtery and **N**erve, which lie between the internal and innermost intercostal muscles. The anatomy of these structures is significant when inserting a chest drain.

The intercostals are supplied by both anterior and posterior intercostal arteries.

Anterior intercostal branches of the internal thoracic artery are responsible for suppling the upper five/six intercostal spaces. The internal thoracic artery finally divides into the superior epigastric artery and musculophrenic artery. The musculophrenic artery supplies the anterior intercostal branches.

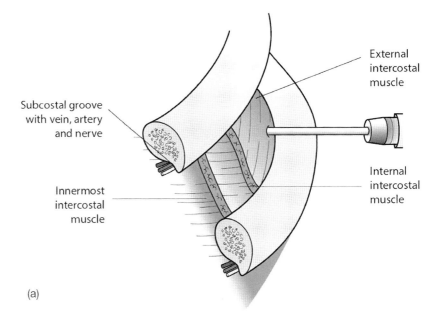

(a)

Figure 4.1 Intercostal space showing the aspirating needle passed just above the rib, thus avoiding the vessels in the subcostal groove above.

The first and second posterior intercostal arteries arise from a branch of the costocervical trunk (the supreme intercostal artery). The lower nine arteries are the aortic intercostals since they arise as branches of the aorta.

THE DIAPHRAGM

The diaphragm is a large, dome-shaped muscle that is innervated by C3, 4 and 5. It has a muscular part and a central aponeurosis. The peripheral portion of the diaphragm receives sensory fibres from the lower intercostal nerves.

Openings within the diaphragm are often asked about in the MRCS exam. These openings, their anatomical levels and the structures which pass through them are as follows:

T8 (CENTRAL TENDON OF THE DIAPHRAGM), TRANSMITS:

1. The vena cava (remember that "vena cava" has eight letters, therefore T8)
2. The right phrenic nerve

T10 (RIGHT CRUS OF THE DIAPHRAGM), TRANSMITS:

1. The oesophagus (remember that "oesophagus" has ten letters, therefore T10)
2. The two vagus nerves
3. Branches of the left gastric vessels

T12, TRANSMITS:

1. The abdominal aorta (remember that "aortic hiatus" has 12 letters, therefore, T12)
2. The azygos vein
3. The thoracic duct

CLINICAL POINTS

Congenital diaphragmatic hernias:
1. *Bochdalek hernia*
   - This is a postero-lateral diaphragmatic hernia.
   - Commonest cause of congenital diaphragmatic hernia.
   - The abnormality is a hole in the postero-lateral corner of the diaphragm which allows passage of the abdominal viscera into the chest cavity.
   - Location—the majority are on the left side of the diaphragm.
   - High mortality.
2. *Morgagni hernia*
   - Rare anterior defect of the diaphragm.
   - Approximately 2% of all congenital diaphragmatic hernia cases.
   - Herniation of abdominal contents through the foramina of Morgagni (located immediately adjacent and posterior to the xiphoid process of the sternum).

THE LOWER RESPIRATORY TRACT

The trachea commences at the C6, i.e. the lower border of the cricoid cartilage (note that the cricoid cartilage is the only complete ring in the respiratory tract). The shape of the trachea is maintained by 15–20 "U"-shaped cartilages. It bifurcates at the angle of Louis (T4/5) into the right and left main bronchi. The right main bronchus is shorter, wider and more horizontal than the left, meaning that aspirated objects or substances (e.g. vomit/nasogastric feed) are more likely to pass into the right bronchus.

The lungs are conical in shape. The right lung has three lobes and two fissures—the oblique and the horizontal fissure. The left lung has only two lobes and one oblique fissure. Each lobe has its own bronchus and its own blood supply, which is clinically important when considering a lobectomy. The lungs are supplied by the bronchial arteries, and venous blood is returned to the lungs by the pulmonary arteries. The bronchial veins drain to the azygos system, whereas the superior and inferior pulmonary veins drain to the left atrium. Lymphatic drainage is centripetal towards the hilum from the pleura. Nerve supply is from both vagus nerves and the sympathetic trunk.

THE MEDIASTINUM

Mediastinum stems from the Latin word *mediastinus*, meaning "midway". It is the space between the two pleural sacs, and it is subdivided anatomically for descriptive purposes. Each part of the mediastinum contains different structures.

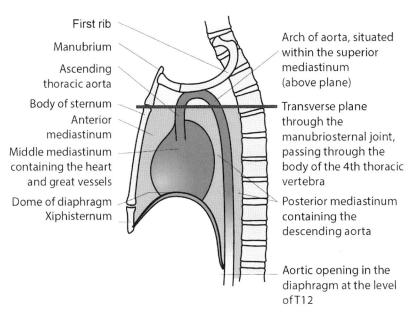

First rib

Manubrium

Ascending thoracic aorta

Body of sternum

Anterior mediastinum

Middle mediastinum containing the heart and great vessels

Dome of diaphragm
Xiphisternum

Arch of aorta, situated within the superior mediastinum (above plane)

Transverse plane through the manubriosternal joint, passing through the body of the 4th thoracic vertebra

Posterior mediastinum containing the descending aorta

Aortic opening in the diaphragm at the level of T12

Figure 4.2 Thorax: sagittal section showing divisions of the mediastinum.

Boundaries and Contents of the Mediastinum

Area of the mediastinum	Boundaries	Contents
Superior	Superiorly by the thoracic inlet, the upper opening of the thorax Inferiorly by the transverse thoracic plane Laterally by the pleurae Anteriorly by the manubrium of the sternum Posteriorly by the first four thoracic vertebral bodies	Thymus, trachea, oesophagus, thoracic duct, aortic arch, veins (superior vena cava, brachiocephalic, left superior intercostal), nerves (vagus, phrenic, left recurrent laryngeal), lymphatics, other small arteries and veins
Anterior	Laterally by the pleurae Posteriorly by the pericardium Anteriorly by the sternum, the left transversus thoracis and the fifth to seventh left costal cartilages	Remnant of the thymus lymph nodes
Middle	Bounded by the pericardial sac	Phrenic nerve, heart, pericardium, ascending aorta, pulmonary trunk, superior vena cava, pericardiophrenic artery
Posterior	Anteriorly by bifurcation of trachea, pulmonary vessels, fibrous pericardium and posterior surface of diaphragm Inferiorly by the thoracic surface of the diaphragm Superiorly by the transverse thoracic plane Posteriorly by the bodies of the vertebral column from the lower border of the fifth to the twelfth thoracic vertebra Laterally—by the mediastinal pleura	Descending thoracic aorta, azygos veins, hemiazygos veins, accessory hemiazygos veins, thoracic duct, cisterna chyli, oesophagus, oesophageal plexus, vagus nerve, greater, lesser and least splanchnic nerves, lymphatics

THE HEART

The heart has a conical shape, and its right border is mainly made up of the right atrium. Its inferior border is mainly the right ventricle. Its base is the left atrium. The heart has four chambers each with certain characteristics which will be considered in the following table.

Features of the Heart Chambers

Chamber	Features
Right atrium	Receives the superior vena cava, the inferior vena cava, the coronary sinus and the anterior cardiac veins
Left atrium	Smaller but has a thicker wall than the right atrium Has openings for the four pulmonary veins Depression for the fossa ovalis of the right atrium Generally smooth except auricular surface
Right ventricle	Tricuspid valve Papillary muscles and chordae tendineae Moderator band—right branch of AV bundle Infundibulum is smooth
Left ventricle	Mitral value Papillary muscles and chordae tendineae Thickest—trabeculae carneae

The blood supply to the heart is from the left and right coronary arteries (which are the first branches of the aorta). The right coronary artery comes from the anterior aortic sinus and runs in the atrioventricular groove whereas the left coronary artery, which is the larger of the two vessels, comes from the posterior aortic sinus. The anterior interventricular branch of the left coronary artery runs in the interventricular groove. The right coronary artery usually supplies the sinoatrial node.

Veins drain to the right atrium, and they accompany the arteries. The venae cordis minimae drain directly into the cardiac cavity. A simplified illustration of the venous drainage of the heart is show in the following figures.

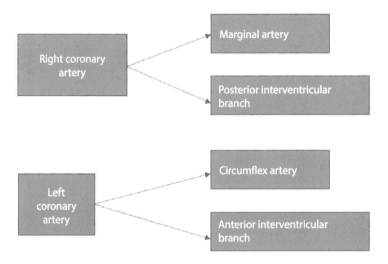

Figure 4.3 Branches of the right and left coronary arteries.

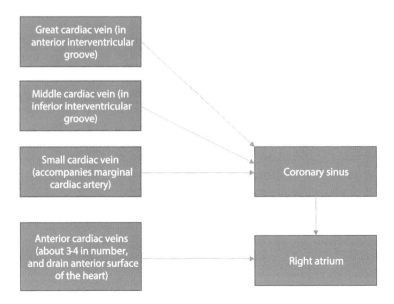

Figure 4.4 Venous drainage of the heart.

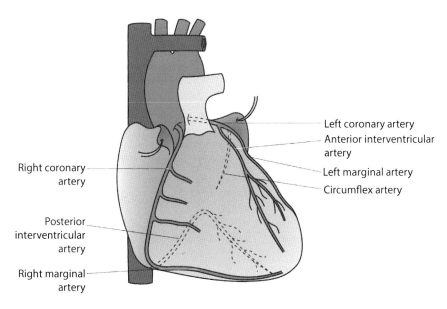

Figure 4.5 Coronary arteries of the heart—those lying posteriorly are shown by dotted lines.

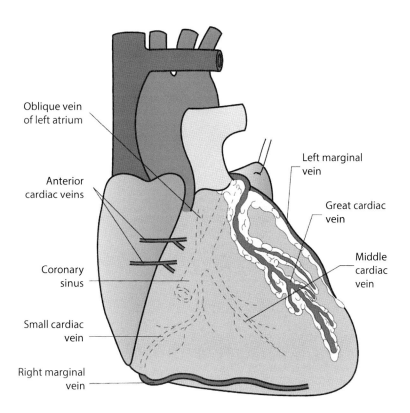

Figure 4.6 Coronary veins of the heart—those lying posteriorly are shown by dotted lines.

EMBRYOLOGY OF THE HEART

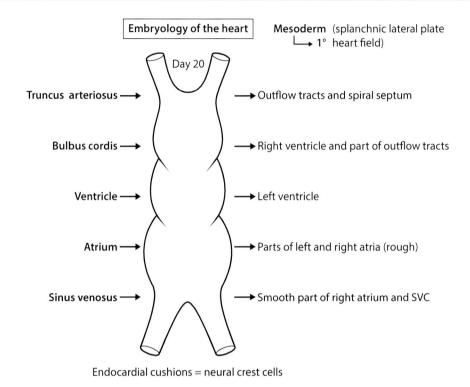

Embryology of the heart		Mesoderm (splanchnic lateral plate

Day 20

Truncus arteriosus ⟶ ⟶ Outflow tracts and spiral septum

Bulbus cordis ⟶ ⟶ Right ventricle and part of outflow tracts

Ventricle ⟶ ⟶ Left ventricle

Atrium ⟶ ⟶ Parts of left and right atria (rough)

Sinus venosus ⟶ ⟶ Smooth part of right atrium and SVC

Mesoderm (splanchnic lateral plate
⟶ 1° heart field)

Endocardial cushions = neural crest cells

Figure 4.7 Cardiac embryology. Derivatives of the heart tube.

THE THYMUS

This bilobed organ plays a role in regulating the immune system. It lies within the superior mediastinum and is related closely to the left brachiocephalic vein.

It receives its blood supply from branches of the internal thoracic and inferior thyroid arteries and sometimes branches from the superior thyroid artery.

Venous blood drains to the left brachiocephalic vein, the internal thoracic vein and the inferior thyroid veins. In some cases, the veins drain directly to the superior vena cava.

Lymphatic drainage accompanies the blood vessels to the brachiocephalic, tracheobronchial and parasternal lymph nodes. Nerve supply arises from the vagus nerve and the cervical sympathetic chain.

THE OESOPHAGUS

The oesophagus commences at C6. It has a connective tissue layer and a muscular layer (external longitudinal muscle, internal circular muscle). This muscle is striated in the upper two-thirds of the oesophagus and smooth in the lower third. The submucosa contains mucous glands. The oesophagus does not have a serosa.

It receives its blood supply from:

- The inferior thyroid artery
- Oesophageal branches of the thoracic aorta
- The left gastric artery

Venous drainage is via:

- The inferior thyroid vein
- The azygos vein
- The left gastric vein

Lymphatic drainage:

- *Proximal third:* deep cervical lymph nodes → thoracic duct
- *Middle third:* to the superior and posterior mediastinal lymph nodes
- *Distal third:* to the gastric and coeliac lymph nodes

CLINICAL POINTS

The oesophagus is narrow at three locations: at the arch of the aorta, the left bronchus and the diaphragm.

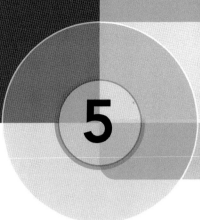

The Head and Neck

5

SURFACE ANATOMY OF THE NECK

C3—the hyoid bone
C4—notch of the thyroid cartilage
C6—the cricoid cartilage

The root of the neck structures anterior to posterior are:

- Subclavian vein
- Phrenic nerve
- Anterior scalene
- Subclavian artery
- Middle scalene

CLINICAL POINTS

C6 is very important to be aware of. It marks:
- The junction of the larynx with the trachea and of the pharynx with the oesophagus
- The level at which the inferior thyroid artery and the middle thyroid vein enter the thyroid gland
- The level at which the vertebral artery enters the transverse foramen in the sixth cervical vertebra
- The level of the middle cervical sympathetic ganglion
- The site at which the carotid artery can be compressed against the transverse process of C6 (the carotid tubercle)

DOI: 10.1201/9781003292005-6

FASCIAL PLANES OF THE NECK

Fascial Compartments of the Neck

Fascia	Location	Contents	Additional information
Superficial cervical fascia	Between the dermis and the deep cervical fascia	Neurovascular supply to the skin Superficial veins (e.g. the external jugular vein) Superficial lymph nodes Fat Platysma muscle	Blends with the "paper thin" platysma muscle Broad, superficial muscle which lies anteriorly in the neck It is innervated by the cervical branch of the facial nerve
Deep cervical fascia	"Deep" to the superficial fascia and platysma muscle	1. *Investing layer*—the most superficial of the deep cervical fascia. It surrounds all the structures in the neck. Where it meets the trapezius and sternocleidomastoid muscles, it splits and envelopes them. 2. *Pre-tracheal layer*—fascia situated in the anterior neck. It spans between the hyoid bone superiorly and the thorax inferiorly. Contains the trachea, oesophagus, thyroid gland and infrahyoid muscles. 3. *Prevertebral fascia*— surrounds the vertebral column and its associated muscles.	Attachments of the investing layer of the deep fascia are: • *Superiorly*—the external occipital protuberance and the superior nuchal line • *Anteriorly*—the hyoid bone • *Inferiorly*—the spine and acromion of the scapula, the clavicle and the manubrium of the sternum • *Posteriorly*—the nuchal ligament Anatomically, the pre-tracheal layer is divided into two parts: 1. *Muscular part*—encloses the infrahyoid muscles 2. *Visceral part*—encloses the thyroid gland, trachea and oesophagus Attachments of the prevertebral fascia are: • *Superiorly*—the base of the skull • *Anteriorly*—transverse processes and vertebral bodies of the vertebral column • *Posteriorly*—the nuchal ligament • *Inferiorly*—the endothoracic fascia of the ribcage An extension of the prevertebral fascia forms the axillary sheath, which surrounds the axillary vessels and the brachial plexus.
Carotid sheath	Either side of the neck as a column	• Common carotid artery • Internal jugular vein • Vagus nerve • Cervical lymph nodes	Extends from the base of the skull to the thoracic mediastinum. Thinnest over the vein. Nerves crossing the sheath: • Glossopharyngeal • Hypoglossal • Spinal part of accessory
Buccopharyngeal fascia	Continuous with the pre-tracheal fascia	• Envelopes the pharynx	

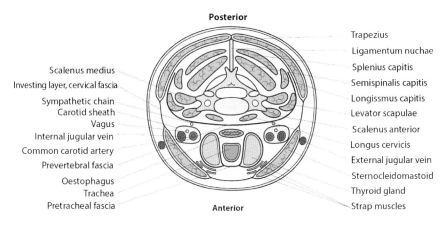

Figure 5.1 Transverse section of the neck showing the fascial planes.

CLINICAL POINTS

- The external jugular vein pierces the deep fascia above the clavicle. If the vein is divided here, it is held open by the deep fascia which is attached to its margins, air is sucked into the vein lumen during inspiration and a fatal air embolism may occur.
- Pus from a tuberculous cervical vertebra may form midline swelling in the posterior wall of the pharynx.

TISSUE SPACES OF THE NECK

1. *The prevertebral space*—this is located behind the prevertebral fascia and is a closed space.
2. *The retropharyngeal space*—located in front of the prevertebral fascia. It is continuous with the parapharyngeal space at the side of the pharynx.
3. *The submandibular space*—this is located between the mylohyoid muscle and the investing layer in between the hyoid and mandible.

CLINICAL POINT

Ludwig's angina is a very rare but severe cellulitis involving the parapharyngeal spaces.

TRIANGLES OF THE NECK

Anatomically, the neck may be split into different triangles. There are many of these, each with different landmarks and each containing different structures that are of importance to the surgeon. Clinically, a greater understanding of these triangles and their contents minimises intra-operative complications.

Broadly speaking, there are two triangles (anterior and posterior) which can be further subdivided.

The boundaries of these two larger triangles will be described and then the table below will outline the other triangles, their boundaries, contents and clinical implications.

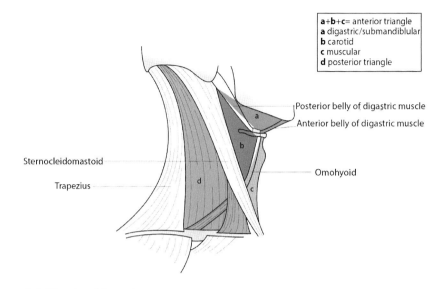

a+b+c= anterior triangle
a digastric/submandiblular
b carotid
c muscular
d posterior triangle

Posterior belly of digastric muscle
Anterior belly of digastric muscle
Sternocleidomastoid
Omohyoid
Trapezius

Figure 5.2 Triangles of the neck.

The Anterior Triangle of the Neck

Borders	• *Superior*—inferior border of the mandible
	• *Medial*—midline of neck
	• *Lateral*—anterior border of sternocleidomastoid muscle
Subdivisions	• Muscular triangle
	• Carotid triangle
	• Submandibular triangle
	• Submental triangle
Contents	• *Muscles*—thyrohyoid, sternothyroid, sternohyoid
	• *Organs*—thyroid gland, parathyroid glands, larynx, trachea, oesophagus, submandibular gland, caudal part of the parotid gland
	• *Arteries*—superior and inferior thyroid, common carotid, external carotid, internal carotid artery (and sinus), facial, submental and lingual
	• *Veins*—anterior jugular veins, internal jugular, common facial, lingual, superior thyroid, middle thyroid veins, facial vein, submental vein and lingual
	• *Nerves*—vagus nerve (CN X), hypoglossal nerve (CN XII), part of sympathetic trunk and mylohyoid

The Posterior Triangle of the Neck

Borders	• *Anterior*—posterior margin of the sternocleidomastoid muscle
	• *Posterior*—anterior margin of the trapezius muscle
	• *Inferior*—middle one-third of the clavicle
Subdivisions	• Occipital triangle
	• Supraclavicular triangle
Contents	• *Vessels*—the third part of the subclavian artery, suprascapular and transverse cervical branches of the thyrocervical trunk, external jugular vein, lymph nodes
	• *Nerves*—accessory nerve (CN XI), the trunks of the brachial plexus, fibres of the cervical plexus

Summary of the Triangular Subdivisions within the Anterior Triangle of the Neck

Subdivision of anterior triangle	Boundaries	Contents	Clinical points
Submandibular (digastric) triangle	• The anterior and posterior borders—anterior and posterior bellies of the digastric muscle, respectively • Base—the inferior border of the mandible • Floor—mylohyoid muscle	• The marginal mandibular branch (MMB) of the facial nerve • The facial and lingual arteries and veins • The submandibular gland and lymph nodes • The nerve to the mylohyoid • The hypoglossal nerve • The lower pole of the parotid gland	• Odontogenic inflammation caused by lower molar tooth infection may spread below the mylohyoid muscle into the submandibular space • Submandibular incision to access this triangle, e.g. abscess drainage and submandibular excision, should be inferior to the marginal mandibular branch of the facial nerve • Three small triangles are included inside the submandibular triangle—Lesser's, Pirogov's and Béclard's triangles
Lesser's triangle	• Bounded by the anterior and posterior bellies of the digastric muscle and the hypoglossal nerve	• Lingual artery	• Location for accessing the lingual artery to control haemorrhage
Pirogov's triangle (This triangle is the posterior part of Lesser's triangle)	• Superiorly—hypoglossal nerve • Inferoposteriorly—intermediate tendon of the digastric muscle • Anteriorly—posterior border of the mylohyoid muscle	• Lingual artery deep to the hyoglossus muscle	• Location for accessing the lingual artery to control severe haemorrhage
Béclard's triangle	• Posterior belly of the digastric muscle • Posterior border of the hyoglossus muscle • Greater horn of the hyoid bone	• Lingual artery • Hypoglossal nerve	• Identification of lingual artery and hypoglossal nerve
Carotid triangle	• The posterior belly of the digastric muscle, the superior belly of the omohyoid muscle and the anterior border of the SCM • Floor and medial wall of this triangle are formed by the hyoglossus, thyrohyoid and inferior and middle pharyngeal constrictor muscles • Inferior border of this triangle reaches the level of the carotid tubercle	• Common carotid artery, its bifurcation into the external carotid artery (ECA) and internal carotid artery (ICA) • Vagus, spinal accessory and hypoglossal nerves • The cervical plexus • Thyroid gland • The larynx • The pharynx • Cervical lymph nodes	• Farabeuf's triangle is a small triangle included within the carotid triangle • The boundaries of this triangle are the IJV, the common facial vein and the hypoglossal nerve

(Continued)

Summary of the Triangular Subdivisions within the Anterior Triangle of the Neck   (Continued)

Subdivision of anterior triangle	Boundaries	Contents	Clinical points
Muscular triangle	• Superior belly of the omohyoid • Anterior border of sternocleidomastoid • Midline of the neck	• Infrahyoid muscles • Thyroid gland • Parathyroid glands • Superior thyroid artery • Anterior jugular and inferior thyroid veins • Ansa cervicalis	• Tracheostomy and thyroidectomy are invasive surgeries that access this triangle • Injury of the superior thyroid artery can result in bleeding during surgery
Submental triangle	• Unpaired triangle • Bounded by the anterior bellies of both digastric muscles and the body of the hyoid bone • Floor consists of the mylohyoid muscle	• Submental lymph nodes • Small veins anastomose in this triangle to form the anterior jugular vein	• Odontogenic infections can spread out into the submental space and form an abscess

Summary of the Triangular Subdivisions within the Posterior Triangle of the Neck

Subdivision of posterior triangle	Boundaries	Contents	Clinical points
Occipital triangle	• *Anteriorly*—posterior border of the sternocleidomastoid • *Posteriorly*—anterior border of the trapezius • *Inferiorly*—inferior belly of the omohyoid	• Spinal accessory nerve • Cutaneous and muscular branches of the cervical plexus • Uppermost part of the brachial plexus • Supraclavicular nerve • Transverse cervical vessels	• Aim to avoid injury to the accessory nerve when working in this triangle • The accessory nerve enters the SCM from behind, approximately 5 cm inferior to the tip of the mastoid process. It emerges between the superficial and prevertebral layers of the deep cervical fascia
Supraclavicular triangle	• *Anteriorly*—posterior border of sternocleidomastoid • *Posteriorly*—anterior border of trapezius • *Superiorly*—inferior belly of omohyoid • *Floor*—first rib, scalenus medius and first slip of serratus anterior • *Roof*—skin, superficial fascia, platysma and investing layer of deep cervical fascia	• Subclavian artery • Subclavian vein • Brachial plexus • Nerve to the subclavius	• This triangle may also harbour the accessory phrenic nerve (APN), which is a common anatomical variant that most often arises from the ansa cervicalis followed by the C5/C6 ventral rami. APN injury can occur with surgical procedures in this region, e.g. scalenectomy • Enlarged left supraclavicular lymph nodes may represent a metastasis

Subdivision of posterior triangle	Boundaries	Contents	Clinical points
Suboccipital triangle	• Bounded by the obliquus capitis superior, the obliquus capitis inferior and the rectus capitis posterior major muscles • Floor is made up of the posterior arch of the atlas and the posterior atlanto-occipital membrane	• V3 segment of the vertebral artery • Vertebral venous plexus • The suboccipital nerve • Greater occipital nerve curves under its base as it ascends onto the occiput	• The vertebral artery may be compressed by ossification of the posterior atlanto-occipital membrane in the floor of this triangle. Ischaemic symptoms result.
Triangle of the vertebral artery	• *Medially*—the anterior scalene muscle, the lateral border of the longus cervicis muscle and the first part of the subclavian artery • *Apex*—the anterior tubercle of the transverse process of the C6 vertebra • *Posteriorly*—the prevertebral fascia and part of the middle scalene muscle	• Vertebral artery • C8 ventral ramus • Ganglionated sympathetic chain • Certain cervical spinal nerves Potentially includes: • Inferior thyroid artery • C7 ventral ramus • Phrenic nerve • Middle and inferior cervical ganglia • Vertebral ganglion • Cervicothoracic (stellate) ganglion	• Osteophytic compression of the vertebral artery may result in vertebral-basilar insufficiency.
Scalene triangle	• Medially—the lateral border of the anterior scalene • Laterally—the medial border of the middle scalene • Inferiorly—the first rib	• The brachial plexus • The third part of the subclavian artery	• Anatomical variations of the scalene muscles can cause compression of neurovascular structures at the thoracic outlet and result in thoracic outlet syndrome

VESSELS OF THE HEAD AND NECK

ARTERIES

COMMON CAROTID ARTERY (CCA):

- Right CCA arises from brachiocephalic artery
- Left CCA arises from the aortic arch
- Extent—sternoclavicular joint to level of upper border of thyroid cartilage
- Branches are external and internal carotid arteries

EXTERNAL CAROTID ARTERY:

- Supplies neck, face, tongue, maxilla and scalp
- Branches include:
  - Superior thyroid artery
  - Ascending pharyngeal artery
  - Lingual artery
  - Facial artery
  - Occipital artery
  - Posterior auricular artery
  - Maxillary artery
  - Superficial temporal artery

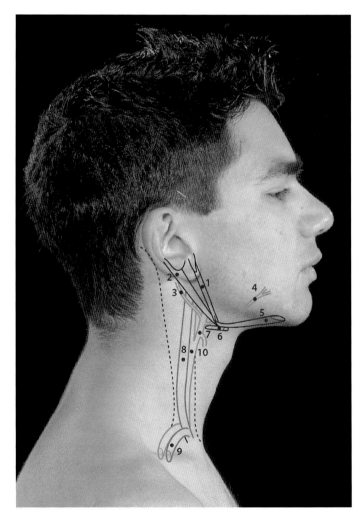

Figure 5.3 Surface anatomy of the lateral neck: 1, stylohyoid; 2, digastric—posterior belly; 3, occipital artery; 4, facial artery; 5, digastric—anterior belly; 6, hyoid bone; 7, external carotid artery; 8, internal jugular vein; 9, subclavian vein; 10, common carotid artery.

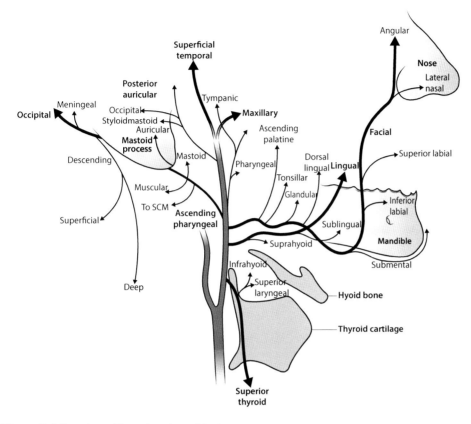

Figure 5.4 Branches of the external carotid artery.

CLINICAL POINT

- The common carotid artery can be exposed over the origin of the sternocleidomastoid immediately above the SC joint.

SUBCLAVIAN ARTERIES:

- The left subclavian artery arises from the arch of the aorta.
- The right subclavian artery is formed by the bifurcation of the brachiocephalic artery.
- Divided in to three parts by the scalenus anterior. Branches include:
  - *First part*—from its origin to the medial border of scalenus anterior
    - The vertebral artery
    - The internal thoracic artery
    - The thyrocervical trunk (inferior thyroid, transverse cervical, suprascapular arteries)
  - *Second part*—posterior to the scalenus anterior
    - The costocervical trunk (deep cervical branch and the superior intercostal artery, which gives off the first and second posterior intercostal arteries)
    dorsal scapular branch
  - *Third part*—from the lateral border of scalenus anterior to the lateral border of the first rib. It has one branch only, the dorsal scapular branch.

CLINICAL POINT

An aneurysm of the subclavian artery is not rare. This usually occurs in the third part of the artery. The symptoms are pain, weakness and numbness in the arm due to its close relationship with the brachial plexus.

VEINS

THE EXTERNAL JUGULAR VEIN:

- *Surface markings*—a line going inferiorly and posteriorly from angle of the mandible to the middle of the clavicle
- Its tributaries are:
  - Posterior auricular vein
  - Retromandibular vein
  - Posterior external jugular vein
  - Oblique jugular vein
  - Transverse cervical vein
  - Suprascapular vein
  - Anterior jugular vein

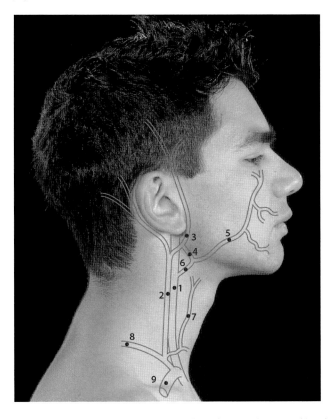

Figure 5.5 Surface anatomy of the neck veins: 1, internal jugular vein; 2, external jugular vein; 3, superficial temporal vein; 4, retromandibular vein, anterior branch; 5, facial vein; 6, retromandibular vein, posterior branch; 7, anterior jugular vein; 8, posterior branch of external jugular vein; 9, subclavian vein.

THE INTERNAL JUGULAR VEIN:

- Commences at the jugular foramen as a continuation of the sigmoid sinus.
- Terminates by joining the subclavian vein to form the brachiocephalic vein.
- Lies in the carotid sheath.
- Its tributaries are:
  - The pharyngeal venous plexus
  - The common facial vein
  - The lingual vein
  - The superior thyroid veins
  - Middle thyroid veins

SUPERFICIAL VEINS:

- The superficial temporal and maxillary veins join to form the retromandibular vein.
- The posterior division of the retromandibular vein joins the posterior auricular vein to form the external jugular vein.
- The anterior division of the retromandibular vein joins the (anterior) facial vein to form the common facial vein and then drains into the internal jugular vein.
- The external jugular vein enters the subclavian vein.
- The subclavian vein is a continuation of the axillary vein and joins the internal jugular vein to form the brachiocephalic vein.

CLINICAL POINTS

- IJV used for central venous catheterisation:
  - To measure CVP
  - To allow rapid blood replacement
  - For long-term intravenous feeding

LYMPH NODES

- Classified into a horizontal group and a vertical group.
- The horizontal nodes drain the superficial tissues of the head and then pass to the deep cervical nodes (note that some lymph vessels drain directly to the cervical nodes and bypass the horizontal nodes).
- The vertical nodes (superficial and deep cervical groups) drain the deep structures of the head and neck.
- The deep cervical group extends along the internal jugular vein from the base of the skull to the root of the neck.
- The superficial cervical nodes lie along the external jugular vein, serve the parotid and lower part of the ear and drain into the deep cervical group.
- The infrahyoid, the pre-laryngeal and the pre- and paratracheal nodes (in the vertical group) drain the thyroid, larynx, trachea and part of the pharynx and drain into the deep cervical group.
- The retropharyngeal nodes drain the back of the nose, pharynx and Eustachian tube. They drain into the upper deep cervical nodes.

MUSCLES OF THE NECK

Summary of Muscles of the Neck, Their Attachments, Innervation and Action

Muscle	Proximal attachment	Distal attachment	Innervation	Action
Sternocleidomastoid	Manubrium and clavicle	Mastoid process and the superior nuchal line	Spinal accessory nerve	Rotates head Laterally flexes and extends the neck
Mylohyoid	Mylohyoid line of the mandible	Mylohyoid raphe and hyoid	Nerve to mylohyoid	Elevates the hyoid
Digastrics	Anterior belly—the mandible Posterior belly—the temporal bone	Intermediate tendon attached to the hyoid bone by connective tissue	Anterior belly—nerve to mylohyoid Posterior belly—the facial nerve	Depresses mandible Elevates the hyoid
Geniohyoid	Inferior mental spine of the mandible	Hyoid	C1 via the hypoglossal nerve	Elevates the hyoid
Stylohyoid	Styloid process	Hyoid	Facial nerve	Elevates the hyoid
Omohyoid	Scapula	Hyoid	Ansa cervicalis	Depresses the hyoid
Sternothyroid	Sternum	Thyroid cartilage	Ansa cervicalis	Depresses the hyoid
Sternohyoid	Sternum	Hyoid	Ansa cervicalis	Depresses the hyoid
Thyrohyoid	Thyroid cartilage	Hyoid	C1 via the hypoglossal nerve	Depresses the hyoid
Longus coli	C1–6 vertebrae	C3–T3 vertebrae	Anterior rami of C2–6	Flexes and rotates neck
Longus capitis	Occipital bone	C3–6 vertebrae	Anterior rami of C1–3	Flexes head
Rectus capitis	Occipital bone	C1 vertebra	Anterior rami of C1–2	Flexes head
Anterior scalene	C4–6 vertebrae	First rib	Anterior rami cervical spinal nerves	Flexes head
Middle scalene	C4–6 vertebrae	First rib	Anterior rami cervical spinal nerves	Laterally flexes head
Posterior scalene	C4–6 vertebrae	Second rib	Anterior rami cervical spinal nerves	Laterally flexes head

THE THYROID GLAND

- The thyroid originates from endodermal cells of the foramen caecum (situated between the tuberculum impar and the copula). It migrates caudally at the beginning of the fifth week of gestation, and during this descent it remains attached to the tongue via the thyroglossal duct. This usually regresses but sometimes persists, presenting as infected or retained tissue.

Parafollicular cells (of the thyroid) secrete calcitonin in response to high calcium levels.

FUNCTIONS OF CALCITONIN:

1. *Bone*—inhibits osteoclasts.
2. *Kidney*—inhibits uptake of calcium and phosphate.

ARTERIAL SUPPLY:

1. *The superior thyroid artery*—this is the first branch of the external carotid artery. It runs close to the superior laryngeal nerve.
2. *The inferior thyroid artery*—a branch of the thyrocervical trunk (from the subclavian). It runs near the inferior laryngeal nerve. It also supplies the inferior and superior parathyroid glands.
3. *Thyroid ima artery*—exists in about 5% of people and is from the brachiocephalic artery.

VENOUS DRAINAGE:

1. Superior thyroid vein drains to the internal jugular vein.
2. Middle thyroid vein drains to the internal jugular vein.
3. Inferior thyroid vein drains to the brachiocephalic vein.

LYMPHATIC DRAINAGE:

- Upper lateral part of the gland drains to the upper deep cervical lymph nodes/ jugulodigastric lymph nodes.
- Lower lateral part of the gland drains to the lower deep cervical lymph nodes/jugulo-omohyoid nodes.
- Upper medial part drains to the pre-laryngeal lymph nodes.
- Lower medial part drains to the pre-tracheal lymph nodes.

NERVE SUPPLY:

- *Sympathetic*—from superior, middle and inferior cervical ganglia.
- *Parasympathetic*—from the vagus and recurrent laryngeal nerves.

CLINICAL POINTS

The thyroid gland moves on deglutition for three reasons:

1. Berry's ligament attaches the thyroid to the cricoid cartilage.
2. The thyroid isthmus is attached to the trachea.
3. The pre-tracheal fascia around the gland is attached to the larynx and the hyoid bone.

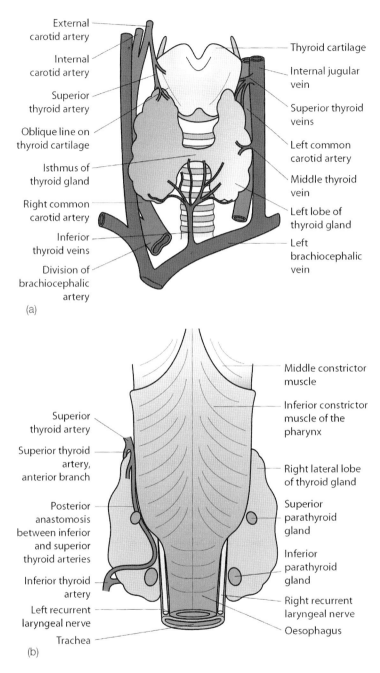

External carotid artery

Internal carotid artery

Superior thyroid artery

Oblique line on thyroid cartilage

Isthmus of thyroid gland

Right common carotid artery

Inferior thyroid veins

Division of brachiocephalic artery

(a)

Thyroid cartilage

Internal jugular vein

Superior thyroid veins

Left common carotid artery

Middle thyroid vein

Left lobe of thyroid gland

Left brachiocephalic vein

Superior thyroid artery

Superior thyroid artery, anterior branch

Posterior anastomosis between inferior and superior thyroid arteries

Inferior thyroid artery

Left recurrent laryngeal nerve

Trachea

(b)

Middle constrictor muscle

Inferior constrictor muscle of the pharynx

Right lateral lobe of thyroid gland

Superior parathyroid gland

Inferior parathyroid gland

Right recurrent laryngeal nerve

Oesophagus

Figure 5.6 Thyroid gland and its relations: (a) anterior view; (b) posterior view.

Complications of thyroidectomy:
- Hypocalcaemia—Hypoparathyroidism is the usual cause of hypocalcaemia; it results from accidental gland injury, removal or devascularisation.
- Wound infection.
- Haematoma—this may cause respiratory compromise.

- Recurrent laryngeal nerve (RLN) injury—if unilateral, hoarseness results. If bilateral, this can result in respiratory compromise due to adduction of the vocal cords. The left recurrent laryngeal nerve is longer and thus more prone to damage.
- Damage to the external laryngeal nerve (this is the only nerve that supplies the crico-thyroid muscle). Damage results in altered pitch.

THE PARATHYROID GLANDS

There are usually four: two superiorly and two inferiorly.

The superior parathyroid glands originate from the fourth pharyngeal pouch and are located posterior and lateral to the recurrent laryngeal nerve. The superior parathyroid glands are usually located near the postero-lateral aspect of the superior pole of the thyroid, about 1 cm superior to the junction of the recurrent laryngeal nerve between the RLN and the inferior thyroid artery. They classically lie deep to the plane of the recurrent laryngeal nerve.

The inferior parathyroid glands originate from the third pharyngeal pouch and are located anterior and medial to the recurrent laryngeal nerve. They classically lie superficial to the plane of the RLN.

Chief cells secrete parathyroid hormone (PTH) in response to low calcium levels.

THE FUNCTIONS OF PTH:

1. *Bone*—binds to osteoblasts, which then stimulate osteoclasts to resorb bone releasing calcium and phosphate.
2. *Kidney*—stimulates calcium uptake from the distal convoluted tubule; inhibits reabsorption of phosphate and bicarbonate; stimulates 25-OH vitamin D to become 1,25-OH vitamin D, which results in increased calcium and phosphate uptake from the gastrointestinal tract.

The glands also contain oxyphil cells. The purpose of these cells is not entirely understood. They are larger than the chief cells and increase in number with advancing age.

ARTERIAL SUPPLY:

The inferior thyroid arteries.

VENOUS DRAINAGE:

Parathyroid veins drain into the thyroid vein plexus.

NERVE SUPPLY:

Branches of the cervical ganglia of the thyroid gland (vasomotor).

LYMPHATIC DRAINAGE:

Drain to the deep cervical and paratracheal lymph nodes.

THE TONGUE

The tongue is composed of intrinsic and extrinsic muscles. The intrinsic muscles are the longitudinalis superior, longitudinalis inferior, transversus linguae and verticalis linguae. The extrinsic muscles are the genioglossus, hyoglossus, styloglossus and palatoglossus.

ARTERIAL SUPPLY:

Lingual branch of the external carotid artery. The lingual artery passes deep to the hyoglossus muscle and superficial to the middle pharyngeal constrictor muscle. It gives rise to the following four arteries:

1. The suprahyoid artery
2. The dorsal lingual artery
3. The sublingual artery
4. The deep lingual artery

VENOUS DRAINAGE:

Lingual vein

Nerve Supply

	Anterior 2/3	Posterior 1/3
General sensation	CNV	CNIX
Taste	CNVII	CNIX
Musculature	CNXII	CNXII

Lymphatic Drainage

Region	Drains to
Tip of tongue	Submental lymph nodes
Anterior two-thirds	Submental lymph nodes
	Submandibular lymph nodes
	(Then to the lower nodes of the deep cervical chain)
Posterior one-third	To the upper nodes of the deep cervical chain
	Parapharyngeal lymph nodes
	Retropharyngeal lymph nodes

THE PHARYNX

ARTERIAL SUPPLY:

Ascending pharyngeal, tonsillar (a branch of the facial artery), maxillary and lingual arteries

VENOUS DRAINAGE:

Pharyngeal veins which drain into the internal jugular vein

NERVE SUPPLY:

Both sensory and motor nerve fibres. Sensory fibres supply the mucous membrane of the three parts of pharynx and transmit common sensation.

Summary of Innervation to the Pharyx

Part of pharynx	Innervation
Nasal pharynx	Maxillary division of the trigeminal nerve CN V2
Oral pharynx	Glossopharyngeal nerve CN IX
Laryngeal pharynx	Internal laryngeal nerve, which is a branch of the superior laryngeal nerve CN X
Muscles of the pharynx except the stylopharyngeus	Vagus CN X
Stylopharyngeus muscle	Glossopharyngeal nerve CN IX

LYMPHATIC DRAINAGE:

Directly to the deep cervical lymph nodes. Indirectly to the deep cervical lymph nodes via the retropharyngeal lymph nodes or to paratracheal lymph nodes.

CLINICAL POINTS

There is a ring of lymphoid tissue that is formed by four lymph groups, called the Waldeyer's ring. This ring protects the entrance of the GIT and the respiratory tract.

The lymph groups involved are: the pharyngeal tonsils superiorly, the palatine tonsils and tubal tonsils laterally and the lingual tonsils inferiorly.

THE LARYNX

The laryngeal skeleton comprises nine cartilages: three paired and three unpaired. The unpaired cartilages are the thyroid cartilage, the cricoid cartilage and the epiglottis. The paired cartilages are the arytenoid cartilages, corniculate cartilages and cuneiform cartilages.

The laryngeal muscles are split into intrinsic muscles, the primary function of which is voice production, and extrinsic muscles which move the larynx. These muscles are summarised in the following tables.

Intrinsic Laryngeal Muscles

Muscles	Attachment	Action
Cricothyroid muscle	Attaches to the cricoid arch, the inferior cornu and lamina of the thyroid cartilage	Elongates the vocal cords, resulting in higher pitch phonation
Posterior cricoarytenoid muscle	Attaches to the posterior cricoid cartilage and to the arytenoid cartilages	Abducts (open) the vocal cords
Lateral or anterior cricoarytenoid muscles	Extend from the lateral cricoid cartilage to the muscular process of the arytenoid cartilage	Adduct the vocal folds
Thyroarytenoid muscles	Originate from the thyroid cartilage and the middle cricothyroid ligaments and insert into the arytenoid cartilages	Relax and approximate the vocal folds
Aryepiglottic muscles	Attach to the arytenoid cartilages and extend to the epiglottis	Adduct the aryepiglottic folds
Arytenoid muscles	Extend to the transverse and oblique portions between the arytenoid cartilages	Adduct the vocal folds

Extrinsic Laryngeal Muscles

Muscles	Attachment	Action
Thyrohyoid muscle	Inserts on the thyroid cartilage and the body of the hyoid bone	Depresses the hyoid bone, thus elevating the larynx
Sternothyroid muscles	Arise from the sternum and first rib and go to the lamina of the thyroid cartilage	Depress the larynx
Inferior pharyngeal constrictor muscles	Extend from the cricoid and thyroid cartilages to the pharyngeal raphe	Narrow the pharynx diameter to contribute to swallowing
Stylopharyngeus muscles	From the styloid process in the temporal bone to the thyroid cartilage	Elevate the larynx and the pharynx
Palatopharyngeus muscles	From the palatine aponeurosis and pterygoid processes and inserts into the thyroid cartilage	Elevate the larynx and pharynx

The extrinsic larynx muscles are paired and allow the movement of the larynx.

ARTERIAL SUPPLY:

Superior and inferior laryngeal arteries from the superior and inferior thyroid arteries respectively.

VENOUS DRAINAGE:

The superior and inferior laryngeal veins. These veins drain into the superior thyroid and inferior thyroids veins, which then drain into internal jugular and subclavian veins respectively.

NERVE SUPPLY:

- *Superior laryngeal nerve*—it has two branches, the internal and the external.
  - The external branch supplies the cricothyroid muscle.
  - The internal branch supplies the mucosa above the vocal cords.
- *Recurrent laryngeal nerve*—innervates all intrinsic muscles of the larynx, except for the cricothyroid muscle. It also supplies the mucosa below the vocal cords.

LYMPHATIC DRAINAGE:

- Above the vocal cords lymph drains to the upper deep cervical lymph nodes and then to the mediastinal lymph nodes.
- Below the vocal cords lymph drains to the lower deep cervical lymph nodes.

THE SALIVARY GLANDS

PAROTID GLAND

Structures passing through the gland: the facial nerve (CNVII), retromandibular vein, external carotid artery and auriculotemporal nerve.

ARTERIAL SUPPLY:

The terminal branches of the external carotid artery:

1. The superficial temporal artery gives off the transverse facial artery which supplies the parotid duct, parotid gland and masseter muscle.

2. The maxillary artery supplies the infratemporal fossa and the pterygopalatine fossa after exiting the medial portion of the parotid.

VENOUS DRAINAGE:

The retromandibular vein.

NERVE SUPPLY:

- *Parasympathetic*—secretomotor
- *Sympathetic*—superior cervical ganglion
- *Sensory*—greater auricular nerve

LYMPHATIC DRAINAGE:

- To the deep cervical lymph nodes.

SUBMANDIBULAR GLANDS

These have two lobes, deep and superficial, which are separated by the mylohyoid muscle.

ARTERIAL SUPPLY:

Submental artery (a branch of the facial artery) and sublingual artery (a branch of the lingual artery).

VENOUS DRAINAGE:

Common facial and sublingual veins drain the gland and flow into the internal jugular vein.

NERVE SUPPLY:

1. Parasympathetic innervation to the submandibular glands is provided by the superior salivatory nucleus via the chorda tympani, a branch of the facial nerve. This synapses to the submandibular ganglion becoming part of the lingual nerve (CNV).
2. Sympathetic nervous system regulates secretions.

LYMPHATIC DRAINAGE:

Drains to the submandibular lymph nodes and then to the jugulodigastric lymph nodes.

CLINICAL POINTS

The facial artery is posterior to the submandibular gland. The cervical branch of the facial nerve is inferior to the submandibular gland. The facial vein is superior to the submandibular gland.

The lingual nerve is medial to the gland but lateral to the duct. The lingual nerve and the hypoglossal nerve are at risk of damage in submandibular gland surgery.

SUBLINGUAL GLANDS

ARTERIAL SUPPLY:

Submental artery (a branch of the facial artery) and sublingual artery (a branch of the lingual artery).

VENOUS DRAINAGE:

The sublingual vein drains into the lingual vein, which then flows into the internal jugular system.

NERVE SUPPLY:

Parasympathetic input via the chorda tympani nerve, which is a branch of the facial nerve via the submandibular ganglion. The chorda tympani nerve then travels with the lingual nerve to synapse at the submandibular ganglion. The postganglionic fibres act on muscarinic receptors to increase salivation.

LYMPHATIC DRAINAGE:

Sublingual glands drain into the submandibular lymph nodes.

THE SCALP AND THE SKULL

The scalp is arranged in five layers that may be remembered by the mnemonic "SCALP":

S—skin
C—connective tissue
A—aponeurosis
L—loose connective tissue
P—periosteum

ARTERIAL SUPPLY:

- External carotid artery. The three branches of the external carotid artery which supply the scalp are as follows:
  - *Superficial temporal*—supplies the frontal and temporal regions
  - *Posterior auricular*—supplies the area superior and posterior to the auricle
  - *Occipital*—supplies the back of the scalp

- Ophthalmic artery. Two branches are involved. These are:

  - The supraorbital arteries
  - The supratrochlear arteries

VENOUS DRAINAGE:

- *Superficial drainage*—follows the named arteries i.e. the superficial temporal, occipital, posterior auricular, supraorbital and supratrochlear veins.
- *Deep drainage*—via the pterygoid venous plexus located between the temporalis and lateral pterygoid muscles. This then drains into the maxillary vein.
- The veins of the scalp connect to the diploic veins of the skull via valveless emissary veins. This provides a connection between the scalp and the dural venous sinuses and is clinically important in the spread of infections.

NERVE SUPPLY:

Branches of the Trigeminal Nerve and Cervical Nerve Roots

Nerve	Branch of	Area supplied
Supratrochlear nerve	Ophthalmic nerve	Anteromedial forehead
Supraorbital nerve	Ophthalmic nerve	Between the anterolateral forehead and the vertex
Zygomaticotemporal nerve	Maxillary nerve	Temple
Auriculotemporal nerve	Mandibular nerve	Skin anterosuperior to the auricle
Lesser occipital nerve	From the anterior ramus (division) of C2	Skin posterior to the ear
Greater occipital nerve	From the posterior ramus (division) of C2	Skin of the occipital region
Great auricular nerve	From the anterior rami of C2 and C3	Skin posterior to the ear and over the angle of the mandible
Third occipital nerve	Posterior ramus of C3	Supplies the skin of the inferior occipital region

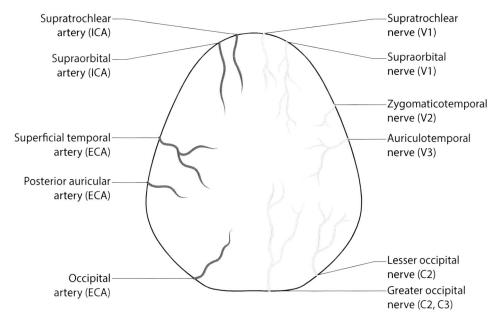

ICA = Internal carotid artery
ECA = External carotid artery

Figure 5.7 Nerve and arterial supply to the scalp.

THE PARANASAL SINUSES

Paranasal Sinuses

Name of sinus	Drains to
Frontal sinus	Frontonasal duct → infundibulum of hiatus semilunaris → middle meatus
Sphenoid sinus	Sphenoethmoidal recess
Anterior ethmoidal cells	Middle meatus
Middle ethmoidal cells	Middle meatus
Maxillary sinus	Middle meatus
Nasolacrimal duct	Inferior meatus

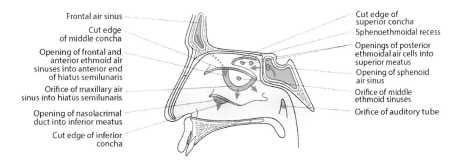

Figure 5.8 Lateral wall of the nasal cavity showing the openings of the paranasal air sinuses (arrows indicate the directions of mucus drainage).

THE VERTEBRAL COLUMN

Summary of Differences between the Types of Vertebrae

Type of vertebrae	Anatomical points
Cervical	There are seven cervical vertebrae. Their distinguishing features are: 1. Bifid spinous processes 2. Triangular foramen 3. Transverse foramina for the vertebral arteries. C1 and C2 are the atlas and the axis, which have a special shape to allow for head movement.
Thoracic	There are 12 thoracic vertebrae. Their distinguishing features are: 1. Two demi facets for articulation with the ribs 2. Inferiorly and obliquely shaped spinous processes 3. Costal facets for articulation with the ribs
Lumbar	There are five lumbar vertebrae. Their distinguishing features are: 1. Large kidney-shaped bodies 2. Shorter and thicker spinous processes
Sacrum and coccyx	The sacrum is fused and looks like an inverted triangle. The coccyx does not have any vertebral arches.

CLINICAL POINTS

Structures punctured by a lumbar puncture from superficial to deep are:

- Skin
- Subcutaneous tissue
- Supraspinous ligament
- Interspinous ligament
- Ligamentum flavum
- Epidural space containing the internal vertebral venous plexus
- Dura
- Arachnoid
- Subarachnoid space

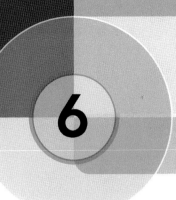

The Nervous System and Special Senses

6

THE BRAIN

Regions of the brain include the following.

FRONTAL LOBE:

- Responsible for motor control of the opposite side of the body i.e. the left frontal lobe controls the right side of the body
- Controls emotion and insight
- Dominant hemisphere is responsible for speech output (Broca's area). Broca's area is located just superior to the lateral fissure
- Primary motor cortex, which plans and executes movement, is located in the posterior portion of the frontal lobe

PARIETAL LOBE:

- Responsible for sensation of the opposite side of the body as well as spatial awareness
- The somatosensory cortex is located in the anterior cortex of the parietal lobe and processes pain, pressure and touch

TEMPORAL LOBE:

- Responsible for memory and emotion
- Wernicke's area is responsible for the comprehension of speech as well as written language and is located just posterior to the superior temporal gyrus
- The primary auditory complex is responsible for hearing and is located within the temporal lobe bilaterally

OCCIPITAL LOBE:

- Responsible for vision
- The primary visual cortex is located here

DOI: 10.1201/9781003292005-7

BASAL GANGLIA:

- Integrates motor and sensory inputs
- It is an interconnection of deep nuclei; the lentiform nucleus, the caudate nucleus, the subthalamic nucleus and the substantia nigra

CEREBELLUM:

- Consists of three lobes, each with its own function
- The paleocerebellum maintains gait
- The neocerebellum maintains postural tone and co-ordinates fine motor skills
- The archicerebellum maintains balance

ARTERIAL SUPPLY:

Blood supply to the brain is normally divided into anterior and posterior segments. These segments are interconnected via the Circle of Willis. The Circle of Willis is important clinically since connections formed here can provide blood to areas that would otherwise be high risk for ischaemia.

VENOUS DRAINAGE:

The superficial venous system is composed of dural venous sinuses, which have walls composed of dura mater. The superior sagittal sinus is the most prominent. The superior sagittal sinus flows in the sagittal plane under the midline of the cerebral vault, posteriorly and inferiorly to the confluence of sinuses. Here the superficial venous system joins the deep venous system. There are two transverse sinuses which bifurcate, traversing laterally and inferiorly in an "S"-shaped curve forming the sigmoid sinuses. This continues to create the jugular veins. The jugular veins drain into the superior vena cava.

The deep venous drainage is composed of veins inside the deep structures of the brain, which join behind the midbrain to form the vein of Galen. This vein merges with the inferior sagittal sinus to form the straight sinus. This joins the superficial venous system at the confluence of sinuses. The following diagram illustrates the superficial and deep venous system.

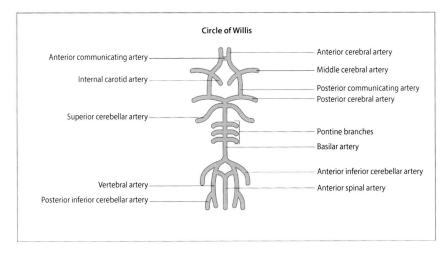

Figure 6.1 The blood supply of the brain.

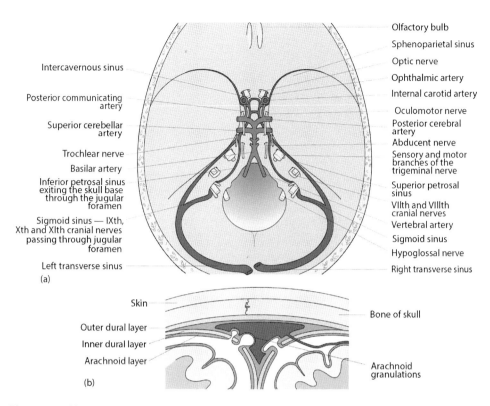

Figure 6.2 (a) Dural venous sinuses. (b) Arachnoid granulations through the inner dural layer meeting endothelium of the venus sinus for the production of cerebrospinal fluid.

Summary of the Cranial Nerves and Their Lesions

Nerve	Sensory or motor	Location	Function	Lesion
I—Olfactory	Sensory	Cribriform plate of the ethmoid bone	Sense of smell	Loss of smell (anosmia)
II—Optic	Sensory	Optic canal	Sight	Different visual field losses depending on the location of the lesion
III—Oculomotor	Motor	Superior orbital fissure	Innervates the superior, medial and inferior rectus muscles as well as the levator palpebrae superioris, inferior oblique and sphincter pupillae	Eye moves down and out due to unopposed action of the superior oblique and lateral rectus muscles Ptosis (drooping eyelid) and mydriasis (dilated pupil)
IV—Trochlear	Motor	Superior orbital fissure	Innervates the superior oblique muscle	Diplopia Eye moves down and in

(Continued)

125

Summary of the Cranial Nerves and Their Lesions   (Continued)

Nerve	Sensory or motor	Location	Function	Lesion
V—Trigeminal	Motor and sensory	V1—ophthalmic nerve: superior orbital fissure V2—maxillary nerve: foramen rotundum V3—mandibular nerve: foramen ovale	Sensation of the face Innervates the muscles of mastication Test corneal reflex	Decreased facial sensation and jaw weakness
VI—Abducens	Motor	Superior orbital fissure	Innervates the lateral rectus muscle	Eye deviates medially
VII—Facial	Motor and sensory	Internal acoustic canal and exits through the stylomastoid foramen	Innervates the muscles of facial expression, stapedius, posterior belly of the digastric muscle, stylohyoid, taste anterior 2/3 tongue, the lacrimal gland and the salivary glands (not parotids)	Upper motor neuron (UMN)— asymmetry of lower face with forehead sparing Lower motor neuron (LMN)— asymmetry of upper and lower face; loss of taste, hyperacusis and eye irritation due to reduced lacrimation
VIII— Vestibulocochlear	Sensory	Internal acoustic canal	Sense of sound and balance	Deafness and vertigo
IX— Glossopharyngeal	Motor and sensory	Jugular foramen	Supplies taste to posterior 1/3 of the tongue and innervates the parotids as well as the stylopharyngeus	Decreased gag reflex Uvular deviation away from lesion
X—Vagus	Motor and sensory	Jugular foramen	Innervates laryngeal and pharyngeal muscles (not stylopharyngeus) and parasympathetic supply to thoracic and abdominal viscera	Dysphagia Recurrent laryngeal nerve palsies and pseudobulbar palsies
XI—Spinal accessory	Motor	Jugular foramen	Innervates trapezius and sternocleidomastoid muscles	Patient cannot shrug and displays weak head movement
XII—Hypoglossal	Motor	Hypoglossal canal	Innervates the muscles of the tongue (except for the palatoglossal, which is supplied by the vagus nerve)	Tongue deviates towards the side of weakness during protrusion

Foramina of the Base of the Skull

Foramen	Contents
Foramen ovale	Remember as "**OVALE**":
	Otic ganglion
	V3 mandibular nerve
	Accessory meningeal artery
	Lesser petrosal nerve
	Emissary veins
Foramen spinosum	Middle meningeal artery
	Meningeal branch of the mandibular nerve
Foramen rotundum	V2 maxillary nerve
Foramen lacerum/carotid canal	ICA
	Nerve and artery to the pterygoid canal
	Greater petrosal nerve
Jugular foramen	Anterior—inferior petrosal sinus
	Inferior—CN IX, X and XI
	Posterior—sigmoid sinus → internal jugular vein (IJV)
	Meningeal branches from the occipital and ascending pharyngeal artery
Foramen magnum	Medulla oblongata
	Vertebral arteries
	Anterior and posterior spinal artery
Stylomastoid foramen	Facial nerve
	Stylomastoid artery
Superior orbital fissure	Lacrimal nerve
	Frontal nerve
	Trochlear nerve
	Superior oculomotor nerve
	Abducens nerve
	Nasociliary nerve
	Inferior oculomotor nerve
	Recurrent meningeal artery
	Superior ophthalmic vein

*Note: T*he cranial nerves which carry parasympathetic fibres are I, IX, VII and III (1973).

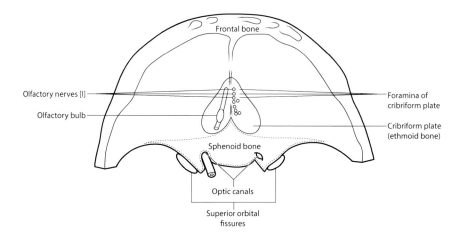

Figure 6.3 Anatomy of the anterior cranial fossa.

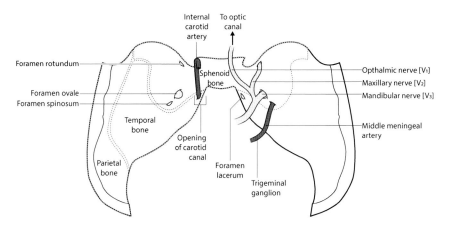

Figure 6.4 Anatomy of the middle cranial fossa.

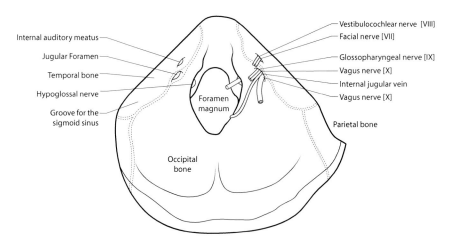

Figure 6.5 Anatomy of the posterior cranial fossa.

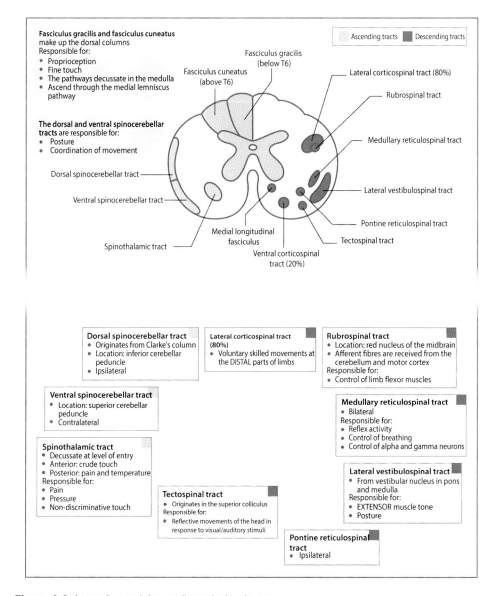

Figure 6.6 Ascending and descending spinal pathways.

It is important to know the ascending and descending spinal pathways for the MRCS examination. The figure summarises these pathways and their functions.

THE CAVERNOUS SINUS

The cavernous sinus is part of the dural venous sinus system. It receives blood from the superior and inferior ophthalmic veins, the sphenoparietal sinus, the superficial middle cerebral veins and the inferior cerebral veins.

Several important structures pass through the sinus, which are summarised in the following table.

Summary of the Structures Passing through the Lateral and Medial Walls of the Cavernous Sinus

Structures passing through the lateral wall from superior to inferior	Structures passing through the medial wall
Oculomotor nerve	Abducens nerve
Trochlear nerve	Internal carotid artery accompanied by the internal carotid plexus
Ophthalmic and maxillary branches of the trigeminal nerve	

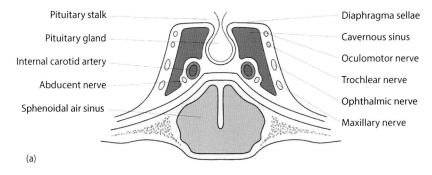

(a)

Figure 6.7 Cavernous sinus—coronal section.

CLINICAL POINT

The cavernous sinus is connected to the facial vein via the superior ophthalmic vein, therefore it is possible to get infections in the cavernous sinus from an external facial injury within the danger area of the face. This danger area of the face encompasses the area within a triangle drawn from the corners of the mouth to the bridge of the nose.

THE NOSE

ARTERIAL SUPPLY:

- *External nose*—the dorsal nasal artery from the ophthalmic artery (supplies the superior superficial aspect of the nose).
- *Lateral nose, ala and columella*—angular and superior labial arteries (from the facial artery).
- *Superior septum*—the anterior and posterior ethmoidal arteries and the sphenopalatine artery. The anterior and posterior ethmoidal arteries are branches of the ophthalmic artery (which is a branch of the internal carotid artery). The sphenopalatine artery is a branch of the maxillary artery (which is a branch of the external carotid artery).
- *Nasal floor*—branches of the superior labial artery.
- *Anterior septum*—the superior labial, anterior ethmoidal, greater palatine and sphenopalatine arteries (a confluence called Kiesselbach's plexus).

VENOUS DRAINAGE:

- Anterior facial vein
- Sphenopalatine vein
- Ethmoid veins

LYMPHATIC DRAINAGE:

- Anteriorly via the upper lip lymphatics
- Posteriorly via the deep cervical and retropharyngeal lymph nodes.

NERVE SUPPLY:

Sensation of the nose comes from the ophthalmic (V1) and maxillary (V2) divisions of the trigeminal nerve.

Summary of Innervation by Region of the Nose

Region of the nose	Nerve
Superior aspect of the external nose	Infratrochlear nerve
Skin of the nasal tip	External nasal nerve (arises from the nasociliary nerve)
Medial aspect of the nasal ala	External nasal nerve
Dorsum of the nose	External nasal nerve
Lateral dorsum and ala	Maxillary division (V2)
Nasal mucosa	Branches of both V1 and V2
Sensation to the anterosuperior aspect of the internal nose and the anterior nasal septal mucosa	Anterior ethmoidal nerve
Nasal septum	Nasopalatine nerve
Lateral nasal sidewall mucosa	Greater palatine nerve and the anterior ethmoidal nerve
Nasal musculature	Facial nerve

THE EXTERNAL EAR

ARTERIAL SUPPLY:

- Branches of the external carotid artery, as follows:
  - Posterior auricular artery
  - Superficial temporal artery
  - Occipital artery
  - Deep auricular branch of the maxillary artery

VENOUS DRAINAGE:

- Posterior auricular vein
- Superficial temporal vein
- Occipital vein
- Deep auricular branch of the maxillary vein

Nerve Supply

Nerve	Region supplied
Greater auricular nerve	Skin of the auricle and ear lobe
Lesser occipital nerve	Skin of the auricle
Auriculotemporal nerve	Skin of the auricle and external auditory meatus
Branches of the facial and vagus nerves	Deeper aspect of the auricle and external auditory meatus

LYMPHATIC DRAINAGE:

- Lateral upper half—superficial parotid lymph nodes
- Cranial surface of upper half—mastoid lymph nodes and deep cervical lymph nodes
- Lower half and lobule—superficial cervical lymph nodes

THE MIDDLE EAR

The middle ear lies within the temporal bone. It extends from the tympanic membrane to the lateral wall of the inner ear. It is divided anatomically into two parts—the tympanic cavity and the epitympanic recess. The tympanic cavity holds the three ossicles: the malleus, incus and stapes, responsible for transmitting vibrations through the middle ear.

The Boundaries of the Middle Ear

Roof	• Petrous part of the temporal bone
Floor	• Jugular wall (a thin portion of bone separating the middle ear from the internal jugular vein)
Lateral wall	• Tympanic membrane and lateral wall of the epitympanic recess
Medial wall	• Lateral wall of the internal ear. The bulge in this wall is created by the facial nerve
Anterior wall	• Thin bone with two openings for 1) the auditory tube and 2) the tensor tympani muscle
Posterior wall	• The mastoid wall which is a layer of bone separating the tympanic cavity and mastoid air cells.

ARTERIAL SUPPLY:

- Maxillary division of the external carotid artery
- Deep auricular artery (from the maxillary artery)
- Tubal artery (a branch of the meningeal accessory artery which originates from the maxillary artery)
- Anterior tympanic artery (arising from the maxillary artery, supplies the ossicles)
- Posterior tympanic branch of the stylomastoid artery (arising from either the occipital or posterior auricular divisions of the external carotid artery)
- Stapedial artery
- The tympanic plexus is formed by contributions of:
  - The inferior tympanic artery (from the ascending pharyngeal artery)
  - The caroticotympanic arteries (branch from the C2 segment of the internal carotid artery)

VENOUS DRAINAGE:

Tympanic veins drain to the superior petrosal sinus and the pterygoid venous plexus.

NERVE SUPPLY:

General sensory innervation to the meatal side of tympanic membrane is provided by the auriculotemporal nerve (branch of CN V3) and the vagus nerve (CN X).

General sensory innervation to the mucosal side of the tympanic membrane is provided by the tympanic branches of the glossopharyngeal nerve (CN IX).

The tympanic cavity is also innervated by CN IX via the tympanic plexus.

CONTAINS TWO MUSCLES:

1. *The stapedius muscle*—controlled by the facial nerve
2. *The tensor tympani muscle*—controlled by the medial pterygoid nerve (a branch of the mandibular nerve of the trigeminal nerve)

These muscles are responsible for the acoustic reflex.

LYMPHATIC DRAINAGE:

Drainage is to the parotid and upper deep cervical lymph nodes.

THE INNER EAR

ARTERIAL SUPPLY:

1. *The bony labyrinth*:
   - Anterior tympanic branch (from maxillary artery).
   - Petrosal branch (from middle meningeal artery).
   - Stylomastoid branch (from posterior auricular artery).
2. *The membranous labyrinth*:
   - Labyrinthine artery, a branch of the inferior cerebellar artery (occasionally, the basilar artery). It has cochlear and vestibular branches.

VENOUS DRAINAGE:

Labyrinthine vein drains to the sigmoid sinus or inferior petrosal sinus.

NERVE SUPPLY:

Vestibulocochlear nerve (CN VIII), which divides into the vestibular nerve (balance) and the cochlear nerve (hearing).

LYMPHATIC DRAINAGE:

The cervical lymph nodes.

THE EYE

The eye is a sensory organ. It has six extraocular muscles which are responsible for the movement of the eye. The four recti of the eye originate from the annular tendon of Zinn. The recti then insert into the sclera at various distances from the limbis. There are two oblique muscles. The superior oblique muscle arises from the inner margin of the optic foramen. It passes through the trochea, which is a fibrous pulley. It is attached to the upper outer part of the sclera. The inferior oblique muscle originates from the orbital floor and inserts onto the outer part of the sclera behind the equator.

Innervation may be remembered by the formula LR6SO4R3:

- Lateral rectus is cranial nerve VI
- Superior oblique is cranial nerve IV
- The rest are innervated by cranial nerve III

ARTERIAL SUPPLY:

Branches of the ophthalmic artery. These branches are summarised in the following table.

A Summary of the Branches of the Ophthalmic Artery and the Areas Supplied

Branches of the ophthalmic artery	Area supplied
Central retinal artery	The inner layer of the retina and all nerve fibres
Lacrimal artery	The eyelids, lacrimal gland and conjunctiva
Ciliary arteries	The choroid and iris
Supraorbital artery	The upper eyelid, levator palpebrae muscle, skin of the forehead and scalp
Ethmoidal arteries	The ethmoid sinuses
Medial palpebral artery	The eyelids
Muscular arteries	The extraocular muscles
Dorsal nasal artery	The lacrimal sac and tip of the nose
Supratrochlear artery	Medial forehead

VENOUS DRAINAGE:

Central retinal vein and vortex veins drain to the superior and inferior ophthalmic veins. These then drain to the cavernous sinus, pterygoid venous plexus and facial vein.

NERVE SUPPLY:

Summary of the Nerve Supply to the Eye

Nerve	Function
Optic nerve (CN II)	Vision
Parasympathetic fibres of short ciliary nerves	Pupillary constriction
Sympathetic fibres of long ciliary nerves	Pupillary dilation
Short ciliary nerves (branch of cranial nerve III)	Ciliary muscles allowing accommodation
Ophthalmic branch (V1) of the CN V	Sensation

LYMPHATIC DRAINAGE:

The conjunctiva is rich in lymphatics, the cornea and the retina are devoid of them. Lymphatic drainage of aqueous from the eye drains to the cervical lymph nodes.

The pupillary light reflex is sometimes asked about in the MRCS examination. The afferent and efferent pathways involved in the pupillary light reflex are outlined here.

AFFERENT PATHWAY:

- *Photoreceptor cells (rods and cones) in the outer layers of the retina convert light stimuli into neuronal impulses. These signals are sent to bipolar cells, which interact with ganglion cells, sending signals to the optic disc and optic nerve (CN II).*
- *The optic nerve then forms the optic chiasm and signals can follow either a left or a right optic tract.*
- *At the optic chiasm, nasal retinal fibres cross to the contralateral side of the optic tract. Temporal retinal fibres continue on the ipsilateral side. (i.e. the left optic tract will contain temporal retinal fibres from the left eye and it will contain nasal retinal fibres from the right eye).*
- *Signals travel to the superior colliculus and send signals to the pretectal region of the midbrain.*
- *Signals are then sent to the Edinger–Westphal nuclei (the preganglionic parasympathetic nuclei in the midbrain).*
- *Some signals also travel to the hypothalamus and the olivary pretectal nucleus.*

EFFERENT PATHWAY:

- *Preganglionic fibres travel on the oculomotor nerve and synapse with the ciliary ganglion.*
- *This sends post ganglionic axons to the sphincter muscles of the iris resulting in constriction of the pupil.*

Due to crossing fibres in this pathway, there is direct pupil constriction of the eye being tested with the light reflex and a consensual pupillary light reflex.

THE LACRIMAL GLAND

ARTERIAL SUPPLY:

Lacrimal branch of the ophthalmic artery.

VENOUS DRAINAGE:

Superior ophthalmic vein.

NERVE SUPPLY:

- Parasympathetics → secretomotor i.e. pterygopalatine (directly or via the zygomatic/lacrimal branches of maxillary nerve).
- Preganglionic fibres travel to the ganglion in the greater petrosal nerve (branch of the facial nerve at the geniculate ganglion).

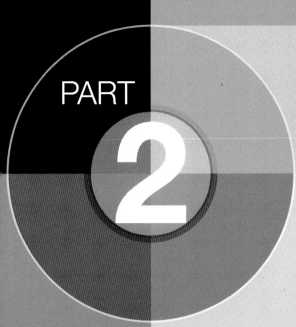

PART

2

PHYSIOLOGY

A–Z of Physiology

7

At the time of writing this book, there are 45 questions related to applied surgical physiology in the MRCS Part A exam. This section is written in an A–Z format and aims to cover key physiological topics that are frequently tested.

ACID–BASE BALANCE

$$pH = -\log_{10} [H^+],\text{ and the normal pH of blood is } 7.36–7.44.$$

Maintaining a normal pH is vital for human survival, and there are numerous buffer systems in the human body to maintain pH. These systems are:

1. The bicarbonate system
2. The phosphate system
3. Plasma proteins
4. The globin component of haemoglobin

H^+ mostly comes from CO_2 via metabolism, e.g. lactic acid from anaerobic metabolism, ketone bodies.

Acid–base balance is maintained by a variety of organ systems—the lungs, the kidneys, the blood, bone and the liver. If the pH is above the normal level this is called alkalosis; if pH falls to its lower limits this is known as acidosis. The following table summarises the causes of acid–base disturbances.

Summary of the Different Types of Acid–Base Disturbances and Their Causes

Type of acid–base disturbance	Cause
Metabolic acidosis	<ul><li>Renal failure</li><li>Hyperkalaemia</li><li>Increased ketone bodies i.e. diabetic ketoacidosis</li><li>Lactic acidosis</li><li>Loss of HCO_3^- through renal excretion e.g. renal tubular acidosis</li></ul>

(Continued)

DOI: 10.1201/9781003292005-9

Summary of the Different Types of Acid–Base Disturbances and Their Causes   (Continued)

Type of acid–base disturbance	Cause
Metabolic alkalosis	• Administration of bases e.g. HCO_3^- infusion • Increased breakdown of organic anions • Loss of H^+ ions due to vomiting • Volume depletion
Respiratory acidosis	• Lung tissue damage e.g. COPD • Impairment of alveolar gas exchange e.g. pulmonary oedema • Paralysis of respiratory muscles • Insufficient respiratory drive e.g. opiate overdose • Reduced chest expansion
Respiratory alkalosis	• Hyperventilation e.g. anxiety attack • High altitude

ACTION POTENTIALS

The resting membrane potential is the potential difference across the cell membrane caused by the movement of Na^+, K^+ and Cl^- ions. The Goldman equation determines the reversal potential across a cell's membrane. A typical value for the resting membrane potential is −70 mV. The Na^+/K^+ ATP-ase pump is vital in maintaining the potential difference across a cell, and it transports three Na^+ out of the cell for every two K^+ pumped into the cell.

An action potential results from changes in the voltage across a cell membrane. This rapid change in membrane potential results in depolarisation, which is an all-or-nothing response, followed by repolarisation. The following figure is an example of neuronal action potential.

The absolute refractory period is a period in which no new action potentials may be generated. The relative refractory period is when an action potential may be generated with a larger than normal stimulus.

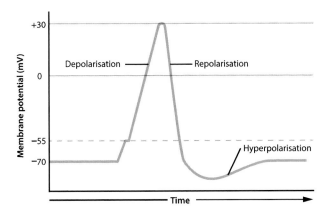

Figure 7.1 Neuronal action potential. A neuronal action potential. The dashed line represents the threshold voltage. (Used with permission from OpenStax under the Creative Commons Attribution 4.0 International license.)

Certain factors may increase the velocity of conduction, e.g. larger fibres in the myelinated neurones due to reduced resistance and saltatory conduction.

Summary of the Types of Peripheral Nerve Fibres

Nerve fibre group	Comment
Group A	The largest group. Subdivided into the following:
	α—motor and proprioceptive
	β—touch, pressure and proprioceptive
	γ—muscle spindle
	δ—pain and pressure
Group B	Autonomic myelinated fibres
Group C	Unmyelinated
	Touch and pain

ACTION POTENTIALS OF THE CARDIAC CELLS

In the MRCS there are often one or two questions related to the action potentials in myocytes. The phases and the cations involved are summarised in the following figures and tables.

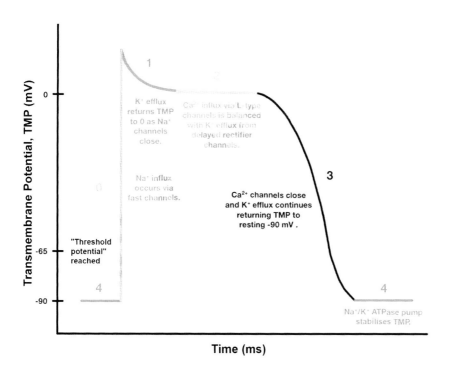

Figure 7.2 Action potential in a cardiac myocyte (This action potential does not apply to the SA node or the AV node).

Summary of the Phases of an Actional Potential within a Myocyte

Phase	Name	Ion involved	Anti-arrhythmic involved
0	Rapid depolarisation	Na^+ influx	Class 1a (moderate) — quinidine
			Class 1b (weak) — lidocaine
			Class 1c (strong) — flecainide
1	Early repolarisation	K^+ efflux	
2	Plateau	Ca^{2+} influx	Class 4 — Ca^{2+} channel blockers, e.g. verapamil
3	Final repolarisation	K^+ efflux	Class 3 — K^+ channel blockers, e.g. amiodarone
4	Restoration	Na^+/K^+ ATPase	Class 2 — beta-blockers, e.g. propranolol

ADRENAL CORTEX AND MEDULLA

The adrenal cortex and the adrenal medulla have different embryological origins. The cortex is derived from the mesoderm, whereas the medulla is from the neuroectoderm.

The adrenal cortex is made up of different layers that are responsible for producing different hormones. These layers are the zona glomerulosa, the zona fasciculata and the zona reticularis. The hormones produced are all steroid hormones and share a common cyclopentanoperhydro-phenanthrene ring.

Conversely, the adrenal medulla, which is derived from the neuroectoderm, is responsible for producing catecholamines from chromaffin cells (80% epinephrine and 20% norepinephrine). The precursor to the catecholamines is tyrosine. Tyrosine is converted to dihydroxyphenylala-nine (DOPA) by tyrosine hydroxylase. DOPA is then converted to norepinephrine by DOPA decarboxylase. Norepinephrine is converted first to dopamine by dopamine β-hydroxylase and then to epinephrine by phenylethanolamine-N-methyltransferase. Acetylcholine is the neu-rotransmitter that stimulates the release of catecholamines.

The hormones released from each layer of the adrenal cortex and adrenal medulla along with some examples are summarised in the following table.

The Different Tissues Areas of the Adrenal Gland and the Hormones Released

Tissue area	Hormones released	Examples
Zona glomerulosa (adrenal cortex)	Mineralocorticoids	Aldosterone
Zona fasciculata (adrenal cortex)	Glucocorticoids	Cortisol
		Cortisone
		Corticosterone
Zona reticularis (adrenal cortex)	Androgens	Dehydroepiandrosterone
Adrenal medulla	Catecholamines	Epinephrine
		Norepinephrine

Main Effects of Mineralocorticoids and Glucocorticoids

Hormone	Action
Aldosterone	• Stimulates reabsorption of sodium in the distal convoluted tubule
	• Induces hypokalaemia
	• Causes metabolic alkalosis (since H^+ may be exchanged with Na^+)
	• Promotes water retention

Hormone	Action
Glucocorticoids	• Anti-inflammatory actions • Immunosuppressant actions • Stimulates the stress response • Promotes Na^+ and water retention • Induces hypokalaemia • Induces hyperglycaemia (antagonises insulin) • Stimulates gluconeogenesis • Stimulates hepatic protein synthesis • Stimulates lipolysis
Catecholamines	• Induces hyperglycaemia • Inhibits the release of insulin • Stimulates lipolysis • Increases basal metabolic rate

ARTERIAL PRESSURE

Blood pressure is defined as a product of cardiac output and systemic vascular resistance (and since cardiac output = heart rate × stroke volume, any changes or influences upon these variables will affect blood pressure).

The mean arterial pressure is the average blood pressure in an individual during a single cardiac cycle. It is calculated by the following formula:

Mean arterial pressure (MAP) = diastolic blood pressure + 0.33 (systolic blood pressure – diastolic blood pressure)

AUTONOMIC NERVOUS SYSTEM

The autonomic nervous system comprises the sympathetic nervous system (SNS) and the parasympathetic nervous system (PNS).

The SNS has myelinated preganglionic and postganglionic cells. The former are found in the lateral horns of the spinal grey matter (T1–L2), whereas the postganglionic cell bodies are situated in the sympathetic chain. The neurotransmitter for preganglionic cells is acetylcholine (ACh), and that for postganglionic cells is noradrenaline. Sympathetic innervation of the chromaffin cells of the adrenal medulla is worth noting since preganglionic sympathetic fibres innervate the adrenal medulla directly.

The PNS differs in the following ways. Firstly, the preganglionic parasympathetic neurones originate from the cranial nerve nuclei (CN III, VII, IX and X). PNS ganglia are located adjacent to near the target organ. ACh is the neurotransmitter used.

Differences between the SNS and PNS

Feature	SNS	PNS
Spinal cord distribution	Thoracolumbar	Craniosacral
Preganglionic neurotransmitter	ACh	ACh
Postganglionic neurotransmitter	Noradrenaline (usually)	ACh
Preganglionic neurone	Short	Long
Postganglionic neurone	Long	Short

BURNS

The Jackson Burn model describes burns as tri-zone injuries. This means that burns have a central zone of coagulative necrosis that is surrounded by a zone of inflammation and ischaemia, which is further surrounded by a zone of hyperaemia.

Burns can be classified in various ways: superficial or deep; partial thickness or full thickness; or by their cause, i.e. flame, chemical, electrical. First-degree burns are confined to the epidermis. Second-degree burns may be superficial or deep. The former affects the papillary dermis and remains painful but typically does not require skin grafts. Deep dermal or reticular second-degree burns are associated with diminished sensation and loss of hair follicles and sometimes do require skin grafts. Third-degree burns penetrate to the subcuticular fat with a leathery appearance. Fourth-degree burns affect the bone.

The layers of the epidermis are as follows: from the innermost layer, they are the stratum basale, stratum spinosum, stratum granulosum, stratum lucidum and stratum corneum.

There are several ways to assess the size of a burn. The commonest is using Wallace's Rule of Nines or a Lund and Browder chart to calculate the total body surface area (TBSA) percentage affected by the burn. Adults with >20% TBSA should receive initial fluid resuscitation and 2 mL Hartmann's solution/kg/%TBSA. This increases to 3 mL/kg/%TBSA for paediatrics and to 4 mL for electrical burns. Half of the calculated fluid is given over 8 hours then the remaining volume is given over 16 hours titrating to maintain urine output of 0.5 mL/hour in adults and 1 mL/hour in the paediatric population who are haemodynamically stable. Boluses may be given if the patient is unstable. Please refer to the most recent ATLS guidance.

Pseudomonas is the commonest organism involved in infected burns, followed by *Staphylococcus* and *E. coli.* HSV is the commonest viral infection.

Acid burns are more painful and are associated with a coagulative necrosis. Alkali burns are less painful but are more concerning as the damage is ongoing, and they are associated with liquefactive necrosis.

The suggested minimum threshold for referral into specialised burn care services can be summarised as:

- All burns ≥3% in adults (over 16 years)
- All full-thickness burns
- All burns to hands, feet, face, neck, perineum or genitalia
- All circumferential burns
- Any chemical or electrical burn
- Any cold injury
- Any burn where there is a suspicion of non-accidental injury or neglect
- Paediatric burns

CARBON DIOXIDE TRANSPORT

Carbon dioxide is transported in three ways in the blood:

1. *As bicarbonate ions:*
   - The following equation describes the carbonic acid–bicarbonate system:

$$CO_2 + H_2O \leftrightarrow H_2CO_3 \leftrightarrow HCO_3^- + H^+$$

The above reaction is catalysed by the enzyme carbonic anhydrase.
   - Le Chatelier's principle states that when a system at equilibrium is disturbed by a change in a property, the system adjusts in a way that opposes the change with corresponding shifts.

- Changes to the system include: (a) a change in concentration, (b) a change in temperature and (c) a change in volume.
- The additional H^+ generated by shifts in this equation is taken up by other buffering systems, e.g. haemoglobin molecules. Bicarbonate diffuses out of the red blood cells and into plasma. This is because the red blood cell membrane is permeable to bicarbonate, whereas it is not permeable to H^+ ions.

2. Dissolved in solution.
3. As carbamino compounds, e.g. plasma proteins, the most significant being haemoglobin.

The above concepts and the production of H^+ are important when considering the oxygen dissociation (sigmoidal) curve. Changes in oxygen affinity for haemoglobin may be seen as shifts on the oxygen dissociation curve. A shift to the right signifies an affinity decrease, and a shift to the left signifies an affinity increase. Causes of these shifts are summarised in the following table. The Bohr effect relates to displacement of the oxygen dissociation curve and changes in pH and P_{CO2}.

Causes of Shifts to the Oxygen Dissociation Curve

Shift to the left (increased affinity)	Shift to the right (decreased affinity)
• Increased pH	• Decreased pH
• Decreased P_{CO2}	• Increased P_{CO2}
• Decreased temperature	• Increased temperature
• Decreased 2,3-bisphosphoglycerate (2,3-DPG)	• Increased 2,3-bisphosphoglycerate (2,3-DPG)

CARDIAC CYCLE, CARDIAC OUTPUT AND THE JVP

The following picture demonstrates the changes that occur during the cardiac cycle. The length of the cycle is typically 0.8–0.9 seconds at rest.

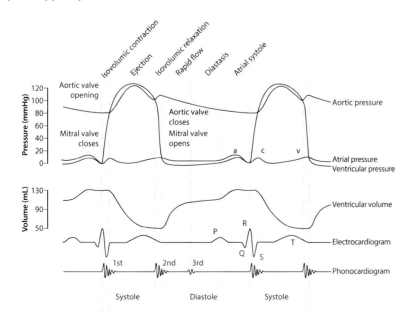

Figure 7.3 The cardiac cycle.

Isovolumetric contraction is the part of the cardiac cycle wherein both the AV and arterial valves are closed, meaning that the ventricles contract against a closed chamber. Closure of the aortic valve results in the dicrotic notch.

The heart sounds are also illustrated on the diagram. The cause of each is summarised in the following table.

Summary of Causes of the Different Heart Sounds

Heart sound	Cause
First	AV (tricuspid and mitral) valve closure
Second	Semilunar (pulmonary and aortic) valve closure
Third	Rapid ventricular filling
Fourth	Associated with cardiac disease

CARDIAC OUTPUT

Cardiac output is the ability of the heart to meet the metabolic demands of the body. It is defined by the following equation:

$$Cardiac\ output = Heart\ rate \times Stroke\ volume$$

Stroke volume is the volume of blood ejected by the ventricles during ventricular systole. It is affected by preload (determined by venous return to the heart), afterload (ventricular wall tension), heart rate and contractility. It may be calculated by the following equation:

$$Stroke\ volume = End\ diastolic\ volume - End\ systolic\ volume$$

FRANK–STARLING CURVE

This curve illustrates how changes in ventricular preload result in changes in stroke volume.

The Frank–Starling law states that the force or tension developed in a muscle fibre depends on the extent to which the fibre is stretched. During systole, the cardiac wall has two important properties—contraction and elastic recoil. When more blood is returned to the heart it stretches the myocardial wall more, and thus preload is increased, and ventricular contraction is increased. In addition to this, the contraction force is greater since the stretched myocardial walls recoil back to their resting position with greater force.

Cardiac contractility is also increased by other intrinsic and extrinsic means: intrinsically by the autonomic nervous system (sympathetic) and extrinsically by catecholamines.

Sympathetic stimulation also increases cardiac output by increasing heart rate and causing vasoconstriction (which increases preload).

JUGULAR VENOUS PRESSURE (JVP)

Jugular venous pressure (JVP) provides an indirect measure of central venous pressure because the internal jugular vein (IJV) connects to the right atrium without any intervening valves.

The following table highlights events that occur throughout the waveform.

Table Illustrating Events throughout the JVP Waveform

Wave	Comment
a	• Right atrium contracts
x	• Right atrium relaxes
c	• Right ventricle contracts
	• Closure of tricuspid valve
x^1	• End of right ventricular contraction
	• Right atrium begins to fill with blood
v	• Right atrium fills with blood against closed tricuspid valve
y	• Opening of tricuspid valve

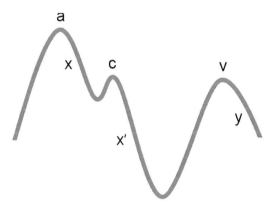

Figure 7.4 JVP waveform.

Pathologies Associated with JVP

JVP wave changes	Pathology
Absent a waves	• Atrial fibrillation
Large a waves	• Tricuspid stenosis
	• Right ventricular hypertrophy
	• Pulmonary hypertension
	• Pulmonary stenosis
Cannon a waves	• Complete heart block
	• Ventricular arrhythmias/ectopics
Prominent v waves	• Tricuspid regurgitation
Slow y descent	• Tricuspid stenosis
	• Right atrial myxoma
Steep y descent	• Right ventricular failure
	• Constrictive pericarditis
	• Tricuspid regurgitation

CELL BIOLOGY

THE CELL CYCLE

G0—quiescent
G1—RNA synthesis, determines the cell cycle length
S—DNA synthesis (p53 prevents cells entering this phase)
G2—RNA synthesis
M—mitosis

STAGES OF MITOSIS

- *Prophase*—centromere attachment, spindle formation
- *Metaphase*—chromosome alignment
- *Anaphase*—chromosomes pulled apart
- *Telophase*—nucleus reforms around each set of chromosomes

DIFFERENT TYPES OF CELLS

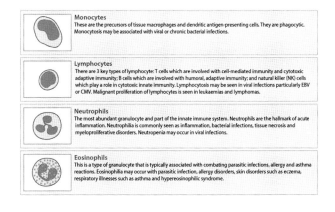

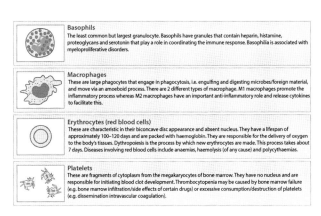

Figure 7.5 Components of a full blood count.

- Basophils release histamine in the blood.
- Mast cells release histamine in the tissue.

CEREBROSPINAL FLUID

Cerebrospinal fluid (CSF) is produced by the choroid plexus and the blood vessels which line the ventricular walls. It is absorbed by the arachnoid villi and the spinal nerve roots. The circulating volume of CSF is approximately 150 mL. The flow of CSF is as follows:

Lateral ventricles → Interventricular foramina of Monro → Third ventricle
→ Cerebral aqueduct of Sylvius → Fourth ventricle → Apertures
→ Subarachnoid space → Dural venous sinuses

The following figure illustrates the ventricular system.

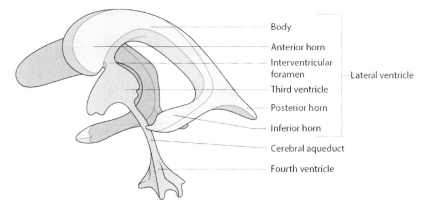

Body
Anterior horn
Interventricular foramen
Third ventricle
Posterior horn
Inferior horn
Cerebral aqueduct
Fourth ventricle
Lateral ventricle

Figure 7.6 The ventricular system through which CSF flows.

CEREBRAL BLOOD FLOW

Blood flow to the brain accounts for 15% of cardiac output. The rate of blood flow is 50 mL per 100 g of brain tissue. The flow of blood to the brain is maintained with changes in arterial blood pressure by a process called autoregulation.

Three principal factors govern cerebral blood flow:

1. *PaCO$_2$ (most important factor)*—increased CO_2 increases the concentration of H$^+$ and thus increases cerebral blood flow.
2. *PaO$_2$*—decreased O_2 causes vasodilatation, thereby increasing cerebral blood flow.
3. *Sympathetic stimulation*—results in vasoconstriction.

Cerebral perfusion pressure = Mean arterial pressure – Intracranial pressure

This is of paramount importance when considering the Monro–Kellie doctrine, which states that the sum of volumes of the brain, CSF and intracranial blood is constant. An increase in one should cause a decrease in one or both of the remaining two. For example, as ICP increases, blood and CSF are displaced as part of the equilibrium to help maintain normal pressure within the fixed cranium, whilst brain tissue remains unchanged.

This is only true to a certain pressure, after which compensation mechanisms are exhausted and herniation results.

FETAL CIRCULATION

Fetal circulation is adapted so that the fetus receives nutrients and oxygenated blood from the placenta via the umbilical cord. The umbilical cord contains 2 umbilical arteries and 1 umbilical vein. The vein carries the oxygenated blood and nutrients whereas waste products are removed via the arteries.

In order to do this effectively, the fetal circulation has 3 shunts that serve to bypass the liver and lungs (although small amounts of blood do go to each). The shunts are; the foramen ovale (blood flows from the right atrium to the left atrium), the ductus arteriosus (blood flows from the pulmonary artery to the aorta) and the ductus venosus (allows blood to bypass the liver to the IVC).

At birth, the umbilical cord is clamped. This initiates change. Nutrients and oxygen are no longer supplied via the placenta. The baby begins to breathe and the lungs expand. This results in several pressure changes. The pulmonary pressures decrease, the blood pressure increases and there is increased pressure within the left artium. These changes result in closure of the afore-mentioned shunts.

At birth, the following changes occur:

1. Decreased pulmonary vascular resistance
2. Closure of the foramen ovale
3. Closure of the ductus venosus
4. Closure of ductus arteriosus
5. Closure of the umbilical vessels

Review of Structures and What They become after Birth

Structure	Becomes the . . .
Ductus arteriosus	Ligamentum arteriosum
Ductus venosus	Ligamentum venosum (usually attached to the left branch of the portal vein within the porta hepatis)
Umbilical vein	Ligamentum teres
Fetal urachus	Median umbilical ligament
Umbilical arteries	Medial umbilical ligament

GASTROINTESTINAL HORMONES

Table to summarise the secretory products from different cells within the gastrointestinal tract

Cells	Secretory products
Surface mucous cells (stomach)	Mucin (in alkaline fluid)
Mucous neck cells (stomach)	Mucin (in acid fluid)
Parietal cells (stomach)	HCl and intrinsic factor
Chief cells (stomach)	Pepsinogen and lipase
G cells (stomach antrum)	Gastrin—gastric acid secretion, increases gastric motility and stimulates exocrine pancreatic secretions
I cells (duodenum and jejunum)	CCK—gallbladder contraction and lipid digestion
S cells (duodenum)	Secretin—stimulates secretion of bicarbonate

Cells	Secretory products
K cells (duodenum and jejunum)	GIP—gastric inhibitory polypeptide, inhibits gastric acid secretion and increases insulin secretion
D cells (pancreatic islet cells)	Somatostatin—inhibitory and an anti-growth hormone

Note: Parietal cells bear receptors for three stimulators of acid secretion: acetylcholine receptors, histamine receptors and gastrin receptors.
- *ACh is derived from the parasympathetic vagal neurones, gastrin is produced by pyloric G cells and histamine is produced by mast cells.*
- *HCl secretion is inhibited by somatostatin, secretin and CCK.*

HAEMATOLOGY/IMMUNOLOGY

The response to vascular injury includes vasoconstriction, platelet adhesion and thrombin generation. Thrombin is vital to coagulation. It:

1. Converts fibrinogen to fibrin
2. Activates factor V and VIII
3. Activates platelets

THE COAGULATION PATHWAY

- *Intrinsic pathway*—activated by exposed collagen, prekallikrein and factor XII
- *Extrinsic pathway*—activated by tissue factor and factor VII
- *PT measurement*—measures factors II, V, VII, X and fibrinogen activity. Best determinant of liver function
- *APTT*—measures most factors except for factors VII and XIII

KEY FACTS:

1. *Factor X*—common to both pathways.
2. *Factor VIII*—helps crosslinks fibrin. It is not synthesised by the liver, it is synthesised by the endothelium.
3. *Fibrin*—binds GP IIb/IIIa linking platelets together to form a platelet plug.
4. *Factor VII*—factor with the shortest half-life.
5. *Factors V and VIII*—most labile factors.
6. *Vitamin K-dependent factors*—II, VII, IX, X, protein C and protein S.
7. *Antithrombin III*—binds to and inhibits thrombin.
8. *Plasmin*—degrades factors V, VIII, fibrinogen and fibrin. This breaks down the platelet plug.
9. *Thromboxane A_2*—released from platelets. It increases platelet aggregation and stimulates vasoconstriction. It stimulates calcium release in platelets, and this exposes the GP IIb/IIIa receptors, which subsequently stimulates platelet binding.
10. *In platelet disorders*, bleeding time is abnormal.

Massive blood transfusion can result in hypocalcaemia. Calcium is required for the clotting cascade. This is because the anticoagulant citrate is in bags of RBCs. This chelates calcium ions.

Platelets are the most common transfusion product that may be contaminated with bacteria, most commonly *E. coli*, since they are not refrigerated.

Hypersensitivity reactions:

- *Type 1*—anaphylactic, IgE
- *Type 2*—cell bound, IgM and IgG
- *Type 3*—immune complex
- *Type 4*—delayed, T-cell

THE SPLEEN

It is the largest reticuloendothelial organ in the body. It comprises two types of pulp:

- Red pulp—filters damaged/old red blood cells
- White pulp—immunologic function

FUNCTIONS OF THE SPLEEN:

- Platelet storage
- Culls damaged or old red blood cells
- Pitting—this is the removal of intracellular products
- Immune function
- Generates proteins, e.g. tuftsin—important for opsonisation

POST-SPLENECTOMY BLOOD FILM CHANGES:

1. *Howell–Jolly bodies*—nuclear remnants
2. *Pappenheimer bodies*—iron deposits
3. *Spurr cells*—deformed membranes
4. *Target cells*—immature red blood cells
5. *Heinz bodies*—intracellular denatured haemoglobin

HYPOTHERMIA

Hypothermia is a core body temperature <35 °C. The severity of hypothermia is categorised using the Swiss Staging System outlined in the following table.

Swiss Staging System of Hypothermia

Stage	Clinical findings	Core temp	Therapy
HT-1	Conscious, shivering	35°C to 32°C	Warm environment, clothing and liquids
HT-II	Impaired consciousness, not shivering	32°C to 28°C	Cardiac monitoring, full body insulation and active external and minimally invasive rewarming techniques (e.g. heating packs, warm parenteral fluids)
HT-III	Unconscious, but vital signs are present	28°C to 24°C	As per HT-II with airway control; if vital signs are unstable, CPB or ECMO
HT-IV	No vital signs		Attempt to restore vital signs with epinephrine, defibrillation, then rewarm with ECMO or CPB

Abbreviations: CPB, cardiopulmonary bypass; ECMO, extracorporeal membrane oxygenation.

Hypothermia may be accidental, induced or therapeutic. The body detects temperature via peripheral receptors in the skin, central thermoreceptors in the hypothalamus and spinal cord as well as higher processing centres. Stimulation of these receptors induces physiological and behavioural responses that aim to increase body temperature.

Those who are at greater risk of hypothermia are listed below:

- *The young*—due to their surface area to body ratio
- *The elderly*—less physiological reserve and influence of chronic disease processes
- *Burn patients*—skin loss
- *Diabetic patients*—autonomic neuropathy
- *Patients following drowning*
- *Social groups*, e.g. homeless
- *Surgical factors*, e.g. the unwarmed surgical patient, anaesthetic, unable to shiver, vasoconstriction, long operative time

Complications of Hypothermia

Complication	Notes
Myocardial ischaemia/arrest	Hypothermia shifts the O_2 curve to the left, meaning that less oxygen is available for use by the tissues.
Interferes with clotting cascade → bleeding	Affects platelets and inhibits enzymes.
Surgical site infections	Inhibits neutrophil function. Vasoconstriction means that it is harder for white cells to get to infected tissues.
Prolongation of drug effects	Hypothermia may increase the concentration of certain drugs thereby prolonging the drug response. Changes in blood flow due to hypothermia may affect drug absorption and clearance systemically.

INTERLEUKINS (IL)

The following table outlines the different interleukins and their function.

IL-1 to IL-10 and Their Function

Interleukin	Function
IL-1	• Induces fever and macrophage release
IL-2	• Proinflammatory
IL-3	• Monocyte production
IL-4	• Production of antibodies
IL-5	• Stimulates eosinophils
IL-6	• Proinflammatory cytokine secreted by macrophages and by muscle in response to trauma, burns and muscle contraction • Increases hepatic acute phase proteins
IL-7	• Aids B cell development
IL-8	• Induces angiogenesis • Attracts neutrophils

(Continued)

IL-1 to IL-10 and Their Function   (Continued)

Interleukin	Function
IL-9	• Stimulates cell proliferation • Prevents apoptosis
IL-10	• "Downregulatory" • It is anti-inflammatory and is expressed mainly by monocytes, type 2 CD4 cells and mast cells

IMMUNOGLOBULINS

- *IgM*—largest, opsonises, fixes complement
- *IgG*—most abundant, crosses placenta, opsonises, fixes complement
- *IgA*—in secretions and breast milk
- *IgE*—allergic and parasitic reactions
- *IgD*—membrane bound receptor on B cells

THE LIVER

The liver has many functions, for example:

- *Detoxification*—of drugs, alcohol, steroid hormones and ammonia
- *Production of cholesterol*
- Metabolism—conversion of T4 to T3
- *Immune function*
- *Storage of micronutrients,* e.g. vitamins A, D, E, K and B12 as well as the minerals copper, zinc, magnesium and iron.
- Role in blood glucose control—stores glycogen
- *Production of bile*
- *Protein synthesis,* e.g. prothrombin, albumin, globulins and lipoproteins

The liver detoxifies many (mostly lipophilic) substances. To do this, the substances undergo bio-transformation wherein reactive OH, NH_2 or COO groups are added to hydrophobic substances enzymatically. The second step in this process is conjugation. Substances are conjugated with glucuronic acid, glutathione, acetate, sulphates, etc. The conjugates are now water soluble and may be secreted into bile by hepatocytes and then excreted in the faeces or processed by the kidneys.

BILE

Bile contains bile salts, cholesterol, lecithin, bilirubin, electrolytes and steroid hormones as well as medications. The liver synthesises the primary bile salts (cholate and chenodeoxycholate) from cholesterol. Hepatocytes secrete bile into biliary canaliculi.

Unconjugated bile salts are reabsorbed from the bile ducts. Conjugated bile salts enter the duodenum and are reabsorbed from the terminal ileum by the apical sodium–bile acid co-transporter.

Bile is stored and concentrated in the gallbladder. It is concentrated because the gallbladder epithelium reabsorbs Na^+, Cl^- and water. Gallbladder contraction is stimulated by cholecystokinin (CCK). CCK is synthesised and released by the I cells (enteroendocrine cells) found within the mucosal lining of the small intestine.

BILIRUBIN METABOLISM

Most bilirubin comes from haemoglobin, and the rest originates from haemoproteins. Haem is cleaved from its globin component and undergoes a variety of enzyme dependent processes, as illustrated by the diagram, to produce conjugated bilirubin. About 80–90% of bilirubin is excreted in the faeces. Gut bacteria break down bilirubin into stercobilinogen, which is partially oxidised into stercobilin; this is brown and colours the stool. Some is excreted by the kidneys as urobilinogen. Another portion of bilirubin is deconjugated by gut bacteria and returns to the liver via enterohepatic circulation.

MUSCLE CONTRACTION

There are three types of muscles within the body—smooth, skeletal and cardiac.

Muscle fibres may be categorised as striated or smooth. Striated muscle contains actin and myosin, which are carefully organised into functioning subunits called sarcomeres. Smooth muscle does not contain sarcomeres, but actin and myosin do contract, e.g. propulsion of food through the GI tract.

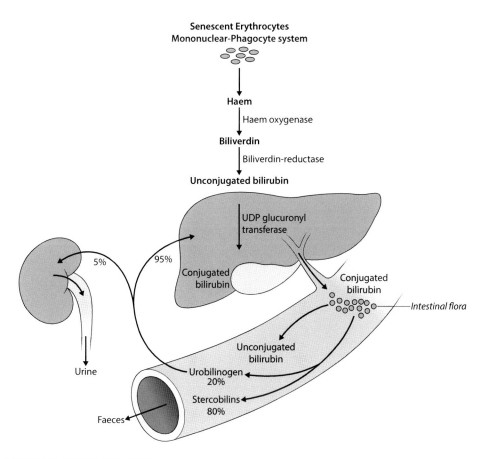

Figure 7.7 Bilirubin metabolism.

STRIATED MUSCLE

Striated muscle, e.g. skeletal and cardiac muscle, is made up of repeating sarcomeres. Sarcomeres consist of thick filaments as well as thin filaments which are made of different proteins and will now be described.

Thick filaments contain the protein myosin, which has one pair of heavy chains and two pairs of light chains. The myosin head binds with ATP.

The thin filaments are composed of actin, tropomyosin and troponin.

The process of excitation–contraction coupling results in an action potential that gives rise to muscle contraction.

Myosin and actin bind together and slide along one another during contraction.

Myosin can only bind with actin in the presence of calcium ions.

SMOOTH MUSCLE

Actin and myosin are also present in smooth muscle; however, they are not organised into sarcomeres. There is a different mechanism for controlling contraction. The steps involved in muscle contraction for both striated and smooth muscle are detailed herein.

MECHANISM OF SKELETAL MUSCLE CONTRACTION

1. An action potential (AP) travels along a motor nerve to its endings on muscle fibres.
2. Acetylcholine (ACh) is released.
3. ACh acts on the muscle fibre membrane and opens ACh-gated cation channels.
4. Na^+ ions diffuse to the interior of the muscle fibre membrane.
5. Local depolarisation occurs, and this causes voltage-gated Na^+ channels to open. This initiates an AP at the membrane.
6. The AP depolarises the muscle membrane, and as a result, the sarcoplasmic reticulum releases Ca^{2+} ions that had been stored within the reticulum.
7. The Ca^{2+} ions produce attractive forces to act between actin and myosin filaments. The filaments slide alongside each other in a contractile process.
8. Ca^{2+} ions are pumped back into the sarcoplasmic reticulum by a Ca^{2+} membrane pump and remain stored in the sarcoplasmic reticulum until the generation of a new AP.

MECHANISM OF SMOOTH MUSCLE CONTRACTION

1. Intracellular Ca^{2+} concentration increases when calcium enters the cell and is released from the sarcoplasmic reticulum (SR).
2. Calcium binds to calmodulin.
3. Ca^{2+}–calmodulin complex activates myosin light chain kinase.
4. Myosin light chain kinase phosphorylates myosin head light chains, thus increasing myosin ATPase activity.
5. Myosin cross-bridges slide along actin, creating muscle tension.
6. Free Ca^{2+} in cytosol decreases when calcium is pumped out of the cell or back into the SR and results in the relaxation of smooth muscle.
7. Ca^{2+} unbinds from calmodulin.
8. Myosin phosphatase removes phosphate from myosin. This reduces myosin ATPase activity and decreases the muscle tension.

DIFFERENCES BETWEEN SKELETAL AND CARDIAC MUSCLE

Sometimes MCQs in the MRCS exam ask about the differences between skeletal and cardiac muscle. The differences are listed here.

- Cardiac muscle is involuntary.
- The cardiac myocytes have centrally located nuclei.
- Myocytes are connected to each other via intercalated disks.
- The T-tubule system is larger in cardiac myocytes.

NEPHRON PHYSIOLOGY

Renal clearance of a substance may be calculated via the following equation:

$$\text{Renal clearance (mL/min)} = \text{(urine concentration} \times \text{urine flow rate)}/\text{plasma concentration i.e. } (U_x \times V)/P_x$$

where U is the urinary concentration of the substance, V is the urine flow rate per minute and P is the plasma concentration of the substance.

When a substance is excreted unchanged, then the clearance of that substance equates to the glomerular filtration rate (GFR). An example of a substance that is excreted in this way is inulin.

Factors a substance must fulfil to measure GFR:

- Freely filtered at the glomerulus
- Is not secreted
- Is not reabsorbed
- Is not metabolised by the kidney

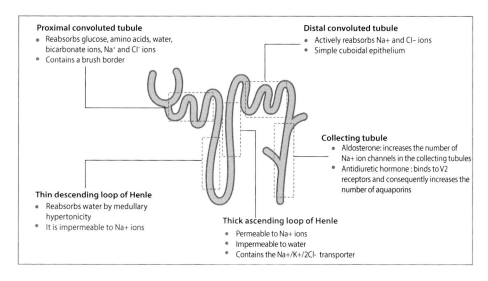

Figure 7.8 Nephron physiology.

NUTRITION

The body enters a catabolic state in response to surgery/stress/injury. The following diagram shows the physiological process in response to stress/injury. Then nutritional strategies will be explored.

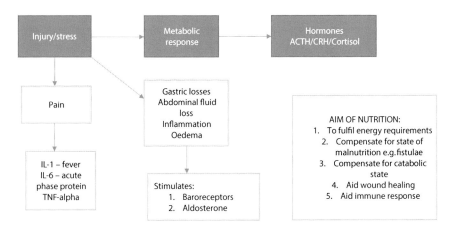

Figure 7.9 The physiologic response of the body to stress/injury.

NUTRITION REQUIREMENTS

Men, 2500 kcal/day; women, 2000 kcal/day. Note that undernutrition is associated with increased risk of infection, increased mortality and increased length of hospital stay.

Recommended Daily Nutritional Component Intake

Nutritonal component	Daily amount required	Additional notes
Carbohydrates	3.5 g/kg/day	Obligatory glucose requirement for the CNS and the haematopoietic cells. Physiologic maximum reached at 4 g/kg (anything not oxidised is then converted to fat).
Fats	1 g/kg/day	Linoleic acid and linolenic acid are "essential" fatty acids because they cannot be synthesised in vivo. Thus, fats need to be given with carbohydrates as a dual-energy supply*.
Protein	0.9 g/kg/day	
Nitrogen	0.1–0.15 g/kg/day	
Water	40 mL/kg/day	

* Providing a dual-energy supply has many benefits, e.g. it reduces the complications associated with TPN, decreases fluid retention, decreases CO_2 production and enhances substrate utilisation.

ASSESSMENT OF NUTRITION

Always seek dietician support and follow guidelines such as those provided by ESPEN.

FACTORS TO CONSIDER ARE:

- General patient appearance
- Hydration status
- Bioimpedance measures
- BMI
- Biochemical measures
- MUST score
- Indirect calorimetry RQ—if RQ >1 = overfed; if RQ <1 = underfed

RQ for Carbohydrates, Protein and Fat

Nutrition	RQ value
Carbohydrate	1.0
Protein	0.8
Fat	0.7

SIGNS OF PATIENTS AT SEVERE RISK OF MALNUTRITION:

- Weight loss >10–15% over 6 months
- BMI <18.5
- SGA grade C
- Pre-op albumin <30

WHAT REPLACEMENT DO INPATIENTS NEED?

Table Highlighting Replacement Requirement of Different Types of Patients

Replacement needed	Type of patient
15–20 kcal/kg/day	Patients at risk of refeeding syndrome*
20–25 kcal/kg/day	Obese adult
25–30 kcal/kg/day	Healthy adult
>30 kcal/kg/day	Burn patient
>40 kcal/kg/day	ICU patient

* Patients at risk of refeeding syndrome, e.g. anorexic patients, liver resection patients.

Refeeding syndrome describes the potentially fatal shifts in electrolytes and fluids that may occur in malnourished patients receiving artificial refeeding. The hallmark biochemical features of refeeding syndrome are: (1) hypophosphataemia, (2) hypokalaemia and (3) hypomagnesaemia. Patients may also experience changes in sodium level and glucose, protein and fat metabolism, as well as thiamine deficiency.

ENTERAL FEEDING V PARENTERAL FEEDING

In general, enteral feeding is preferred. It is inexpensive, it maintains the gastrointestinal tract mucosa and is physiological; however, it cannot be used if the gastrointestinal tract is compromised, e.g. via an enterocutaneous fistula or if the patient has an aspiration risk.

Examples of Enteral Feeding Methods and Complications

Method	Complication
Tube feeding, e.g. NG tube	Tube-related complications, e.g. malposition, blockage, displacement, erosions
Gastrostomy/PEG	Procedure-related complications, e.g. infection, abdominal wall abscess, necrotising fasciitis, migration
Jejunostomy	Leakage, displacement

Parenteral nutrition means that all nutrition needs are met intravenously, either peripherally or centrally. Risks associated with a peripheral line include thrombophlebitis. If peripheral access is used, guidance is that the location should be changed every 24 hours. Therefore, central access is preferred, and some centres do not offer peripheral access for this purpose at all. Central access may be via the SCV, IJV or EJV. Hickmann lines are preferable.

SIDE EFFECTS OF PARENTERAL NUTRITION:

- Fluid overload
- Abnormal LFTs
- Hyperglycaemia
- Electrolyte abnormalities—low phosphate, low calcium, low potassium and low magnesium
- Vitamin deficiencies

INDICATIONS FOR TPN:

- Short gut syndrome
- Massive small-bowel resection because it results in short gut
- Malabsorption
- High-output enterocutaneous fistula
- Inability to obtain enteral access
- Severe catabolism

COMPLICATIONS OF TPN:

- Complications related to the catheter—infection, pneumothorax
- Refeeding syndrome
- Electrolyte disturbances—low phosphate, low calcium, low potassium and low magnesium
- Abnormal LFTs and jaundice
- Folate deficiency

THE PANCREAS

The pancreas is a mixed exocrine and endocrine gland.

Summary of Cells and Hormones Secreted by the Pancreas

Cell of the pancreas	Substance secreted
α cells	Glucagon
β cells	Insulin
δ cells	Somatostatin

About 1–1.5 litres of pancreatic juice is produced per day. This has an aqueous and enzymatic component. Enzymes are proteases, e.g. trypsinogen, proelastase; lipolytics, e.g. lipases; phospholipases, e.g. A_2; and amylases.

Inactive zymogens, e.g. trypsinogen, are activated by the enteropeptidase enzyme.

Pancreatic juice secretion is stimulated by:

- Secretin
- Gastrin
- CCK
- Vagal stimulation

MECHANISM OF ACTION OF INSULIN

Insulin binds to tyrosine kinase receptors and initiates two pathways by phosphorylation:

1. *The MAPK signalling pathway*—this is responsible for cell growth and proliferation.
2. *The PI-3K signalling pathway*—this is responsible for the transport of GLUT-4 receptors to the cell surface membrane; GLUT-4 transports glucose into the cell. This pathway is also responsible for protein, lipid and glycogen synthesis.

RENIN–ANGIOTENSIN–ALDOSTERONE SYSTEM

The release of aldosterone is controlled by the renin angiotensin-aldosterone system (RAAS). Angiotensinogen is released from the liver and is converted to angiotensin I by renin. Renin is produced by the cells of the juxtaglomerular apparatus. Several factors may stimulate renin release, e.g. hypotension, low sodium levels, increased sympathetic drive, catecholamines and erect posture. Angiotensin I is converted to angiotensin II by angiotensin-converting enzyme (ACE). ACE is produced by the endothelium in the lungs and kidney.

Angiotensin II stimulates several pathways:

1. Production of aldosterone from the zona glomerulosa, which in turn results in sodium and water retention and an increase in blood pressure.
2. Increases sympathetic activity.

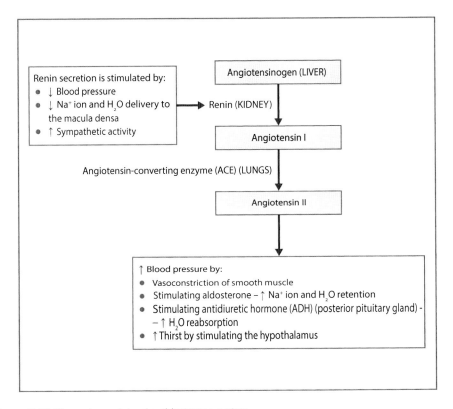

Figure 7.10 The renin–angiotensin–aldosterone system.

3. Increases Na$^+$ and Cl$^-$ reabsorption, K$^+$ excretion and water retention.
4. Vasoconstriction.
5. Stimulates the posterior pituitary gland to produce antidiuretic hormone and thus increases water reabsorption from the collecting ducts of the kidney.

These pathways are summarised in the diagram above.

VENTILATION

Ventilation is controlled by:

1. *The brainstem*—involuntary control.
   a. *The medullary respiratory centre*—located in the reticular formation. Responsible for inspiration (dorsal) and expiration (ventral).
   b. *The apneustic area*—located in the pons. Responsible for prolongation of the inspiratory phase of respiration.
   c. *The pneumotaxic area*—located in the pons. Responsible for the rate, rhythm and depth of respiration.
2. The cerebral cortex—voluntary control.

Compliance of the lungs is the change in lung volume per unit change in pressure. Surfactant, produced by type 2 pneumocytes, increases compliance of the lungs by decreasing surface tension.

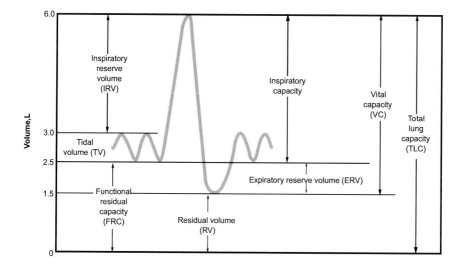

TLC = VC + RV.
TLC = TV + RV + IRV + ERV.
VC = maximal exhalation after maximal inhalation.
RV = lung volume after maximal exhalation.
TV = volume of air with normal inhalation and exhalation.
FRC = ERV + RV. This is the lung volume after normal exhalation. It is decreased with atelectasis, sepsis (ARDS) and trauma.
ERV = the volume of air that can be forcefully expired after normal expiration.
FEV_1 = forced expiratory volume in I second.
Dead space = the area of the lung that is ventilated but not perfused. This is increased with pulmonary embolism, pulmonary hypertension and ARDS.
Ageing decreases FEV, and VC but increases FRC.
Ventilation/perfusion mismatch is greatest in the upper lobes of the lung.
Compliance = change in volume/change in pressure.

Patterns in restrictive lung disease = FEV_1 is normal or increased. TLC, RV and FVC are decreased.

Patterns in obstructive lung disease = FVC is normal or decreased. FEV_1 is decreased. TLC and RV are increased.

Figure 7.11 Respiratory function tests.

WOUND HEALING

There are four stages of wound healing: haemostasis, inflammation, proliferation and remodelling. Each will be outlined in turn.

1. Haemostasis
   - Stimulation of the coagulation cascade results in stimulation of fibrinogen.
   - This stimulates platelets and the formation of the fibrin scaffold.
   - Platelets help to form a haemostatic plug, and they have alpha granules that release growth factors and cytokines, e.g. PDGF and TGF-β, that attract neutrophils, monocytes and fibroblasts.
   - Platelets are the critical cells in this step.
2. Inflammation
   - Days 1–6.
   - Coagulation cascades, complement and bacterial degradation stimulate chemotactic factors, e.g. TGF-β, C3a and C3b, which attract inflammatory cells to the scaffold.

- Neutrophils phagocytose debris.
- Monocytes transform into macrophages and bind to the extracellular matrix, releasing mediators.
- Fibroblast infiltration is stimulated.
- Macrophages are the critical cells in this step.

3. Proliferation
   - Day 4–week 3.
   - Keratinocytes migrate and form the epithelial layer.
   - Fibroblasts produce collagen to act as a scaffold.
   - Fibroblasts and macrophages replace the fibrin mesh to form granulation tissue.
   - Granulation tissue comprises hyaluronic acid, procollagen, elastin and prostaglandins as well as new blood vessels.
   - Some fibroblasts become myofibroblasts.
   - Wound contraction occurs due to myofibroblasts.

4. Remodelling
   - Months to years.
   - Many cells within the wound undergo apoptosis.
   - Type III collagen is turned into the more organised type I collagen by matrix metalloproteinases (MMPs).
   - MMPs are produced by fibroblasts.

FACTORS THAT AFFECT WOUND HEALING

1. *Mechanical forces*—tension, shear forces, gravity and osmosis.
2. *Patient factors*—immunosuppression, diabetes, poor nutrition, steroids, smoking.
3. *Infection/biofilms*—biofilms are adherent populations of microbes that form 3D populations and re-organise on extracellular polymers.
4. *Surgical techniques*—excess tension on the wound, wrong suture material.
5. *Negative pressure wound devices*—may promote wound healing by draining the wound, stimulating granulation tissue development and by expediting wound contraction.

TYPES OF GRAFTS:

1. *Autograft*—tissue transplanted from one location to another on the same individual
2. *Allograft*—tissue transplanted between separate individuals of the same species
3. *Xenograft*—tissue transplanted between different species
4. *Split-thickness skin graft*—contains varying amounts of dermis
5. *Full-thickness skin graft*—contains the entire dermis

PHASES OF GRAFT TAKE:

1. Fibrin adhesion
2. Plasmatic imbibition
3. Inosculation
4. Revascularisation and remodelling

FACTORS THAT AFFECT GRAFT TAKE:

1. *Patient factors*—comorbidities like immunosuppression, diabetes, poor nutrition, steroids, smoking
2. *Graft factors*—inappropriate preparation, traumatic tissue handling
3. *Recipient site factors*—inappropriate preparation, irregular surface, shear force, infection
4. *Surgical technique*—graft not secured appropriately, compromise to local blood supply
5. *Bandages*—excessive pressure on the graft, friction

General Surgery

8

HERNIAS

Definition: a hernia is a protrusion of a viscus, or part of a viscus, through the wall of its containing cavity into an anatomically abnormal position.

There are many different types of hernias with respect to the anterior abdominal wall. Broadly speaking, there are groin hernias (inguinal, femoral) and ventral hernias. For further information related to the anatomy of groin hernia please see the Anatomy section.

The rest of this section will focus on abdominal wall hernias specifically.

CAUSES:

- Weakness in abdominal wall
- Developmental failures
- Collagen disorders
- Weakness related to pregnancy
- Weakness related to ageing
- Increased intra-abdominal pressure, e.g. obesity, chronic cough
- Associations with neuromuscular disorders and muscle weakness

SIGNS AND SYMPTOMS:

- Bulge that may be reducible or irreducible
- Skin colour changes
- Pain/tenderness
- Cough impulse
- If related to an incisional hernia, there may be a bulge located at the site of a previous surgical incision
- Scrotal content for groin hernia

INVESTIGATIONS:

- *USS*—low cost but operator-dependent
- *CT scan*—increasingly used in the management of incisional hernia and in complex abdominal wall reconstruction

DOI: 10.1201/9781003292005-11

MANAGEMENT:

Depends on the type of hernia, location, patient factors and symptoms.

Not all hernias require surgical repair. It is worth noting that hernias with a small neck are at greater risk of strangulation, as are femoral hernias, and femoral hernias should always be repaired operatively. If skin colour changes have occurred, it is likely the hernia is already strangulated.

A precise definition of complex abdominal wall hernia (CAWH) is still lacking. In general, common unfavourable factors are quoted as affecting the complexity of CAWH and operative repair. These are:

- The need for a tailored approach to abdominal wall repair
- Learning curve of specific complex procedures such as component separation
- CAWH requiring emergency repair
- Obesity (BMI ≥ 30)
- Recurrence
- Large defects
- Age ≥ 80 years
- Specific comorbidities, e.g. airway disease, diabetes, aortic aneurysm, immunosuppression, smoking, coagulopathy or concurrent anticoagulant/antiplatelet therapy

As discussed, hernia and CAWH can be treated in one of two ways—as an emergency that requires an immediate life-saving procedure, or electively in a planned manner. The preference for both patients and surgeons is the latter. Whilst waiting for an elective procedure, CAWH patients in particular need to undergo optimisation, e.g. weight loss management, nutritional support and improving muscle tonality. CAWH cases are typically joint general surgery and plastic surgery cases.

EPONYMOUS HERNIA NAMES

- *Amyand's hernia*—presence of the appendix within the hernial sac.
- *Barth's hernia*—hernia of the loops of intestine between the serosa of the abdominal wall and that of a persistent vitelline duct.
- *Cooper's hernia (bilocular femoral hernia)*—femoral hernia with two sacs, the first being in the femoral canal and the second passing through a defect in the superficial fascia and appearing immediately beneath the skin.
- *Gibbon's hernia*—hernia with hydrocoele.
- *Hesselbach's hernia*—hernia of a loop of intestine through the cribriform fascia presenting lateral to femoral artery.
- *Littre's hernia*—hernia containing Meckel's diverticulum.
- *Pantaloon hernia*—a combined direct and indirect hernia, where the hernial sac protrudes on either side of the inferior epigastric vessels.
- *Spigelian hernia*—occurs through congenital or acquired defects in the spigelian fascia.
- *Canal of Nuck hernia*—continued outpouching of the parietal peritoneum through the inguinal canal to the labia major. This is caused by the incomplete closure of the processus vaginalis in females.

THE OESOPHAGUS

Causes of dysphagia are summarised by the following table and are important to consider in differential diagnoses.

Causes of Dysphagia

Area of compression	Differential diagnosis
Extrinsic compression	Mediastinal masses
	Cervical spondylosis
Problems related to the oesophageal wall	Achalasia
	Oesophageal spasm
Intrinsic compression	Tumours
	Strictures
	Schatzki rings
Neurological issues	CVA
	Parkinson's disease
	Multiple sclerosis

BARRETT'S OESOPHAGUS

DEFINITION:

- This is a premalignant condition that is characterised by the metaplastic replacement of the normal squamous epithelium of the lower oesophagus by columnar epithelium.
- This is a risk factor for the development of adenocarcinoma.

CAUSES:

Prolonged gastro-oesophageal reflux disease (GORD).

INVESTIGATIONS:

- *H. pylori* test.
- Endoscopy—suspected Barrett's metaplasia if an abnormal-looking salmon-coloured mucosa is seen extending above the oesophagogastric junction into the distal oesophagus; four-quadrant biopsy.

MANAGEMENT:

- Treatment of GORD, conservative treatment, e.g. lifestyle modifications like weight loss, smoking cessation, reduction in alcohol intake; medical therapy, e.g. proton pump inhibitors.
- Follow endoscopic screening programme to check for resolution/progression of disease.

BENIGN NEOPLASMS OF THE OESOPHAGUS

Generally rare. These include polyps, adenomas and papillomas. They tend not to be epithelial in origin.

MALIGNANT NEOPLASMS OF THE OESOPHAGUS

OESOPHAGEAL CARCINOMA—KEY POINTS:

- Squamous cell carcinoma and adenocarcinoma are the commonest
- Dysphagia is the most common presenting symptom

SQUAMOUS CELL CARCINOMA—KEY POINTS:

- Usually affects the upper two-thirds of the oesophagus, whereas adenocarcinoma affects the lower third
- Risk factors—tobacco and alcohol
- Geography—Transkei region of South Africa and in the Asian "cancer belt" particularly Henan province in China

ADENOCARCINOMA—KEY POINTS:

- Usually affects the lower third of the oesophagus
- Risk factors—GORD and obesity
- Geography—more common in Western countries

SIGNS AND SYMPTOMS:

- Mechanical symptoms—dysphagia, regurgitation, vomiting, odynophagia
- Weight loss
- Metastases—recurrent laryngeal nerve palsy, Horner's syndrome, chronic spinal pain, diaphragmatic paralysis, enlarged supraclavicular lymph nodes

INVESTIGATIONS:

- Endoscopy is the first line of investigation, with biopsies for cytology and/or histology
- CT scan/MRI for metastasis

MANAGEMENT:

- Depends on patient factors and pathological factors, e.g. TMN staging. Options include chemotherapy, radiotherapy and surgery. The treatment option chosen depends on whether the intent is curative or palliative. This is an overly simplistic description, and the management of such patients involves an MDT discussion and often multimodal therapies.

TNM Staging Scheme for Oesophageal Cancer

Classification	Definition
Tis	High-grade dysplasia
T1	Tumour invading lamina propria or submucosa
T2	Tumour invading muscularis propria
T3	Tumour invading beyond muscularis propria
T4a	Tumour invading adjacent structures (pleura, pericardium, diaphragm)
T4b	Tumour invading adjacent structures (trachea, bone, aorta)
N0	No lymph node metastases
N1	Lymph node metastases in 1–2 nodes
N2	Lymph nodes metastases in 3–6 nodes
N3	Lymph node metastases in seven or more lymph nodes
M0	No distant metastases
M1	All other distant metastases

- Surgical options include the following.

A Summary of Surgical Options for Oesophageal Carcinoma

Type of operation	Comment
Endoscopic mucosal resection	Treatment for early localised adenocarcinoma of the distal oesophagus
Transhiatal oesophagectomy	Most used for junctional (type II) tumours
Ivor Lewis oesophagectomy	Two-stage approach for middle and distal tumours
	Lower incidence of recurrent laryngeal nerve injury
McKeown oesophagectomy	May be useful for proximal tumours
	Higher incidence of recurrent laryngeal nerve injury

- Neoadjuvant treatments may improve survival in a select group of patients.
- Chemoradiotherapy alone may be curative in a select group of squamous cell carcinoma patients.
- Palliation may be achieved by chemo-/radiotherapy or endoscopic treatments.
- Trastuzumab may improve survival in patients with HER2-positive tumours.
- Oesophageal intubation with self-expanding metal stents is the treatment of choice in patients with occluding tumours >2 cm from the cricopharyngeus.

OESOPHAGEAL MOTILITY DISORDERS

The following table outlines the Chicago Classification of Oesophageal Motility Disorders. Key high-yield examinable points of certain conditions will be outlined.

The Chicago Classification of Oesophageal Motility Disorders

Achalasia and EGJ outflow obstruction	Criteria
Type I achalasia (classic achalasia)	Elevated median IRP (>15 mmHg), 100% failed peristalsis (DCI <100 mmHg-s-cm). *Premature contractions with DCI values <450 mmHg-s-cm satisfy criteria for failed peristalsis.*
Type II achalasia (with oesophageal compression)	Elevated median IRP (>15 mmHg), 100% failed peristalsis, panoesophageal pressurisation with ≥20% of swallows. *Contractions may be masked by oesophageal pressurisation and DCI should not be calculated.*
Type III achalasia (spastic achalasia)	Elevated median IRP (>15 mmHg), no normal peristalsis, premature (spastic) contractions with DCI >450 mmHg-s-cm with ≥20% of swallows. *May be mixed with panoesophageal pressurisation.*
EGJ outflow obstruction	Elevated median IRP (>15 mmHg), sufficient evidence of peristalsis such that criteria for types I–III achalasia are not met.

(Continued)

The Chicago Classification of Oesophageal motility disorders   (Continued)

Achalasia and EGJ outflow obstruction	Criteria
Major disorders of peristalsis (not encountered in normal individuals)	
Absent contractility	Normal median IRP, 100% failed peristalsis. *Achalasia should be considered when IRP values are borderline and when there is evidence of oesophageal pressurisation. Premature contractions with DCI values <450 mmHg-s-cm meet criteria for failed peristalsis.*
Distal oesophageal spasm	Normal median IRP, ≥20% premature contractions with DCI >450 mmHg-s-cm. Some normal peristalsis may be present.
Hypercontractile oesophagus (jackhammer)	At least two swallows with DCI >8000 mmHg-s-cm. *Hypercontractility may involve, or even be localised to the LES.*
Minor disorders of peristalsis (characterised by contractile vigour and contraction pattern)	
Ineffective oesophageal motility (IEM)	≥50% ineffective swallows. *Ineffective swallows can be failed or weak (DCI <450 mmHg-s-cm). Multiple repetitive swallow assessment may be helpful in determining peristaltic reserve.*
Fragmented peristalsis	≥50% fragmented contractions with DCI >450 mmHg-s-cm.
Normal oesophageal motility—not fulfilling any of the above classifications	

ACHALASIA:

- Failure of the lower oesophageal sphincter to relax due to loss of the ganglion cells in the myenteric (Auerbach's) plexus. The cause is unknown, but Chagas' disease (caused by infection with parasite *Trypanosoma cruzi*) has a similar appearance.
- Symptoms include dysphagia; therefore, it is vital to exclude carcinoma.
- *Investigations*—barium swallow (bird beak appearance) and fluid level, elevated median integrated relaxation pressure (IRP) (>15 mmHg), endoscopy.
- *Management*—endoscopic dilatation, endoscopic or surgical Heller's myotomy.

OESOPHAGEAL SPASM:

- Uncoordinated contraction of the oesophagus that may be dramatic. The Chicago Classification grades the spasm based on the mmHg.
- Symptoms include dysphagia; therefore, it is vital to exclude carcinoma.
- Investigations—barium swallow (corkscrew appearances).
- Management—no firm management. Trials of calcium channel blockers, vasodilators and endoscopic dilatation have been used to variable effect.

OTHER OESOPHAGEAL CONDITIONS

PLUMMER–VINSON SYNDROME:

- Symptoms—dysphagia.
- Consists of the following triad:

  1. Post-cricoid web
  2. Iron-deficiency anaemia
  3. Glossitis

SCHATZKI'S RING:

A circular ring in the distal oesophagus typically located at the squamocolumnar junction. Some require endoscopic dilation.

PHARYNGEAL POUCH/ZENKER'S DIVERTICULUM:

- *Definition*—this is an outpouching between the upper border of the cricopharyngeal muscle and the lower border of the inferior constrictor muscle of the pharynx in an area of weakness known as Killian's dehiscence.
- *Signs and symptoms*—palpable lump to the left of the neck, regurgitation of food, halitosis, gurgling sounds. The pouch might be emptied by applying external pressure.
- *Note that endoscopy can risk perforating this diverticulum.*
- *Management*—excision of the pouch.

EOSINOPHILIC OESOPHAGITIS:

- Typically occurs in children or young adults, 50% of whom have a history of atopy.
- The exact cause is unclear but is likely allergic or idiopathic in origin.
- Endoscopy confirms the diagnosis. Mucosal rings may be present. Patients have the propensity to form deep ulcers, and these may stricture.
- Treatment is usually via the use of steroids and elimination diets.

THE STOMACH AND GI TRACT

GASTRITIS

Definition—any histologically confirmed inflammation of the gastric mucosa.

1. Autoimmune gastritis
   a. Due to antibodies to the parietal cell.
   b. The result eventually is achlorhydria.
   c. Gastric antrum is unaffected, and the hypochlorhydria leads to the production of high levels of gastrin from the antral G cells.
   d. Risk of pernicious anaemia and gastric cancer.
2. *H. pylori* gastritis
   a. Associated with *H. pylori* infection.
   b. This is a Gram-negative, microaerophilic, spiral (helical) bacterium.

c. Predisposes to peptic ulcer disease.

  d. Treatment: triple eradication therapy, i.e. 2× antibiotics and 1× proton pump inhibitor (PPI).

3. Erosive gastritis

  a. Associated with NSAIDS and alcohol.

  b. NSAIDS inhibit COX-1 which is responsible for generating gastric protecting prostaglandins.

4. Reflux gastritis

  a. More common after gastric surgery.

PEPTIC ULCERS

PEPTIC ULCER DISEASE:

- Common anatomical locations—first part of the duodenum and the lesser curve of the stomach. Duodenal ulcers are more common than gastric ulcers.
- Most can be healed with the use of proton pump inhibitors and eradication of *H. pylori* (if indicated).
- Elective surgery is very rarely performed. Operative options for duodenal ulceration include Billroth II gastrectomy, gastrojejunostomy, truncal vagotomy and drainage.
- An operative option for gastric ulceration is Billroth I gastrectomy. Complications of peptic ulcer disease include perforation, bleeding and stenosis.

PERFORATED PEPTIC ULCER:

- Sudden onset of pain (usually epigastric). Often preceding history of upper abdominal pain/GORD.
- Anterior perforation—causes peritonitis via contamination. Requires laparoscopy (not laparotomy) for omental patch repair. Conversion to laparotomy only if unable to complete laparoscopically. Most important part of this procedure is the washout.
- Posterior—causes haemorrhage, e.g. first part of the duodenum into the gastroduodenal artery. This is treated by gastroenterology via OGD. If they are unable to gain control, then general surgery will do laparotomy and underrun the ulcer.
- Complications of peptic ulcer surgery include recurrent ulceration, small stomach syndrome, early and late dumping syndrome, vitamin B12 deficiency and gallstones.

Features of Early and Late Dumping Syndrome

	Early	Late
Incidence	5–10%	5%
Relation to meals	Within 10–30 minutes after a meal	1–3 hours after a high carbohydrate meal
Relief	Lying down	Food
Aggravated by	More food	
Precipitating factor	Food, especially carbohydrate-rich	As early dumping
Major symptoms	Epigastric fullness, sweating, tachycardia, colic, diarrhoea	Tremor, lightheadedness and a desire to lie down

UPPER GI BLEEDING

A Non-Exhaustive List of Causes of Upper GI Bleeding

Cause	Symptoms
Oesophagitis	Small volume of fresh blood, often streaking vomit
	History of GORD symptoms
Cancer	Small volume of blood (except as pre-terminal event with erosion of major vessels)
	Dysphagia and constitutional symptoms such as weight loss
Mallory Weiss tear	Brisk small-to-moderate volume of bright red blood following bout of repeated vomiting
Varices	Large volume of fresh blood
	Haemodynamic compromise
	Liver disease
Gastric cancer	May be frank haematemesis or altered blood mixed with vomit
	Dyspepsia, may have constitutional symptoms
Dieulafoy lesion	An arteriovenous malformation that may result in significant haemorrhage
Gastric ulcer	May be insidious in onset
	Iron-deficiency anaemia
	Erosion into a significant vessel may produce considerable haemorrhage and haematemesis
Duodenal ulcer	Posteriorly sited

MANAGEMENT:

Depends on the cause of the bleeding. Approach using A–E principles and resuscitate the patient. Early control of airway is vital (e.g. encephalopathic patient with liver failure), and patient likely will need blood; therefore, initiate the major haemorrhage protocol early. Blood tests would include a cross match, FBC, LFTs, U+E and clotting and a blood gas (involving a lactate).

Patients with suspected varices should receive terlipressin prior to endoscopy but check your local hospital policy. Ideally all patients admitted with upper gastrointestinal haemorrhage should undergo upper GI endoscopy within 24 hours of admission.

Treatment of varices includes banding or sclerotherapy. Should this fail, a Sengstaken–Blakemore tube may be inserted. This tube has two balloons—a gastric one and an oesophageal one. The gastric balloon should be inflated first.

Portal pressure may be lowered by a combination of medical therapy +/– TIPSS.

Commence patients on IV PPI since this helps to reduce the risk of rebleeding. Bleeding ulcers that cannot be controlled endoscopically may require laparotomy and under-running of the ulcer.

The Rockall Score for Upper GI Bleeding is a score that is used in patients with clinical upper GI bleeding who have undergone endoscopy. It helps to stratify which patients need endoscopy and intensive care. It is less accurate at identifying low-risk patients.

GASTRIC OUTLET OBSTRUCTION

CAUSES:

- Gastric cancer and pyloric stenosis secondary to peptic ulceration
  - Metabolic abnormality seen—hypochloraemic alkalosis
  - Endoscopic biopsy needed to exclude malignancy

MANAGEMENT:

Correct electrolyte abnormalities, medical therapy for peptic ulcer disease, endoscopic dilatation, appropriate resection if cancer.

GASTRIC CANCER

Prognosis tends to be poor since it is often detected late. Sixth commonest cancer in the UK.

CELL TYPE:

* Majority are adenocarcinoma.

RISK FACTORS:

* *H. pylori*, blood group A, smoking, nitrate containing foods, pernicious anaemia and previous gastric surgery.

SYMPTOMS:

* Epigastric pain, weight loss, nausea and vomiting, GI bleeding and gastric perforation.

SIGNS:

* Epigastric mass, ascites, hepatomegaly, Virchow's node, acanthosis nigricans.

HISTOLOGY:

* Intestinal or diffuse (linitis plastica).

SPREAD:

* Transcoelomic throughout peritoneal cavity; predilection for the ovaries (Krukenburg tumour).

INVESTIGATIONS:

* Blood tests (FBC, U&E, LFTs, coag), endoscopy and biopsy, CT scan.

STAGING:

* TNM, outlined here.

TNM Staging Scheme Gastric Cancer

Classification	Definition
Tis	Tumour "in situ"
T1	Tumour grown through lining and into connective tissue
T2	Tumour invading into thick inner muscle
T3	Tumour invading beyond outer lining but not into nearby organs
T4	Tumour invading adjacent organs or structures
N0	No lymph node metastases
N1	Lymph node metastases in 1–6 nodes
N2	Lymph nodes metastases in 7–15 nodes
N3	Lymph node metastases >15 nodes
M0	No distant metastases
M1	All other distant metastases

Management involves discussion in the MDT and will depend on the stage of cancer, patient factors and treatment intent (i.e. palliative vs curative). Options include chemotherapy; medical palliation, e.g. pyloric stenting; argon plasma coagulation; and surgery, e.g. total or subtotal gastrectomy with a Roux-en-Y anastomosis to prevent bile reflux.

GASTROINTESTINAL STROMAL TUMOURS

DEFINITION:

Mesenchymal tumours of the GI tract which originate within the bowel wall.
They are divided into three groups:

1. *Leiomyomas and leiomyosarcomas*—express markers of smooth muscle differentiation.
2. *Neurofibromas*—positive for S100, indicating a neural origin.
3. *Gastrointestinal stromal tumours (GISTs)*—positive for CD34 and CD117, c-Kit protein, and originate from the interstitial cells of Cajal.

LOCATION:

Stomach (70%), but leiomyomas predominate in the oesophagus.
About 75% are benign, but there are some features of malignancy to be aware of:

1. Extragastric location
2. High mitotic index
3. Tumour size >10 cm

SIGNS AND SYMPTOMS:

- Abdominal pain, GI bleeding, obstructive symptoms

INVESTIGATION:

- Endoscopy

TREATMENT:

- Imatinib may be used in c-Kit positive GISTs, surgical resection

ZOLLINGER–ELLISON SYNDROME

DEFINITION:

Hypersecretion of gastric acid due to a gastrinoma (gastrin-producing tumour).

LOCATION:

Usually gastrinomas are found in the pancreas but they may also be found in the stomach, duodenum and ovaries; 60% are malignant. Most gastrinomas are found within the gastrinoma triangle. The boundaries of this triangle are:

- *Superiorly*—cystic and common bile ducts
- *Inferiorly*—second and third part of the duodenum
- *Medially*—neck and body of pancreas

They are associated with multiple endocrine neoplasia (MEN) type 1.

SIGNS AND SYMPTOMS:

- Refractory peptic ulceration, diarrhoea, GORD, GI bleed.

INVESTIGATIONS:

Gastrin levels (post-secretin), endoscopy, CT, MRI, radionucleotide scanning.
Diagnosis is based on the following three criteria:

1. Fasting hypergastrinaemia
2. Increased basal acid output
3. Secretin stimulation test positive

MANAGEMENT:

- Surgical resection.

THE APPENDIX

ACUTE APPENDICITIS

PATHOPHYSIOLOGY OF APPENDICITIS:

- Appendicitis is the inflammation of the vermiform appendix. The pathophysiology of appendicitis likely stems from obstruction of the appendiceal orifice. The obstruction may be caused by lymphoid hyperplasia, infections (parasitic), faecaliths and benign or malignant tumours.
- The obstruction causes an increase in intramural and intraluminal pressure. Subsequently, this results in lymphatic stasis and small vessel occlusion. With vascular and lymphatic compromise, the appendix wall becomes ischaemic and necrotic.

INVESTIGATIONS:

- Diagnosis is clinical
- Blood tests: FBC, U&Es and CRP
- USS may be useful in some cases
- Pregnancy test in females of childbearing age to exclude ectopic pregnancy
- CT scan if >50 years old to exclude caecal tumour (follow Trust guidelines)

ALVARADO SCORE FOR ACUTE APPENDICITIS:

- A score of 5 or 6 is compatible with the diagnosis of acute appendicitis; a score of 7 or 8 indicates probable appendicitis; a score of 9 or 10 indicates very probable appendicitis.
- The components comprising this score include right lower quadrant tenderness, elevated temperature, rebound tenderness, migration of pain to the right iliac fossa, anorexia, nausea and vomiting, leucocytosis and leukocyte left shift. The scoring system may be found here: www.mdcalc.com/alvarado-score-acute-appendicitis. MANTRELS is a helpful mnemonic to remember these parameters - Migration of pain to the right iliac fossa, Anorexia, Nausea/vomiting, Tenderness in the right iliac fossa, Rebound pain, Elevated temperature, Leukocytosis and Shift of leukocytes to the left.

TREATMENT:

- Typically, management is surgical—laparoscopic or open appendicectomy.
- Sometimes patients may be treated conservatively with analgesia and antibiotics depending on certain risk factors e.g. multiple comorbidities with high anaesthetic risk but this is a consultant surgeon decision.

DIFFERENTIAL DIAGNOSIS OF RIGHT ILIAC FOSSA PAIN:

1. Appendix mass/appendicitis
2. Mesenteric adentitis
3. Gynaecological mass (e.g. ovarian cyst, ecoptic pregnancy)
4. Caecal cancer
5. Inflammatory bowel disease
6. Soft tissue tumour, e.g. sarcoma
7. TB
8. Actinomycosis
9. Aneurysm

BOWEL AND RECTUM

INFLAMMATORY BOWEL DISEASE

Inflammatory bowel disease is a chronic inflammatory disease of the gastrointestinal tract. It is subdivided into Crohn's disease and ulcerative colitis. The CARD15 gene has been associated with IBD but the exact cause remains unclear. There is often a positive family history and Crohn's disease has a strong link with tobacco smoking. Age distribution is bimodal usually presenting in those aged 15–30 years and there is another peak in those >60 years old. Crohn's disease and ulcerative colitis will now be explored in greater detail.

CROHN'S DISEASE

This is a disordered response to intestinal bacteria with transmural inflammation. It may affect any aspect of the GI tract but often targets the terminal ileum. It is associated with granuloma formation.

SIGNS AND SYMPTOMS:

- *These include*—weight loss, abdominal pain (sometimes with a palpable mass in the right iliac fossa), diarrhoea (+/– mucous), fever, skip lesions, clubbing, cobblestone mucosa, fistula formation and linear ulceration.
- *Extraintestinal manifestations*—arthritis, aphthous stomatitis, uveitis, erythema nodosum, ankylosing spondyloarthropathy and gallstones.

INVESTIGATIONS:

- *Bloods*: FBC, U&Es, LFTs, albumin, ESR and CRP
- *Faecal calprotectin*
- *Colonoscopy with biopsy*: diagnostic
- *Histology*: transmural inflammation with granuloma formation and lymphocytic infiltrate
- *Radiology*: small-bowel MRI

TREATMENT:

- *Conservative*: smoking cessation
- *Medicinal*: corticosteroids may be required in acute flares. Immunomodulating agents like 6-mercaptopurine, azathioprine or low-dose methotrexate may be used. Anti-tumour necrosis factor/biologics may be initiated in some cases at the discretion of the gastroenterology team
- *Surgical*: resection of strictured or obstructed region of bowel

ULCERATIVE COLITIS

This is a relapsing remitting autoimmune condition that is not associated with granuloma formation. It is contiguous, usually involves the rectum and may involve the terminal ileum (backwash ileitis).

SIGNS AND SYMPTOMS:

- These include—weight loss, pyrexia, pseudopolyps, lead pipe appearances of bowel on radiographs, bloody diarrhoea, proctitis
- Extraintestinal manifestations: inflammatory arthropathies and primary sclerosing cholangitis

Investigations—the same as Crohn's disease.

TREATMENT:

- *Conservative*: patient education. Smoking has been shown by some studies to be protective but is not advised.
- *Medicinal*: Depends on the extent of the disease and if there are any extraintestinal aspects of the disease. Corticosteroids may be required in acute flares. Immunomodulating agents like 6-mercaptopurine, azathioprine or low-dose methotrexate may be used. Anti-tumour necrosis factor/biologics may be initiated in some cases at the discretion of the gastroenterology team. In patients with moderate disease limited to the rectum, aminosalicylate agents like rectal mesalamine are the mainstays.
- *Surgical*: Proctocolectomy with ileal pouch-anal anastomosis or colectomy.

SMALL-BOWEL OBSTRUCTION

CAUSES:

Adhesions and hernia are the commonest. Causes may be intraluminal, intramural or extramural.

- *Intraluminal causes include*—polyps, foreign body, intussusception
- *Intramural causes include*—tumours, benign/malignant strictures, Crohn's disease
- *Extramural causes include*—adhesions, extrinsic masses, volvulus, hernia

SYMPTOMS:

- Pain (colicky), vomiting, abdominal distension, absolute constipation.

INVESTIGATIONS:

- Blood tests (FBC, U&E, LFTS, coag, group and save), CT scan.

MANAGEMENT:

- Depends on underlying cause, "drip and suck" regime—use of NG tube to decompress the bowel and give IV fluids to avoid dehydration, surgery +/− stoma.

LARGE-BOWEL OBSTRUCTION

CAUSES:

- Colon cancer, diverticular stricture, volvulus

SYMPTOMS:

- Pain (colicky), vomiting, abdominal distension, absolute constipation, peritonitis (perforation—usually occurs at the caecum).

INVESTIGATIONS:

- Blood tests (FBC, U&E, LFTS, coag, group and save), CT scan.

MANAGEMENT:

- Depends on underlying cause, "drip and suck" regime—use of NG tube to decompress the bowel and give IV fluids to avoid dehydration. Other options include self-expanding metallic stents under radiological guidance and surgery +/− stoma depending on the case.

COLON CANCER

Colorectal cancer (CRC) is cancer of the colon and the rectum. It is the third most common malignancy. Usually adenocarcinoma on histology.

CAUSE:

Multifactorial and often unknown. There are risk factors that predispose an individual to CRC. These risk factors will now be considered.

- Smoking
- Increasing age
- Family history of CRC
- Inflammatory bowel disease
- Streptococcus bovis bacteraemia
- Congenital polyposis syndromes
  - Juvenile polyposis syndrome—autosomal dominant, usually not malignant
  - Peutz–Jegher's syndrome—autosomal dominant, melanosis present on oral mucosa, increases risk of CRC
- Genetic predisposition
  - Hereditary nonpolyposis colon cancer (HNPCC)

Hereditary nonpolyposis colon cancer (HNPCC), also known as Lynch syndrome, is an autosomal dominant syndrome associated with mutations in a number of DNA mismatch repair (MMR) genes. This places individuals at an increased risk for synchronous and metachronous colorectal cancer. It is characterised by a strong family history. The Amsterdam Criteria for HNPCC are a set list of criteria that help clinicians identify families at risk of HNPCC. It can be thought of as the 3–2–1 rule, as follows:

1. At least three relatives with histologically confirmed colorectal, one of whom is a first-degree relative of the other.
   a. Familial adenomatous polyposis should be excluded.
2. At least two successive generations involved.
3. At least one of the cancers diagnosed before age 50.
   • Familial adenomatous polyposis (FAP)Autosomal dominant mutation of the APC gene on chromosome 5. Results in the formation of thousands of polyps within the bowel and 100% lead to CRC.

INVESTIGATIONS:

- Bowel cancer screening programme
- Bloods: FBC for iron deficiency anaemia, LFTs for liver metastasis, carcinoembryonic antigen (CEA) tumour marker
- Colonoscopy/sigmoidoscopy
- Imaging: CT scan, double contrast barium enema (apple core sign), virtual colonoscopy.

Management: depends on the extent of the disease and the intent of treatment e.g. curative or palliation. The extent of the disease is assessed using the TNM system. All cases are discussed at MDT.

Medical therapy may include: chemotherapy (oxaliplatin, folinic acid and 5-fluorouracil) and sometimes radiotherapy (extraperitoneal rectum).

Surgical resection is usually the treatment of choice and a summary of these resections is considered in the following table.

Summary of Resections Considered in Colorectal Cancer

Site of cancer	Type of resection	Anastomosis
Right colon	Right hemicolectomy	Ileo-colic
Transverse	Extended right hemicolectomy	Ileo-colic
Splenic flexure	Extended right hemicolectomy	Ileo-colic
Splenic flexure	Left hemicolectomy	Colo-colon
Left colon	Left hemicolectomy	Colo-colon
Sigmoid colon	Sigmoid colectomy	Colorectal
	>10 cm from the peritoneal reflection = high anterior resection	
	6–10 cm from the peritoneal reflection = low anterior resection	
	<6 cm from the peritoneal reflection = ultra-low anterior resection	
Upper rectum	Anterior resection (TME)	Colorectal
Low rectum	Anterior resection (low TME)	Colorectal (+/− Defunctioning stoma)
Anal verge	Abdomino-perineal excision of colon and rectum	None

TNM Staging Scheme CRC

Classification	Definition
Tis	Tumour "in situ"
T1	Into (but not through) submucosa
T2	Into (but not through) muscularis propria

Classification	Definition
T3	Through muscularis propria into the subserosa, or into non-peritonealised pericolic/perirectal tissues
T4a	Penetration of the visceral peritoneal layer
T4b	Penetration or adhesion to adjacent organs
N0	No lymph node metastases
N1a	Involvement of 1 regional node
N1b	Involvement of 2–3 regional nodes
N1c	Deposits involving serosa or non-peritonealised pericolic/perirectal tissues without regional nodal metastasis
N2a	Involvement of 4–6 nodes
N2b	Involvement of >7 nodes
M0	No distant metastases
M1	Distant metastasis confined to one organ
M2	Distant metastasis involving more than one organ

DIVERTICULAR DISEASE/DIVERTICULOSIS/DIVERTICULITIS

DEFINITION:

It is important to differentiate between diverticular disease, diverticulosis and diverticulitis.

- *Diverticular disease*—presence of diverticula but no symptoms.
- *Diverticulosis*—symptoms present, e.g. painless PR bleeding.
- *Diverticulitis*—infection present.

CAUSES:

The exact cause is unknown, but it is thought to be linked to decreased fibre in the Western diet.

LOCATION:

More common in the left/sigmoid colon, but can be found anywhere in the large bowel.

SIGNS AND SYMPTOMS:

- Asymptomatic, abdominal pain (gripey), diarrhoea. Where the diverticulum becomes inflamed there is often LIF pain, fever, diarrhoea and blood in the stool. Perforated diverticular disease may have signs of peritonitis.
- Diverticulitis and diverticulosis both may present with haemorrhage which can be sudden and painless.

INVESTIGATIONS:

- Blood tests (FBC, U&E, LFTS, coag, cross match), CT scan.
- The Hinchey classification for acute diverticulitis (anywhere along the bowel, not just the colon) is useful in outlining successive stages of severity. In general, abscesses in stages Ib and II may be drained by interventional radiology, and stage III and IV disease is managed with emergency surgery.

The Hinchey Classification for Acute Diverticulitis

Stage	Clinical findings	CT findings
0	Mild clinical diverticulitis	Diverticula with colonic wall thickening
Ia	Confined pericolic inflammation or phlegmon	Pericolic soft tissue changes
Ib	Pericolic or mesocolic abscess	Ia changes and pericolic or mesocolic abscess
II	Pelvic, distant intra-abdominal or retroperitoneal abscess	Ia changes and distant abscess, usually deep pelvic
III	Generalised purulent peritonitis	Localised or generalised ascites, pneumoperitoneum, peritoneal thickening
IV	Generalised faecal peritonitis	Same as stage III

MANAGEMENT:

- Depends on the presentation and severity of diverticulitis and whether or not the patient is systemically well or requires resuscitation. Some patients may be able to be managed with PO antibiotics alone, others require admission, IV fluids and IV antibiotics +/– radiological guided drainage +/– surgery (Hartmann's procedure—sigmoid colectomy with end colostomy).

LOWER GI BLEEDING

Causes of lower GI bleeding include:

1. Haemorrhoids
2. Carcinoma
3. Diverticular disease
4. Angiodysplasia
5. Infective colitis
6. Polyps
7. Anal fissure
8. Ulcerative colitis
9. Crohn's disease

HAEMORRHOIDS

DEFINITION:

- A vascular cushion that is covered with a layer of mucosa. It contains a branch of the superior rectal artery and a tributary of the superior rectal vein.

CAUSES:

- The exact cause is unclear. Multiple factors have been implicated including constipation and prolonged straining.

POSITION:

At 3, 7 and 11 o'clock.

GRADING:

Internal haemorrhoids are graded based on the Goligher's classification:

- *First-degree haemorrhoids (grade I)*—the anal cushions bleed but do not prolapse.
- *Second-degree haemorrhoids (grade II)*—the anal cushions prolapse through the anus on straining but reduce spontaneously.
- *Third-degree haemorrhoids (grade III)*—the anal cushions prolapse through the anus on straining or exertion and require manual replacement into the anal canal.
- *Fourth-degree haemorrhoids (grade IV)*—the prolapse always stays out and is irreducible.

MANAGEMENT:

Multiple factors proposed including:

- *Conservative*—dietary and lifestyle modification.
- *Medical*—topical medications can contain various ingredients such as local anaesthesia, corticosteroids, antibiotics and anti-inflammatory drugs.

NON-OPERATIVE INTERVENTION:

- Sclerotherapy is currently recommended as a treatment option for first- and second-degree haemorrhoids.
- Rubber band ligation may be used to treat first- and second-degree haemorrhoids and selected cases of third-degree haemorrhoids.
- Infrared coagulation.
- Radiofrequency ablation.
- Cryotherapy.

OPERATIVE INTERVENTION:

- Stapled haemorrhoidectomies are not recommended.
- Banding can be used for early-grade haemorrhoids.
- Then, first line is haemorrhoidal artery ligation with Doppler guide, and the second line is open haemorrhoidectomy.

FISSURE IN ANO

DEFINITION:

A linear/oval tear in the anal canal starting just below the dentate line extending to the anal verge. May be acute or chronic. Chronic fissures are present for >6 weeks and are associated with a sentinel skin tag.

MANAGEMENT:

- *Conservative*—lifestyle and laxatives.
- *Medical*—GTN or diltiazem topical treatment.
- Botox.
- *Surgical*—lateral sphincterotomy (incomplete cut of the internal sphincter at 3 o'clock). This would not be done for a female patient as the combination of sphincterotomy with the potential for obstetric injury would be catastrophic for continence.

Aim of management is to relax the internal sphincter, which is hypothesised to be the cause.

FISTULA IN ANO

A fistula is an abnormal connection between two epithelial surfaces.

DEFINITION:

A fistula in ano has an opening internally to the anal canal and another
opening externally onto the skin.

CAUSES:

Perianal abscess, Crohn's disease, tuberculosis, radiotherapy, sexual transmitted diseases, leukaemia.

GOODSALL'S RULE:

- Anterior fistulae will tend to have an internal opening opposite the external opening.
- Posterior fistulae will tend to have a curved track that passes towards the midline.
- Fistula in ano may be classified as "low" when they do not cross the sphincter muscles above the dentate line and "high" when they cross the sphincter above the dentate line. When treating high fistula in ano there is a risk of damaging the sphincter mechanism and this may result in incontinence.

INVESTIGATIONS:

EUA is used to assess the fistula. If unable to delineate anatomy, MRI is useful.

MANAGEMENT:

Depends on whether there is concurrent infection. Infected fistula should be treated with antibiotics and seton to drain the sepsis. Low fistulae may be laid open. High fistulae may need to be treated with a seton.

THE PANCREAS, LIVER AND GALLBLADDER

PANCREATITIS

ACUTE PANCREATITIS:

Typically due to gallstones, or alcohol-induced in the UK.

- The ATLANTA classification for post pancreatitis fluid collections—split into either necrotising or non-necrotising.
1. Necrotising
   a. <4 weeks = acute necrotic
   b. >4 weeks = walled off necrosis
2. Non-necrotising
   a. <4 weeks = acute peripancreatic fluid
   b. >4 weeks = pseudocyst

Mnemonic for the assessment of the severity of pancreatitis: "**PANCREAS**" (which equates to the Glasgow IMRIE criteria)

P—$P_a0_2 < 60$ mmHg
A—**A**ge > 55 years

N—**N**eutrophils >15 × 10³/μL (10⁹/L)
C—**C**alcium < 2 mmol/L
R—**R**aised urea > 16 mmol/L
E—**E**nzyme (lactate dehydrogenase) > 600 units/L
A—**A**lbumin < 32 g/L
S—**S**ugar (glucose) > 10 mmol/L

More than three positive criteria indicates severe pancreatitis.

There is a new criterion which many UK hospitals are using called HAPS (harmless acute pancreatitis score). HAPS identifies patients who do not require intensive care for their first episode of acute pancreatitis and comprises three parameters:

1. Absence of abdominal tenderness or rebound
2. Normal haematocrit
3. Normal creatinine level

CHRONIC PANCREATITIS:

Usually secondary to multiple, recurrent episodes of pancreatitis that is associated with alcohol use, autoimmune disease, biliary disease or cystic fibrosis. This results in pancreatic insufficiency, malabsorption, diabetes, weight loss and abdominal pain. A CT scan confirms gland fibrosis/atrophy and calcification in some cases. The condition increases the risk of pancreatic cancer.

Acute management is supportive. IV fluids, analgesia, anti-emetics. May require ITU management for pain/respiratory support. Extensive third spacing in pancreatitis and reduced tidal volumes secondary to pain can cause respiratory compromise.

For alcohol-induced pancreatitis, abstinence is advised.

For gallstone cases, ERCP if a stone is blocking CBD (assess with MRCP) and then laparoscopic cholecystectomy.

Replacement of pancreatic enzymes is for severe pancreatitis in the acute setting (but not common as most cases only last a few days), more for chronic—Creon is the medication, taken with meals/snacks.

NEUROENDOCRINE TUMOURS OF THE PANCREAS

About 60–90% of these are malignant. They can result in typical symptoms that will be described in greater detail below. If present in the head of the pancreas there may be compressive effects.

1. *Insulinoma*—this is the commonest functioning neuroendocrine tumour.
   a. About 90% are benign.
   b. *Location*—evenly distributed throughout the pancreas.
   c. *Symptoms*—Whipple's triad
      1. Fasting hypoglycaemia.
      2. Neuroglycopenic symptoms, e.g. confusion, seizures.
      3. Symptoms are relieved by glucose.
   d. *Investigations*—serum glucose, insulin levels, c-peptide, pro-insulin levels, beta-hydroxybutyrate and glucose level after administration of glucagon.
   e. *Imaging*—pancreas protocol CT/MRI, endoscopic USS.
   f. *Treatment*—depends on the location and if other tumours are present. If solitary and benign, typically the treatment is enucleation of the cyst.

2. *Gastrinoma*—majority are malignant.
   a. *Location*—two-thirds are found in the gastrinoma triangle.
   b. The gastrinoma triangle is bounded by:
      1. Junction of the cystic duct and common bile duct
      2. Junction of D2 and D3
      3. Junction of neck and body of the pancreas
   c. *Symptoms*—the gastrinoma triad
      1. Abdominal pain
      2. Diarrhoea
      3. Weight loss
      Gastrinoma are often associated with peptic ulcer disease.
   d. *Investigations*—gastrin levels, gastric pH. Stop PPI before checking gastrin levels since they falsely increase this reading.
   e. *Imaging*—pancreas protocol CT/MRI, endoscopic USS, somatostatin scintigraphy.
   f. If the gastrin level is <1000, then perform a secretin test. Gastrinomas will respond paradoxically to secretin and gastrin will increase.
   g. *Treatment*—depends on the location and if other tumours are present as well as tumour size. May undergo enucleation with paraduodenal lymph node dissection if <5 cm. If distally located, consider distal pancreatectomy. If >5 cm and invasive, then consider Whipple's procedure.

3. *Glucagonoma*—90% malignant.
   a. *Location*—tail of the pancreas.
   b. *Symptoms*—the "**4 D's**":
      D—Dermatitis
      D—Diabetes
      D—Depression
      D—Deep vein thrombosis (due to a factor X-like antigen that is secreted)
   c. *Investigations*—glucose tolerance test, fasting glucagon level.
   d. *Imaging*—pancreas protocol CT/MRI, endoscopic USS, somatostatin scintigraphy.
   e. *Treatment*—do NOT enucleate. Requires resection with regional lymphadenectomy. Cholecystectomy may be required due to prolonged need for somatostatin therapy.

4. *Somatostatinoma*—tumour of the delta cells of the pancreas. Mostly malignant.
   a. *Location*—head of the pancreas.
   b. *Symptoms*—steatorrhoea, malabsorption, cholecystitis, diabetes.
   c. *Investigations*—pancreas protocol CT/MRI, endoscopic USS, somatostatin scintigraphy, selective visceral angiography.
   d. *Treatment*—requires resection with regional lymphadenectomy and usually cholecystectomy.

5. *VIPoma*—malignant.
   a. *Location*—body/tail of the pancreas. However, they can also be present elsewhere, e.g. retroperitoneally or in the adrenals.
   b. *Symptoms*—watery diarrhoea, hypokalaemia and achlorhydria.
   c. *Investigations*—fasting VIP level.
   d. *Imaging*—pancreas protocol CT/MRI, endoscopic USS, somatostatin scintigraphy, selective visceral angiography.
   e. *Treatment*—radical dissection with regional lymphadenectomy. Cholecystectomy may be required due to prolonged need for somatostatin therapy.

PANCREATIC ADENOCARCINOMA

RISK FACTORS:

Smoking, alcohol, chronic pancreatitis, diabetes, increased BMI.

SYMPTOMS:

Painless jaundice, epigastric/back pain, vomiting (compressive effects causing gastric outlet obstruction), generic symptoms, e.g. weight loss, lethargy, etc.

INVESTIGATIONS:

CA19.9, pancreas protocol CT, endoscopic USS, lymph node biopsy, +/– PET CT.

TREATMENT:

Depends on the TNM grading, size and extent of spread. If for curative treatment (note this is only 10–15% of patients), optimise patients for theatre, offer nutritional support, involve MacMillan nursing staff and palliative care team if indicated. Surgery—primary surgery may be used if it is a distal tumour and amenable to resection with splenectomy. If located at the pancreatic head, Whipple's is the preferred operation. If there is superior mesenteric vein or portal vein involvement, these may require reconstruction. Neoadjuvant and adjuvant therapy (oxiplatin, 5-FU, etc.) may be considered. If palliative, will still require biliary drainage and stenting. Self-expanding metal stents are preferred.

GALLSTONES

This is a common pathology that may be asymptomatic. There are different types of gallstones—cholesterol and pigmented gallstones. Cholesterol stones are the commonest, whereas pigmented stones are smaller and are associated with high turnover of haem, such as in cirrhosis or chronic haemolysis.

RISK FACTORS FOR GALLSTONE DEVELOPMENT:

- Classic = fat, female, forty, fertile
- Obesity
- Certain medications (oestrogens, fibrates, somatostatin analogues)
- Stasis of the gallbladder
- Female gender
- Metabolic syndrome
- Rapid weight loss
- Prolonged fasting
- Bariatric surgery
- Crohn's disease
- Ileal resection

BILIARY COLIC

SIGNS AND SYMPTOMS:

- Asymptomatic
- RUQ pain, particularly after eating
- Murphy's sign

INVESTIGATIONS:

- Blood tests—FBC, U&E, LFTs, cholesterol, coag, group and save for theatre, only if considering theatre, which you may not at the first presentation of biliary colic. Amylase if considering pancreatitis as a differential.
- USS/MRCP/ERCP are considered if the LFTs are deranged. Depending on the results of the USS +/– MRCP, then the gold standard is an ERCP to extract the stones affecting the common bile duct +/– perform sphincterotomy.

MANAGEMENT:

1. ERCP + laparoscopic cholecystectomy (as per local department protocol)

or

2. Laparoscopic cholecystectomy with intra-operative cholangiogram +/– bile duct exploration

COMPLICATIONS:

- Cholecystitis
- Common bile duct blockage resulting in cholangitis and jaundice
- Pancreatic duct blockage which can cause pancreatitis
- Gallstone ileus
- Cancer of the gallbladder
- Mirizzi syndrome

MIRIZZI SYNDROME

This is a rare condition caused by the obstruction of the common bile duct or common hepatic duct by external compression from multiple impacted gallstones or a single, large, impacted gallstone in Hartmann's pouch.

If the disease progresses, then fistulas from the gallbladder into the common bile duct, common hepatic duct (CHD) and the duodenum can develop.

The following grading system has been developed for Mirizzi syndrome:

Type I—no fistula present
Type IA—presence of the cystic duct
Type IB—obliteration of the cystic duct
Types II to IV—fistula present
Type II—defect smaller than 33% of the CHD diameter
Type III—defect 33% to 66% of the CHD diameter
Type IV—defect larger than 66% of the CHD diameter

SIGNS AND SYMPTOMS:

These are similar to acute or chronic cholecystitis with the addition of jaundice.

INVESTIGATIONS:

- Blood tests—FBC, U&Es, LFTs and coag.
- Imaging—initially abdominal USS. If a stone is suspected in the common bile duct based on ultrasound results, MRCP is the next step.
- If a common duct stone is identified on the MRCP, then the gold standard next step is ERCP.

MANAGEMENT:

- Depends on whether a fistula is present.
- Usually, in patients without a fistula, management consists of an ERCP + laparoscopic cholecystectomy (as per local department protocol).
- For patients with a small-to-moderate-sized fistula, management may involve T-tube placement or biliary diversion with a choledochoduodenostomy. For large fistulas, patients may require a Roux-en-Y choledochojejunostomy.

JAUNDICE

Jaundice (icterus) is the yellow discolouration of mucous membranes, sclera and skin. This happens due to the accumulation of bilirubin. Jaundice may be seen at a bilirubin concentration >2.5–3.0 mg/dL (42.8–51.3 mmol/L).

- *Causes*: causes are usually split into pre-hepatic, hepatic and post-hepatic causes. These will be explored in the following table.

Causes of Jaundice (a Non-Exhaustive List)

Category	Cause	Examples
Pre-hepatic	Haemolytic disease	Sickle cell G6PD deficiency Malaria
Hepatic	Hepatic cell failure or intrahepatic obstruction	Viral hepatitis Alcoholic cirrhosis Hepatocellular cancer
Post-hepatic	Biliary duct obstruction Extrinsic compression of the biliary system	Gallstones Biliary strictures Pancreatic masses

Investigations: aim to identify the underlying cause.

- Urine dip/stool sample
- Bloods: FBC, U&Es, LFTs, hepatitis serology +/– HIV in at risk individuals, non-invasive liver screen, coagulation profile (PT best test of liver synthetic function)

Different Blood Tests Results for the Different Categories of Jaundice

Investigation	Pre-hepatic	Hepatic	Post-hepatic
Urine appearance	Normal	Dark	Dark
Stool appearance	Normal	Normal/Pale	Pale
Conjugated bilirubin	Normal	Increased	Increased
Unconjugated bilirubin	Normal/increased	Increased	Decreased
Alkaline phosphatase	Normal	Increased	Increased
ALT/AST	Normal	Increased (viral hepatitis)	Increased
Conjugated bilirubin in urine	No	Yes	Yes

- *Radiology:* USS, MRCP +/– ERCP
- *Management:* depends on the underlying causes

MULTIPLE ENDOCRINE NEOPLASIA

Multiple endocrine neoplasia typically involves neoplasia in at least two endocrine glands. These growths can be benign or malignant. The following provides a summary of the different types of multiple endocrine neoplasia and the tumours associated with them.

MEN 1:

- Also known as Wermer syndrome
- Mutated MEN 1 gene

Diagnostic criteria include:

- Age <40 years
- Positive family history
- Multifocal or recurrent neoplasia
- Two or more organ systems affected

MEN 2A:

- Also known as Sipple syndrome
- Variation in the RET proto-oncogene (for cells of neural crest origin)
- Autosomal dominant

MEN 2B:

- Also known as Wagenmann–Froboese syndrome
- Variation in the RET proto-oncogene (for cells of neural crest origin)
- Autosomal dominant
- "Marfanoid" body habitus

Summary Highlighting the Associations with Each MEN Syndrome

Syndrome	Association
MEN I	- Parathyroid hyperplasia - Pituitary tumours - Pancreatic island cell tumours
IIa	- Parathyroid hyperplasia - Phaeochromocytoma - Medullary thyroid cancer
IIb	- Marfanoid habitus - Phaeochromocytoma - Medullary thyroid cancer

Breast and Endocrine Surgery

9

Benign breast disease and breast cancer are frequently asked about in the MRCS examination. Some causes of benign breast disease will now be explored.

Benign Breast Disease

Benign breast disease	Characteristics	Investigations	Treatment
Mastalgia	Very common Can be cyclical and occurs predominantly in the reproductive years Breast cancer often does not present with breast pain Risk factors include: OCP, HRT, pregnancy, increased caffeine intake	Women >35 years typically have a mammogram that is normal Ultrasound scan (USS) of area of nodularity +/– biopsy	There is no definitive treatment available for breast pain. Options include reducing caffeine intake, decreasing dietary fat and treatment with danazol and tamoxifen
Fibroadenoma	Considered an aberration of normal development Peak incidence in the third decade Discrete, highly mobile, non-tethered and smooth lesions Also known as "breast mouse disease" Develops from a lobule in the breast and demonstrates high levels of oestrogen and sulphates Usually solitary but sometimes patients present with multiple lesions	Mammogram— popcorn calcification in association with a soft tissue mass is pathognomonic for fibroadenoma USS +/– biopsy	Usually watchful waiting If very large may proceed to surgical excision

(Continued)

DOI: 10.1201/9781003292005-12

Benign Breast Disease   (Continued)

Benign breast disease	Characteristics	Investigations	Treatment
Phyllodes tumour	Tumours on a spectrum from benign to malignant and often clinically mimic a fibroadenoma Leaf-like projections	Mammogram—calcification is rarely seen unlike fibroadenomas USS +/− biopsy	Surgical excision due to malignant potential
Hamartoma	Rare Patients present with a discrete mobile lesion May be impalpable and an incidental finding on screening mammography	Mammogram—"breast within a breast" appearance with a capsule Hamartomas appear histologically as disorganized lobules and adipose tissue. USS +/− biopsy	Leave alone If the lesion undergoes rapid progressive growth, surgical excision would be indicated
Cysts	Common Peak incidence in fifth to sixth decade Can be single or multiple May be completely asymptomatic, detected on screening mammogram or become tender, painful or infected Patients may present with well-circumscribed, discrete, mobile lesions	Mammogram USS	Aspiration
Duct ectasia	Benign condition with loss of elastin in the ducts Associated with chronic inflammatory cell infiltrate Patient presents with cheesy nipple discharge	Mammogram USS +/− biopsy to exclude any underlying malignancy	If the patient has troublesome discharge, then total duct excision with nipple eversion
Mammary duct fistula	A fistula is an abnormal communication between two epithelial surfaces. Here it is an abnormal connection between the subareolar duct and the skin. This typically occurs in the periaerolar region following periductal mastitis. It is more common in smokers	USS	Antibiotic therapy as per local Trust guidelines if in the presence of infection Surgical options include complete duct excision with excision of mammary duct fistula

Benign breast disease	Characteristics	Investigations	Treatment
Solitary intraductal papilloma	Benign lesion arising from a single central duct Patients present with spontaneous nipple discharge Conversely, multiple papillomas typically occur in peripheral ducts and patients present with a palpable mass associated rarely with nipple discharge. Associated with an increased risk of subsequent ipsilateral breast carcinoma	Mammogram USS +/− biopsy	Duct excision Long-term follow-up with mammogram screening in patients with multiple papillomas
Mastitis	This is inflammation of the breast tissue. Milk stasis or overproduction causes regional infection of the breast parenchyma with *Staphylococcus aureus*, which enters the breast via trauma to the tipple. This in turn causes mastitis. Signs and symptoms include heat, pain, erythema, swelling of the breast tissue, nipple discharge, fever	It is a clinical diagnosis. USS may be used to delineate abscess	Antibiotics as per local policy Encourage mother to continue to breastfeed since this will help to overcome obstruction

BREAST CANCER

DEFINITION:

Breast cancer arises in the terminal duct-lobular unit. It affects 1 in 8 women in the UK, where there are 55,000 women who are diagnosed with breast cancer each year. The most common type of breast malignancy is invasive ductal carcinoma not otherwise specified (NOS).

CAUSES:

The exact cause and sequencing of breast cancer is incompletely understood. However, there are several risk factors which are detailed here.

- Genetic risk factors
  - BRCA 1 (chromosome 17)
  - BRCA 2 (chromosome 13)
  - Cowden's disease (p10 mutation)
  - Li Fraumeni syndrome (p53 mutation)

- Peutz–Jegher's disease (STK11/LKB1 mutation chromosome 19)
- Breast cancer and gastric cancer (CDH1 mutation)
- The Gail Model for Breast Cancer Risk estimates the absolute 5-year risk and lifetime risk of developing breast cancer. Factors include age, age at menarche, age at first live birth, family history of breast cancer, previous breast biopsies and race/ethnicity.
- Other factors
  - Female sex
  - Family history
  - Alcohol use
  - Smoking history
  - Nulliparity
  - Not breastfeeding
  - Oral contraceptive pill (OCP)
  - Hormone replacement therapy (HRT)

SIGNS AND SYMPTOMS:

1. Breast lump
2. Nipple discharge
3. Inverted nipple
4. Inflamed breast skin
5. Axillary lump (lymph node)
6. Peau d'orange
7. Asymptomatic at screening

INVESTIGATIONS:

All patients undergo triple assessment, which includes:

1. Examination
2. Imaging
3. Biopsy +/– staging of the axilla

Patients are discussed at MDT with their results including receptor status, i.e. ER/PR/HER2 status as well as CT and MRI reports (if relevant) looking for metastases and the stage of the disease. Prognosis of disease can be assessed using the Nottingham prognostic index (NPI):

$$NPI = (0.2 \times invasive\ size) + Lymph\ node\ stage + Grade\ of\ tumour$$

TNM FOR BREAST CANCER

Breast Cancer TNM Classification

		Stage	Primary tumour (T)*	Regional lymph node status (L)	Distant metastasis (M)
T—Tumour		0	Tis	N0	M0
T1	Tumour ≤ 2 cm	I	T1	N0	M0
T2	Tumour ≥ 2 cm but < 5 cm		T0	N1	M0

		Stage	Primary tumour (T)*	Regional lymph node status (L)	Distant metastasis (M)
T3	Tumour ≥ 5 cm	**II A**	T1	N1	MO
T4	Tumour of any size with direct extension to chest wall or skin		T2	NO	MO
N—Lymph node		**II B**	T2	N1	MO
NO	No cancer in regional node		T3	NO	MO
N1	Regional movable metastasis	**III A**	TO	N2	MO
N2	Non-movable regional metastases		T1	N2	MO
N3	Cancer in the internal mammary lymph nodes		T2	N2	MO
M—Metastasis			T3	N1/N2	MO
MO	No distant metastases	**III B**	T4	Any N	MO
MI	Distant metastases	**III C**	Any T	N3	MO
		IV	Any T	Any N	MI

* Size measurements are for the tumour's greatest dimension.

Source: Criteria for staging breast tumours according to the UICC ICD-10 TNM classification.

TREATMENT

- **Conservative**—patient and family education, involve breast cancer specialist nurses, referral to Macmillan nurses, referral to fertility services, provide psychological assessment and support, offer genetic counselling e.g. for BRCA 1 and 2 pathway (refer those with unilateral breast cancer <30 years old, bilateral breast cancer <50 years old, those <60 years old with triple negative breast cancer, male breast cancer at any age, those with non-mucinous ovarian cancer at any age, breast cancer in a patient <45 years old, who has a first-degree relative with breast cancer <45 years old, patients with Ashkenazi Jewish ancestry and breast cancer, patients with a pathology adjusted Manchester score >15).
- **Medical**—split into hormonal therapy, HER2 directed therapy and chemo/radiotherapy.

HORMONAL THERAPY:

- *Tamoxifen*—a selective oestrogen receptor modulator (SERM). It has antioestrogen affects in the breast but estrogenic effects in the uterus and liver. Side effects include endometrial cancer, DVT, PE and hepatotoxicity. Premenopausal women are treated with tamoxifen; postmenopausal women are treated with anastrozole/letrozole (aromatase inhibitors). This is because trials such as the ATAC trial have suggested that aromatase inhibitors are superior to tamoxifen in postmenopausal women. If a woman becomes menopausal during treatment, she will benefit from switching medications.
- *Letrozole*—an aromatase inhibitor. Prevents conversion of oestrogens in the peripheral fat. Side effects include arthralgia, fatigue and perimenopausal symptoms such as hot flushes and sweating. Osteoporosis with long-term use. Therefore, patients are often commenced on bone protective agents such as bisphosphonates.

HER2 DIRECTED THERAPY:

- *Trastuzumab (herceptin)*—a monoclonal antibody. The HER2 gene (tyrosine kinase protein) is amplified up to 30% in breast cancer that is HER2 positive. Herceptin targets HER2, causing an immune mediated response that results in internalisation and recycling of HER2. The HER2 pathway promotes cellular growth. Side effects include fever, cough, headaches, poor sleep, rash, cardiotoxicity, heart failure and allergic reactions.

CHEMO/RADIOTHERAPY:

- The precise regime is discussed with an oncology specialist. Chemotherapy and radiotherapy regimens vary depending on tumour type. Clips are placed within the cavity after wide local excision procedures for targeted post-operative radiotherapy. Chemotherapy can be adjuvant or neoadjuvant. Some regimes used are as follows:

  - AC (doxorubicin and cyclophosphamide)
  - EC (epirubicin, cyclophosphamide)
  - AC or EC followed by T (paclitaxel or docetaxel), or the reverse
  - CAF (cyclophosphamide, doxorubicin and 5-FU)

SURGERY:

- The primary aim of surgery is to remove the invasive and non-invasive cancer with clear margins. The surgery offered depends on the type of cancer, the location within the breast, the degree of spread, whether the axillary lymph nodes are involved, the tumour-to-breast-size ratio, patient preference and whether plastic surgery reconstructive options are being considered immediately or later.

- Some examples of procedures are listed here, but the ultimate decision is taken at the surgical MDT in line with the patient's oncology results and preferences. Clinical staging of the axilla should also be assessed by sentinel lymph node biopsy. The reason for this is to avoid unnecessary axillary clearance.

  - Wide local excision +/– sentinel lymph node biopsy
  - Wide local excision +/– axillary node clearance
  - Radical or simple mastectomy +/– sentinel lymph node biopsy
  - Radical or simple mastectomy +/– axillary node clearance
  - Oncoplastic procedures, e.g. therapeutic mammoplasty +/– sentinel lymph node biopsy

- Reconstruction options include but are not limited to:

  - Implants
  - Tissue flap procedures, e.g. transverse rectus abdominis muscle (TRAM) flap, deep inferior epigastric artery perforator (DIEP) flap, latissimus dorsi flap

COMPLICATIONS:

- Death
- *Metastases*—brain, bone, liver, lungs
- Depression
- Side effects of treatment

Breast Cancer

Breast cancer	Characteristics
Lobular carcinoma in situ	Proliferative lesion confined to the lobules +/– terminal ductal lobular unit
	Tends to be an incidental diagnosis
	Increased risk of multicentric breast cancer
	This increased risk is distributed evenly between both breasts
Ductal carcinoma in situ	Abnormal proliferation of mammary epithelium that has not invaded the basement membrane; precursor to invasive ductal carcinoma
	Heterogenous group of lesions including several different types, e.g. comedo, cribriform, papillary, micropapillary and solid
	Microcalcifications are seen on mammogram
Invasive ductal carcinoma	Most common type of breast malignancy
	Graded based on tubular formation, nuclear hyperchromatism, mitotic rate and differentiation: 1 = well differentiated; 2 = intermediated; 3 = poorly differentiated
Invasive lobular carcinoma	Malignant transformation of lobular epithelium that has invaded the breast stroma
Inflammatory	Invades the dermis and lymphatic system
	Peau d'orange appearance
	Retracted nipple
Paget's disease of the breast	Epidermal infiltration of ductal carcinoma
	Eczematoid nipple changes

ENDOCRINE

HYPERTHYROIDISM

This occurs when there is too much circulating thyroid hormone in the body. There are many different causes of hyperthyroidism.

Causes of Hyperthyroidism

Cause	Comment
Graves' disease	• Commonest cause
	• Autoimmune condition
	• Ocular changes e.g. exophthalmos
	• Associated with other autoimmune conditions e.g. pernicious anaemia
	• It is caused by thyroid stimulating immunoglobulin (TSI). This binds to the thyroid stimulating hormone receptor on the thyroid cell membrane and stimulates the action of the thyroid stimulating hormone
Toxic multinodular goitre and toxic solitary nodule	• Second commonest cause
	• Increased risk with age
	• More common in females
De Quervain's thyroiditis	• Transient hyperthyroidism following a viral infection
	• Painful goitre
	• A period of hypothyroidism may follow

SIGNS AND SYMPTOMS:

- Weight loss
- Heat intolerance
- Diarrhoea
- Exopthalmos (Graves' disease)
- Lid lag
- Palpitation/atrial fibrillation
- Anxiety
- Tremor
- Goitre +/– bruit
- Brisk reflexes

INVESTIGATIONS:

- TFTs—decreased TSH, increased T3 and T4
- USS of nodules
- Fine needle aspiration of nodules to exclude malignancy
- Isotope scan to assess hot and cold nodules

MANAGEMENT:

Medical

- Symptomatic control: beta-blockers (palpitations and tremor), lubricating eye drops (ocular symptoms)
- Anti-thyroid medications: carbimazole, propylthiouracil. Side effects include agranulocytosis
- Radioactive iodine ablation: patients must be euthyroid before commencing treatment

Surgical

- Subtotal thyroidectomy

HYPOTHYROIDISM

This occurs when there is too little circulating thyroid hormone in the body. There are many different causes.

Causes of Hypohyroidism

Cause	Comment
Primary hypothyroidism	<ul><li>Iodine deficiency</li><li>Hashimoto's autoimmune thyroiditis</li><li>Post-thyroidectomy/radioactive iodine therapy</li><li>Drug induced e.g. lithium</li></ul>
Secondary	<ul><li>Dysfunction of hypothalamic-pituitary axis</li><li>Pituitary adenoma</li><li>Sheehan's syndrome (ischaemic necrosis of the pituitary gland that typically occurs after childbirth)</li><li>Infiltrative disease e.g. TB</li></ul>

SIGNS AND SYMPTOMS:

- These include—weight gain, cold intolerance, constipation, dry skin, thinning of hair, bradycardia, depression, delayed reflexes.

INVESTIGATIONS:

- TFTs—increased TSH, decreased T3 and T4
- Cholesterol levels (often increased)
- USS of nodules
- Fine needle aspiration of nodules to exclude malignancy
- Isotope scan to assess hot and cold nodules
- CT/MRI if secondary hypothyroidism
- Guthrie test for congenital screening

MANAGEMENT:

- *Medical:* Lifelong replacement of thyroid hormone with levothyroxine.

THYROID CANCER

This is cancer that originates from follicular or parafollicular cells.

CAUSES:

Malignant neoplasm. Increased risk with childhood neck irradiation. Thyroid carcinomas may be classified histopathologically as shown in the table here.

Defining the Histological Appearance of Different Types of Thyroid Cancer

Histological appearance	% of thyroid cancer		Comment
Papillary	70%	• Affects younger patients • Spreads to cervical lymph nodes	• Good prognosis. • Microscopic findings—Orphan Annie nuclei and psammoma bodies.
Follicular	20%	• More common in low iodine areas • Spreads to bone and lungs	• Good prognosis
Medullary	5%	• Arises from parafollicular cells • Calcitonin is a biochemical marker	• Associated with MEN syndrome • Spreads to lymph nodes
Anaplastic	<5%	• Affects older patients • Aggressive	• Spreads to lymph nodes • Poor prognosis • p53 gene mutation is the commonest gene mutation found in anaplastic thyroid cancer. Others include, RAS, BRAF, APC, PTEN and Axin
Other	–	• Lymphoma of the thyroid • Sarcoma of the thyroid	• Hurthle cell carcinoma. Hurthle cell carcinoma was considered a variant of follicular carcinoma however, it is now defined as a follicular thyroid cell derived cancer. It is more common in females >40 years. Polymorphisms of ATPase 6 gene may be implicated in the pathogenesis of Hurthle cell tumours. On histopathology there is a presence of Hurtle cells (also known as Askanazy cells)—eosinophilic oxyphilic cells with round/oval nuclei and packed mitochondria

SIGNS AND SYMPTOMS:

- Thyroid nodules
- Signs and symptoms of hyperthyroidism (rarely)
- Signs and symptoms of hypothyroidism (rarely)

INVESTIGATIONS:

- Bloods: TFTs to assess thyroid status
- Fine needle aspiration cytology
- Diagnostic lobectomy
- Radiology: Ultrasound scan of thyroid/Thyroid isotope scan (hot nodules are less likely to indicate malignancy)

Management: depends on histological subtype and extent of spread of the disease. All cases are discussed at MDT. The following table provides an outline regarding treatments for thyroid cancer.

Treatment of Thyroid Cancer Depending on Histological Subtype

Histological appearance	Treatment
Papillary	<ul><li>Lesion <1 cm: thyroid lobectomy, then lifelong levothyroxine and annual thyroglobulin measurements</li><li>Lesion >1 cm: total thyroidectomy, radio-iodine ablation then lifelong levothyroxine and annual thyroglobulin measurements</li></ul>
Follicular	<ul><li>Lesion <1 cm: thyroid lobectomy, then lifelong levothyroxine and annual thyroglobulin measurements</li><li>Lesion >1 cm: total thyroidectomy, radio-iodine ablation then lifelong levothyroxine and annual thyroglobulin measurements</li></ul>
Medullary	Total thyroidectomy then lifelong levothyroxine; screen family members for multiple endocrine neoplasia (MEN) syndrome and thyroid cancer
Anaplastic	Debulking surgery and palliative care

DIABETES INSIPIDUS

This is a disorder caused by low levels of or insensitivity to antidiuretic hormone (ADH) leading to polyuria. This can be cranial or nephrogenic in origin.

CAUSES:

1. *Cranial:* decreased ADH is released by the posterior pituitary gland. Remember this as **CIVIT**:
   - **C**ongenital defect in ADH gene.
   - **I**diopathic.
   - **V**ascular.
   - **I**nfection: meningoencephalitis.
   - **T**umour (e.g. pituitary adenoma), **T**uberculosis and **T**rauma.
2. *Nephrogenic:* the kidney does not respond to ADH. Remember this as **DIMC**:
   - **D**rugs, e.g. lithium.
   - **I**nherited.

- **M**etabolic low potassium, raised calcium.
- **C**hronic renal disease.

SIGNS AND SYMPTOMS:

- *These include*—Polydipsia, polyuria and dehydration.
- *Investigations*—these are summarised in the table here.

Summary of Investigations to Differentiate Cranial and Nephrogenic Diabetes Insipidus

Investigation	Cranial cause	Nephrogenic cause
Plasma osmolality	↑	↑
Urine osmolality	↓	↓
Plasma Na$^+$	↑	↑
24-h urine volume	>2 L	>2 L
Water deprivation test	Urine does not concentrate	Urine does not concentrate
After treatment with desmopressin	Urine becomes concentrated	Urine does not concentrate
MRI scan	Look for abnormality of the pituitary gland, e.g. tumour	

Management: Depends on the underlying cause.

- *Medicinal*
  - Cranial: desmopressin: a synthetic replacement for vasopressin; it increases the number of aquaporin-2 channels in the distal convoluted tubules and the collecting ducts. This increases water reabsorption
  - Nephrogenic: high-dose desmopressin, correction of electrolyte imbalances, thiazide diuretics, prostaglandin synthase inhibitors
- *Surgical:* excision of tumour if indicated

HYPOPARATHYROIDISM

This occurs when too little PTH is produced from the parathyroid gland. It may be categorised into congenital, acquired, transient and inherited causes.

Different Causes of Hypoparathyroidism

Type	Cause
Congenital	DiGeorge syndrome (chromosome 22q11.2 deletion)
Acquired	Complication of parathyroidectomy or thyroidectomy
Transient	Neonates born prematurely
Inherited	Pseudohypoparathyroidism and Pseudopseudohypoparathyroidism

SIGNS AND SYMPTOMS:

These depend on the cause and include—abdominal pain, myalgia, muscle spasm, seizures, fatigue, headaches, carpopedal spasm, Chvostek's sign, Trousseau's sign.

INVESTIGATIONS:

- *Bloods:* PTH level, serum calcium, serum phosphate, FBC, U&Es, LFTs, creatinine, urea.
- *ECG:* arrhythmias.
- *ECHO:* cardiac structural defects (DiGeorge syndrome).
- *Radiology:* X-ray of hand (pseudohypoparathyroidism patients have shorter 4th and 5th metacarpals).

The biochemical differences between hypoparathyroidism, pseudohypoparathyroidism and pseudopseudohypoparathyroidism are outlined in the following table.

Biochemical Differences between Hypoparathyroidism, Pseudohypoparathyroidism and Pseudopseudohypoparathyroidism

Investigation	Hypoparathyroidism	Pseudohypo-parathyroidism	Pseudopseudo-hypoparathyroidism
PTH level	↓	↑	Normal
Serum calcium	↓	↓	Normal
Serum phosphate	↑	↑	Normal

MANAGEMENT:

- *Conservative*: diet high in calcium and low in phosphate. Support for parents.
- *Medicinal*: calcium and vitamin D supplements.

Hyperparathyroidism

This occurs when too much parathyroid hormone (PTH) is produced from the parathyroid gland. It may be categorised into primary, secondary and tertiary causes.

Causes of Primary, Secondary and Tertiary Hyperparathyroidism

Type	Cause
Primary	Parathyroid adenoma
	Parathyroid hyperplasia
	Parathyroid carcinoma
	Drug induced e.g. lithium
Secondary	Vitamin D deficiency
	Chronic kidney injury
Tertiary	Prolonged secondary hyperparathyroidism

Signs and symptoms: asymptomatic or "bones (pain, osteoporosis), moans (depression, fatigue), groans (myalgia) and stones (renal stones)."

INVESTIGATIONS:

- Bloods: PTH level, serum calcium, serum phosphate, FBC, U&Es, LFTs, creatinine.
- Urine calcium level.
- Dual-energy X-ray (DEXA) scan. Radiology:
  - Ultrasound scan of kidneys and neck.
  - Plain X-ray (for bone changes).
  - Parathyroid gland biopsy.

Biochemical Differences between Primary, Secondary and Tertiary Hyperparathyroidism

Investigation	Primary	Secondary	Tertiary
PTH level	↑	↑	↑
Serum calcium	↑	↓	↑
Serum phosphate	↓	↑	↓

Management: Depends on cause.

Types of Treatment Available for the Different Types of Hyperparathyroidism

Type of treatment	Primary	Secondary	Tertiary
Conservative	Monitoring increase oral fluid intake	Diet low in phosphate and high in calcium	–
Medical	Bisphosphonates	Calcimimetics, e.g. cinacalcet	–
Surgical	Parathyroidectomy	Parathyroidectomy if unresponsive to medical therapy	Parathyroidectomy

CUSHING'S SYNDROME

This is a collection of signs and symptoms that occur when a patient has long-term exposure to cortisol. There are many causes of Cushing's syndrome and they may be classified as exogenous or endogenous causes.

The Different Causes of Cushing's Syndrome

Type	Cause
Exogenous	Iatrogenic e.g. prescription glucocorticoids
Endogenous	This may be split into adrenocorticotropic hormone (ACTH) dependent and ACTH independent causes:

ACTH dependent

- Cushing's disease: this occurs when ACTH is produced from a pituitary adenoma. Use a low-dose dexamethasone test to confirm.
- Ectopic ACTH production (usually from small cell lung cancer).

ACTH independent: **CARS**

- **C**ancer: adrenal adenoma.
- **A**drenal nodular hyperplasia.
- **R**are causes: McCune–Albright syndrome.
- **S**teroid use

SIGNS AND SYMPTOMS:

These include—Moon face, central obesity, buffalo hump, acne, hypertension, hyperglycaemia, striae, vertebral collapse, proximal muscle wasting and psychosis.

INVESTIGATIONS:

- *Diagnostic tests:* urinary free cortisol, low-dose and high-dose dexamethasone suppression test.
- *Bloods:* FBC, U&Es, LFTs, glucose, lipid levels.
- *Radiology:* CXR (look for lung cancer and vertebral collapse).
- *Other:* dual-energy X-ray (DEXA) scan.

MANAGEMENT:

- *Conservative*: advise patient to decrease alcohol consumption since alcohol increases cortisol levels.
- *Medicinal*: ketoconazole, metyrapone, mitotane. Treat complications such as hypertension and diabetes mellitus.
- *Surgical*: trans-sphenoidal surgery to remove pituitary adenoma or bilateral adrenalectomy to remove adrenal adenoma, if indicated.

ADRENAL INSUFFICIENCY

This occurs when the adrenal glands fail to produce sufficient steroid hormone. The causes of adrenal insufficiency may be categorised into primary and secondary adrenal failure.

Table Illustrating the Causes of Adrenal Insufficiency

Type	Cause
Primary	<ul><li>Addison's disease: causes = MAIL</li></ul>**M**—Metastases from breast, lung and renal cancers **A**—Autoimmune **I**—Infections e.g. TB, CMV **L**—Lymphomas<ul><li>Idiopathic</li><li>Post-adrenalectomy</li></ul>
Secondary	<ul><li>Prolonged prednisolone use</li><li>Pituitary adenoma</li><li>Sheehan's syndrome</li></ul>

SIGNS AND SYMPTOMS:

These include—unintentional weight loss, myalgia, weakness, fatigue, postural hypotension, abdominal pain, skin pigmentation, body hair loss, diarrhoea, nausea, vomiting and depression.

INVESTIGATIONS:

- *Diagnostic tests*
  - Adrenocorticotropic hormone (ACTH) and cortisol measurements.
  - Insulin tolerance test.
  - Short tetracosactide test aka Short Synacthen test.
- *Bloods:* FBC, U&Es (low Na^+, high K^+), LFTs, glucose, lipid levels, serum calcium.
- *Radiology:* CXR (look for lung cancer)/CT and MRI scan of the adrenal glands.

MANAGEMENT:

- *Conservative*: patient education. Patient must carry a steroid alert card.
- *Medicinal*: replace glucocorticoids and mineralocorticoids with hydrocortisone and fludrocortisone; treat complications.
- *Surgical*: surgical excision of tumour, if indicated.

ACROMEGALY

Acromegaly is a syndrome that results from excessive growth hormone (GH) production after fusion of the epiphyseal plates. Excess GH produced before epiphyseal plate fusion causes gigantism.

CAUSES:

- Pituitary adenoma (most common).
- GH releasing hormone (GHRH) production from bronchial carcinoid.

SIGNS AND SYMPTOMS:

- These include—increased jaw size, increased hand size, macroglossia, lower pitch of voice, carpal tunnel syndrome.
- Ask to see old photographs of the patient and note changes in appearance.

INVESTIGATIONS:

- *Bloods:* FBC, U&Es, creatinine, LFTs, glucose, lipid levels, GH levels, glucose tolerance test, insulin-like growth factor (IGF)-1 levels (raised), prolactin levels.
- *Radiology:* CXR/CT/MRI scan.
- *ECG and ECHO:* assess for cardiac complications, e.g. cardiomyopathy.
- *Visual field testing:* bilateral hemianopia.

MANAGEMENT:

- *Conservative*: patient education. Inform the patient that bone changes will not revert after treatment.
- *Medicinal*
  - Somatostatin analogues, e.g. octreotide.
  - Dopamine agonists, e.g. cabergoline.
  - GH receptor antagonists, e.g. pegvisomant.
- *Surgical*: trans-sphenoidal surgical excision of the adenoma is the treatment of choice.

Vascular Surgery

10

ATHEROSCLEROSIS

Atherosclerosis is a slowly progressive disease and is the underlying cause of ischaemic heart disease and peripheral artery disease.

There are three stages of atheroma formation:

1. *Fatty streak formation*—lipids are deposited in the intimal layer of the artery. This, coupled with vascular injury, causes inflammation, increased permeability and white blood cell recruitment. Macrophages phagocytose the lipids and become foam cells. These form the fatty streak.
2. *Fibrolipid plaque formation*—lipids within the intimal layer stimulate the formation of fibrocollagenous tissue. This eventually causes thinning of the muscularis media.
3. *Complicated atheroma*—this occurs when the plaque is extensive and prone to rupture. The plaque may be calcified due to lipid acquisition of calcium. Rupture activates clot formation and thrombosis.

ANEURYSMS

DEFINITION:

An aneurysm is a permanent, abnormal dilatation of an artery to 50% greater than its normal diameter. Aneurysms are further classified as true or false, where true aneurysms involve all three layers of the arterial wall. They may also be defined in terms of their shape, e.g. saccular, fusiform, berry, etc., as well as their anatomical location, e.g. aortic, femoral, popliteal.

Note that Berry aneurysms are found in within the circle of Willis and can cause subarachnoid haemorrhages when they rupture. Berry aneurysms are associated with polycystic kidney disease.

ABDOMINAL AORTIC ANEURYSMS

CAUSES:

- Atherosclerosis; connective tissue disorders, e.g. Ehlers–Danlos syndrome, Marfan's syndrome; syphilis. Other, rarer causes, include syphilis and HIV.
- Risk factors include hypertension, diabetes, smoking, increasing age and male sex.

DOI: 10.1201/9781003292005-13

INVESTIGATIONS:

- National screening programme (may pick up the aneurysm incidentally). In the UK, this is a one-off abdominal USS for all men at age 65 years
- Blood tests—FBC, U&Es, LFTs, cross match, coag, cholesterol and HBA1c
- ECG, ECHO, cardiopulmonary exercise testing
- Radiology: CT, USS

ELECTIVE SETTING:

- Watchful waiting (surveillance with USS as per national guidance which is based on size)
- Management of cardiovascular risk factors
- Endovascular repair
- Open repair

EMERGENCY SETTING:

- Medical resuscitation with permissive hypotension
- Major haemorrhage protocol
- Intervention (open or endovascular) v palliation

COMPLICATIONS OF ANEURYSMS:

1. Rupture and death - this is due to the Law of Laplace (see Physiology section). The stress placed on the wall of an aneurysm is proportional to the aneurysm's radius. Therefore, larger aneurysms are more prone to rupture
2. Thrombosis
3. Embolism
4. Pressure on adjacent structures
5. Fistula into adjacent structures (vena cava or intestine)
6. Infection of the aneurysm thrombus

CLINICAL POINT

The main differential for AAA is renal colic, and all men aged >60 who attend with abdominal/flank pain should be considered to have AAA until proven otherwise.

BUERGER'S DISEASE (THROMBOANGIITIS OBLITERANS)

DEFINITION:

This is a progressive, segmental inflammatory disease that affects the small to medium sized arteries of the upper and lower limbs. It is not related to atherosclerosis. Usually present in males around 30 years old who are smokers. Angiography may show corkscrewing of the arteries.

HISTOLOGY:

Inflammatory changes that result in thrombosis and thus, ischaemic signs/symptoms to the fingertips/toes. The exact etiology is unclear.

MANAGEMENT:

Smoking cessation.

RAYNAUD'S DISEASE

DEFINITION:

Abnormal arteriolar response to the cold. Usually affects young women.

SIGNS AND SYMPTOMS:

Fingers turn from white to red to blue.

TREATMENT:

Calcium antagonists.

RAYNAUD'S PHENOMENON

DEFINITION:

Raynaud's phenomenon may be categorised as primary or secondary. Primary Raynaud's is a vasorestrictive response in the absence of disease whereas secondary Raynaud's is a peripheral arterial manifestation of a collagen disease e.g. SLE, rheumatoid arthritis, antiphospholipid syndrome. Sometimes it is related to certain drugs e.g. cyclosporine and certain infections like hepatitis B and C.

TREATMENT:

Treatment of the underlying condition. Nifedipine, steroids and vasospastic antagonists may play a role.

CAROTID ARTERY DISEASE/CAROTID ARTERY STENOSIS

DEFINITION:

Narrowing of the carotid artery, usually due to atherosclerosis.

RISKS FACTORS:

Smoking, hyperlipidaemia, male gender and age.

SIGNS AND SYMPTOMS:

TIA/stroke symptoms (slurred speech, cranial nerve deficits, limb weakness, or visual disturbances) which either have resolved or should be expected to improve within 48 hours. Strokes may also improve in this timeframe and, therefore, this is not a diagnostic factor.

INVESTIGATIONS:

- Blood tests (FBC, U&Es, HbA1c, LFTs, coag, cross match, cholesterol).
- Radiology: carotid duplex, magnetic resonance arteriography (MRA), or computed tomographic (CT) arteriography.
- As per guidelines, diagnosis is done via 2× imaging formats, i.e. USS then either CTA or MRA.

MANAGEMENT:

Reduction of cardiovascular risk factors and carotid endarterectomy. The percentage of stenosis is measured. Depending on whether using North American or European guidelines, intervention is considered at 50% or 70% stenosis (slightly different measuring techniques).

COMPLICATIONS OF ENDARTERECTOMY:

- Damage to hypoglossal nerve
- Damage to the vagus nerve
- Damage to the glossopharyngeal nerve
- Damage to the facial (marginal mandibular) nerve
- Damage to the greater auricular nerve
- Myocardial Infarction
- Hyperperfusion syndrome
- Perioperative stroke
- Restenosis
- Death
- Transient ischaemic attack
- Bleeding
- Infection

DEEP VEIN THROMBOSIS (DVT)

A DVT is a clot that usually develops in one of the deep veins. It usually occurs in the leg. The pathophysiology of DVT may be summarised by Virchow's triad. This comprises predisposing factors for DVT formation (the causes of each factor are listed):

1. *Hypercoagulability*
   - Malignancy
   - Surgery
   - Trauma
   - Oral contraceptive pill
   - Clotting abnormalities
2. *Venous stasis*
   - Immobility, e.g. after surgery
   - Pregnancy
   - Heart failure
3. *Trauma*
   - Inflammation
   - Previous thrombosis

SIGNS AND SYMPTOMS:

- Asymptomatic
- Pain
- Oedema

- Erythema/discolouration
- Increased temperature of symptomatic leg
- Engorgement of surface veins

Differential diagnosis: remember as ABC = **A** musculoskeletal injury. **B**aker's cyst rupture. **C**ellulitis.

INVESTIGATIONS:

- D-dimer: this is sensitive but not specific, i.e. if the result is negative then the cause is unlikely to be DVT.
- B-mode venous compression ultrasonography: for DVT above the knee.
- Investigations to uncover cause of DVT.
- The Modified Wells Score may be used to calculate probability of DVT.

MANAGEMENT:

Anticoagulation therapy with unfractionated heparin or a low molecular weight heparin, e.g. dalteparin, and secondary management with a vitamin K antagonist, e.g. warfarin.

PULMONARY EMBOLISM (PE)

This is occlusion of the pulmonary vasculature by a clot. Often it occurs from a deep vein thrombosis (DVT) that has become dislodged and forms an embolus that lodges in the pulmonary arterial vasculature, blocking the vessels.

The extent of thrombus may be classified into small-medium, multiple and massive PE. Symptom correlation depends on where the pulmonary circulation is occluded. There are three pathways involved in the pathophysiology of PE:

1. *Platelet factor release:* serotonin and thromboxane A2 cause vasoconstriction.
2. *Decreased alveolar perfusion:* lung is underperfused and this leads to diminished gas exchange.
3. *Decreased surfactant:* this leads to ventilation/perfusion mismatch, hypoxaemia and dyspnoea.

SIGNS AND SYMPTOMS:

- Breathlessness: this may be of sudden onset or progressive
- Tachypnoea
- Pleuritic chest pain
- Cyanosis
- Haemoptysis

INVESTIGATIONS:

- D-dimer: sensitive but not specific; negative result used to rule out PE
- Thrombophilia screening: in patients <50 years with recurrent PE
- CXR: usually normal

- ECG: sinus tachycardia, S1Q3T3 pattern is classical but rare; excludes MI
- ABG: hypoxaemia
- CT pulmonary angiography
- V/Q scan
- The Wells Score may be used to calculate risk of PE

MANAGEMENT:

Acute management

- Oxygen
- IV fluids
- Thrombolysis therapy if indicated, e.g. alteplase if massive PE or haemodynamically unstable
- Low molecular weight heparin

Long-term management

- Anticoagulation
- Inferior vena cava filter

11

Urology

URINARY TRACT INFECTIONS

This is an infection of the urinary tract with typical signs and symptoms. It may be classified as either a lower or upper (acute pyelonephritis) UTI.

- Signs and symptoms of lower UTI include dysuria, frequency, urgency and suprapubic pain.
- Signs and symptoms of upper UTI include fever/chills, flank pain and haematuria.

The urinary system has many defences to prevent UTI such as:

- Micturition.
- Urine: osmolarity, pH and organic acids are antibacterial.
- Secreted factors:
  - Tamm–Horsfall protein: binds bacteria non-specifically; produced by cells of the thick ascending loop of Henle; mutations in the gene that codes for this protein are associated with progressive renal failure and medullary cysts.
  - IgA: against specific bacteria.
  - Lactoferrin: hoovers up free iron.
- Mucosal defences: mucopolysaccharides coat the mucosal surfaces of the bladder.

If these defence mechanisms are overcome by bacterial virulence factors, then the patient is prone to developing a UTI. Some virulence factors are:

- For uropathogenic *E. coli* (UPEC):
  - Type 1 fimbriae: binds to mannose residues; associated with cystitis.
  - Type P fimbriae: binds to glycolipid residues; associated with pyelonephritis.
  - Bacterial capsule: aka antigen K, resists phagocytosis; associated with pyelonephritis.
- For *Proteus mirabilis*:
  - Produces urease.
  - Increases pH of urine.
  - *Proteus mirabilis* is associated with staghorn calculi.

Risk factors for the development of UTI include: Female gender, sexual intercourse, catheterisation, pregnancy, menopause, diabetes, genitourinary malformation, immunosuppression and urinary tract obstruction, e.g. stones.

DOI: 10.1201/9781003292005-14

KEY FACTS ABOUT COMMON CAUSATIVE ORGANISMS:

- *Escherichia coli*: leading cause of UTI in the community and also nosocomial infection. Metallic sheen on eosin methylene blue (EMB).
- *Staphylococcus saprophyticus*: 2nd leading cause in sexually active females.
- *Klebsiella pneumoniae*: 3rd leading cause. Viscous colonies.
- *Proteus mirabilis*: produces urease. Gram-negative bacterium.
- *Pseudomonas aeruginosa*: bile green pigment and fruity odour. Usually nosocomial and drug resistant.
- Adenovirus: haemorrhagic cystitis.
- BK and JC viruses: associated with graft failure after transplant.
- *Schistosoma haematobium*: parasitic infection.

INVESTIGATIONS:

- *Urine dipstick*: positive for leucocytes and nitrites.
- *Urine culture*: for diagnosis for causative organism (>10^5 organisms per mL of midstream urine).
- *Radiology*: consider ultrasound scan or cystoscopy if UTI occurs in children, in men or if UTI is recurrent.

MANAGEMENT:

- Conservative: education about the condition and avoidance of predisposing risk factors.
- Medicinal: check local hospital guidelines regarding first-line treatment of UTI. Usually, treatment is with trimethoprim or nitrofurantoin. Consider prophylactic antibiotics if UTI is recurrent.
- If recurrent, i.e. >4 UTIs per year, seek to exclude anatomical variant or abnormality of the renal tract.

RENAL CALCULI

Renal calculi (urolithiasis) are stones that form within the renal tract. There are many different types of renal stone, which will be outlined below. The exact cause of stone formation is not always clear but there are certain factors that may promote development such as urinary stasis, urinary tract infections, certain medications (e.g. indinavir, atazanavir, loop diuretics) and sometimes genetic diseases.

Types of renal calculi and key facts pertaining to them are as follows:

1. Calcium stones—radiopaque
2. Struvite stones—staghorn calculi, associated with Gram-negative urease-producing organisms e.g. *Proteus*
3. Uric acid stones—radiolucent. Associated with gout
4. Cystine stones—associated with renal tubular disease

SIGNS AND SYMPTOMS:

- Asymptomatic

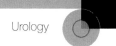

- Renal colic pain—colicky pain that is severe in nature. Loin to groin pain. Associated with nausea and vomiting. May come on suddenly or wake the patient from sleep
- Obstructive pyelonephritis—the patient may be septic, presenting with the above symptoms as well as fevers/rigors. This is a urological emergency that may require urgent decompression of an infective obstructive system
- Haematuria (frank or microscopic)

INVESTIGATIONS:

- Bloods—FBC, U&E, coagulation (in preparation for nephrostomy, which may be required in the event of an infected obstructed system)
- Urinalysis—haematuria, leukocytosis. Note however that up to 15% of renal stone patients do not present with haematuria.
- CT KUB—will pick up significant urolithiasis but may miss small stones
- USS—may be useful in cases where CT is contraindicated e.g. pregnancy
- Chemical analysis of stone composition may be useful in some cases

MANAGEMENT:

Management depends on patient presentation and whether there is infection present/the patient is septic.

Acute management of renal colic (without infection) usually requires good analgesia, antiemetics +/– rehydration. Follow-up may be arranged as per local hospital policy in urology stone clinic.

Small stones <5 mm may be management conservatively and usually pass on their own. Medical expulsion therapy e.g. tamsulosin, may sometimes be helpful in facilitating expulsion. The following table summarises how renal stones of different sizes may be managed electively.

Management of Different-Sized Ureteric and Renal Stones

Location and size of stone	Management
Ureteric stone <5 mm	• Watchful waiting if asymptomatic
Ureteric stone <10 mm	• Consider SWL • Consider URS if there are contraindications to SWL, or if the stone is not targetable with SWL, or previous SWL has failed
Ureteric stone 10-20 mm	• Offer URS • Consider SWL if local facilities allow up to 2 SWL sessions within 4 weeks of the decision to treat • Consider PCNL for impacted proximal stone when URS has failed
Renal stone <10 mm	• Offer SWL • Consider URS if there are contraindications for SWL, or if a previous course of SWL has failed, or if there are anatomical anomalies • Consider PCNL if SWL and URS have failed to treat the current stone or if SLW and URS are contraindicated
Renal stone 10-20 mm	• Consider URS or SWL • Consider PCNL if URS or SWL have failed
Renal stone >20 mm including staghorn calculi	• Offer PCNL • Consider URS if PCNL is contraindicated

Some cases require emergency intervention e.g. infective obstructive system, an obstructed solitary kidney, obstruction resulting in elevated creatinine / renal failure.

Patients should be admitted and treated urgently as per the septic six guidelines with early involvement of the urology and medical teams. Follow local guidance with regard to antibiotics. Ultimately the decision regarding which treatment modality is best suited to relieve the obstructed system is taken by urology but options include the placement of a nephrostomy (by interventional radiology) or a J stent. Renal function should be closely monitored.

ACUTE KIDNEY INJURY

Acute kidney injury (AKI) is the sudden reduction in renal function (days to weeks) and is characterised by a rapid fall in glomerular filtration rate and an increase in creatinine and urea levels. It may be reversible.

According to NICE, AKI can be detected using any of the following KDIGO (Kidney Disease: Improving Global Outcomes) criteria:

- A rise in serum creatinine of 26 µmol/L within 48 hours.
- A 50% rise in serum creatinine known or presumed to have occurred within the past 7 days.
- A fall in urine output to <0.5 mL/kg/h for more than 6 hours.

AKI may be subdivided into pre-renal, intrinsic renal and post-renal failure. There are many different causes of acute renal failure within these subdivisions, which are outlined in the table below.

CAUSES:

Outline of Some of the Causes of AKI

Types of AKI	Cause
Pre-renal failure	1. Hypovolaemia—haemorrhage, diarrhoea, vomiting 2. Hypotension—septic shock, anaphylactic shock, cardiogenic shock 3. Renal vasoconstriction—NSAIDS, contrast agents
Intrinsic failure	1. Glomerular disease—glomerulonephritis (e.g. IgA nephropathy, anti-glomerular basement membrane disease), vasculitis, immune complex disease (e.g. SLE) 2. Vascular lesions—bilateral renal artery stenosis, malignant hypertension 3. Tubulointerstitial disease—acute tubular necrosis (rhabdomyolysis, vancomycin, aminoglycosides), acute interstitial nephritis (penicillin, NSAIDs), multiple myeloma, nephrotoxic drugs
Post-renal failure	Any cause of obstruction of the ureter, urethra and bladder neck e.g. stones, tumours, strictures, benign prostatic hypertrophy/prostatic, blood clots, phimosis

SIGNS AND SYMPTOMS:

The exact signs and symptoms depend on the underlying cause. All patients require a top to toe examination with an assessment of fluid balance and volume status.

- Oliguria
- Anuria
- Cardiovascular examination—assessment of volume status, pericardial rub (uraemic pericarditis), elevated JVP in fluid overload
- Skin—skin changes indicative of underlying disease e.g. butterfly rash in SLE, maculopapular rashes in drug-induced acute interstitial nephritis, purpuras in vasculitis.
- Eye examination—jaundice (liver disease), retinopathy (diabetes), iritis/uveitis (autoimmune disease)
- Cognitive assessment—confusion, encephalopathy
- Abdominal examination—flank pain may be present in some cases

INVESTIGATIONS:

Specific investigations may be related to the underlying cause.

- Bloods: FBC and platelets, U&Es, GFR, calcium and phosphate levels, ESR, CRP, immunology, virology
- Urinalysis: blood, protein, glucose, leucocytes and nitrites, Bence Jones protein. Muddy brown casts are seen in ATN and white blood cell casts are seen in AIN
- Serum and urine protein electrophoresis: may be required when investigating monoclonal gammopathy and multiple myeloma
- Imaging: ultrasound scan (+/− biopsy)

MANAGEMENT:

Depends on the underlying cause.

- Fluid challenge—To determine whether the cause is pre-renal in nature patients often undergo a fluid challenge. If the renal function improved with fluid challenge, then this is indicative of a pre-renal AKI
- Stop nephrotoxic drugs
- Daily U&Es
- Careful monitoring of fluid balance
- Early referral to renal team
- Referral to dietician re renal diet
- Management of complications e.g. hyperkalaemia (follow local guidelines).
- Short term renal replacement may be required (initiated by the renal team). Some indications for renal replacement therapy include: acidaemia, electrolyte disturbances, uremic pericarditis, and pulmonary oedema
- Immunosuppressants/steroids may be required for various causes of glomerulonephritis/vasculitis (again to be discussed with the renal team)

RENAL CELL CANCER

This is a type of malignant tumour of the kidney. There are fourteen different cell types of renal cell cancer (RCC) described; clear cell RCC, multilocular cystic renal neoplasm of low malignant potential, papillary RCC, hereditary leiomyomatosis RCC, chromophobe RCC, collecting duct carcinoma, renal medullary carcinoma, MiT family translocation carcinomas, succinate dehydrogenase (SDH) deficient RCC, mucinous tubular and spindle cell carcinoma, tubulocystic RCC, acquired cystic disease-associated RCC, clear cell papillary RCC and unclassified RCC.

For the MRCS examination, the key points of the most common subtypes asked about in the examination will be outlined in the following table.

Cell type	Key points
Clear cell carcinoma	Commonest Usually single and unilateral Macroscopically the cut surface looks yellow due to lipid laden cells Microscopically appearances are trabecular and there are clear cells
Papillary carcinoma	Second commonest Can be multifocal and bilateral Histologically there are two subtypes: 1. Papillae and tubular structures, small cells, oval nuclei and basophilic cytoplasm 2. Papillae, large cells, spherical nuclei and eosinophilic cytoplasm (more aggressive)
Chromophobe carcinoma	From the intercalated cells of collecting ducts Microscopically there are basic chromophobe polygonal cells and perinuclear halos
Collecting duct carcinoma	From the medullary cells of collecting ducts Microscopically there are irregular channels lined with atypical epithelium and fibrotic stroma

CAUSES:

The exact cause of RCC is not known. However, there are some risk factors and hereditary associations.

Risk factors include; smoking, chemical exposure e.g. benzene, herbicides and vinyl chloride. Hereditary associations include:

- Von Hippel-Lindau syndrome: VHL gene mutation chromosome 3
- Hereditary papillary carcinoma: MET gene mutation chromosome 7
- Tuberous sclerosis: Autosomal dominant condition. The genes involved are as follows. TSC1 gene (chromosome 9) codes for tumour growth suppressor protein hamartin and TSC2 gene (chromosome 16) codes for tumour growth suppressor protein tuberin.

INVESTIGATIONS:

- Bloods—FBC, U&E, LFTs, Coagulation, calcium
- Blood tests based on paraneoplastic syndromes sometimes associated with RCC—secretion of adrenocorticotrophic hormone (ACTH): may produce symptoms of hypercalcaemia. Secretion of erythropoietin (EPO): may produce symptoms of polycythaemia
- Radiology—USS, CT, MRI

MANAGEMENT:

Management of RCC depends on the stage of the disease, the presence of metastasis and the intention of treatment i.e. curative v palliative. All cases are discussed within a multi-disciplinary team meeting.

Examples of treatment depending on stage are outlined in the following table.

Treatment Options of the Different Stages of RCC

Stage of RCC	Treatment
1a	Tumour is confined to the kidney therefore aim to treat with curative intent Partial nephrectomy
1b	Partial or radical nephrectomy
2 and 3	Radical nephrectomy
4	Systemic targeted molecular therapies Nephrectomy +/– immunotherapy

BLADDER CANCER:

A neoplasm of the urinary bladder. The most common cell type is urothelial carcinoma (this term has replaced transitional cell carcinoma). The exact cause of urothelial carcinoma is unknown however it is associated with several risk factors such as smoking, chemical exposure e.g. aniline dyes and drugs like cyclophosphamide. Schistosomiasis infection is associated with an increased risk of squamous cell cancer of the bladder.

SIGNS AND SYMPTOMS:

- Microscopic or macroscopic haematuria (usually painless)
- Symptoms of urinary infection
- Symptoms of bladder outflow obstruction
- Suprapubic tenderness/palpable mass
- Constitutional symptoms e.g. fatigue and weight loss

INVESTIGATIONS:

- Bloods: FBC, U&E, LFTs, coagulation, group and save (in case transfusion required)
- Imaging: USS, CT, intravenous urography (IVU)
- Cystoscopy and ureteroscopy with biopsy – gold standard for diagnosis

MANAGEMENT:

Management of bladder cancer depends on the stage of the disease, whether there is high- or low-grade disease, if the muscle is invaded, the presence of metastasis and the intention of treatment i.e. curative v palliative. All cases are discussed within a multi-disciplinary team meeting.
   Examples of treatment include the following:

- For non-muscle invasive bladder cancer—endoscopic resection/ trans urethral resection of bladder tumour (TURBT) and risk-based intravesical therapy e.g. bacillus Calmette–Guérin (BCG).
- For muscle invasive bladder cancer—cystectomy with or without chemotherapy (+/– neo-adjuvant / adjuvant therapy)

PROSTATE CANCER

Prostate cancer tends to be an adenocarcinoma affecting the peripheral zone of the prostate gland. It metastasises to the bone and lymph nodes.
   The exact cause of prostate cancer is unknown however it is associated with increasing age, a positive family history and African ethnicity. Mutations in BRCA1 and BRCA2 have been associated with prostate cancer as well as breast cancer.

SIGNS AND SYMPTOMS:

- Some cases may be asymptomatic.
- Symptoms of bladder outflow obstruction—frequent urination, nocturia, terminal dribbling, dysuria
- Haematuria
- Erectile dysfunction / painful ejaculation
- History of colon cancer (suggestive of Lynch syndrome)
- Digital rectal examination—an enlarged prostate gland that may be uninodular or multinodular. The midline sulcus is usually no longer palpable.
- Symptoms of metastasis—bone pain, back pain, neurological symptoms in the legs indicative of spinal cord compression, weight loss, fatigue

INVESTIGATIONS

- Urine dipstick, microscopy and culture.
- Bloods: FBCs, U&Es and creatinine (renal function), LFTs.
- Prostate specific antigen (PSA)—usually raised.
- Radiology: transrectal ultrasound and biopsy. If this procedure diagnoses a malignancy, then the patient should be sent for an MRI and bone scan to look for distant metastases. Prostate cancer is staged using the TMN system. Since there may also be symptoms of bladder outflow obstruction an ultrasound scan of the urinary tract may also be required.

MANAGEMENT:

Depends on the stage of the disease, degree of spread and intent of treatment i.e. curative v palliative. All cases are discussed with a multi-disciplinary team.

Examples of treatment include:

- Radiation oncology treatments—external beam radiotherapy, stereotactic ablative radiotherapy, brachytherapy (radioactive seed implants)
- Hormone therapy—LHRH agonists preceded by anti-androgen therapy or LHRH antagonists
- Radical prostatectomy—robotically or laparoscopically +/– lymph node dissection
- Salvage radiotherapy post radical prostatectomy
- Chemotherapy—to be discussed with oncology. Often docetaxel is used.

TESTICULAR CANCER

There are many different types of testicular cancer. They are defined based on their cell type:

1. **Germ cell tumours**
   a. Germ cell neoplasia in situ (GCNIS)
2. **Derived from germ cell neoplasia in situ (GCNIS)**
   a. Seminoma
   b. Embryonal carcinoma
   c. Yolk sac tumour, post-pubertal type
   d. Trophoblastic tumour
   e. Teratoma, post-pubertal type
   f. Teratoma with somatic-type malignancies
   g. Mixed germ cell tumours

3. **Germ cell tumours unrelated to GCNIS**
   a. Spermatocytic tumour
   b. Yolk sac tumour, pre-pubertal type
   c. Mixed germ cell tumour, pre-pubertal type
4. **Sex cord/stromal cell tumours**
   a. Leydig cell tumour
      - Malignant Leydig cell tumour
   b. Sertoli cell tumour
      - Malignant Sertoli cell tumour
      - Large cell-calcifying Sertoli cell tumour
      - Intratubular large cell-hyalinising Sertoli cell neoplasia
   c. Granulosa cell tumour
      - Adult type
      - Juvenile type
   d. Thecoma/fibroma group of tumours
   e. Other sex cord/gonadal stromal tumours
      - Mixed
      - Unclassified
   f. Tumours containing both germ cell and sex cord/gonadal stromal
      - Gonadoblastoma
5. **Miscellaneous non-specific stromal cell tumours**
   a. Ovarian epithelial tumours
   b. Tumours of collecting ducts and rete testes
      - Adenoma
      - Carcinoma
   c. Tumours of paratesticular structures
      - Adenomatoid tumour
      - Mesothelioma (epithelioid, biphasic)
      - Epididymal tumours
   d. Cystadenoma of the epididymis
   e. Papillary cystadenoma
   f. Adenocarcinoma of the epididymis
   g. Mesenchymal tumours of the spermatic cord and the testicular adnexa

RISK FACTORS FOR THE DEVELOPMENT OF TESTICULAR CANCER:

- Cryptorchidism—2–4-fold increase in risk
- Family history—relative risk increased 6–10-fold
- Infections—human papillomavirus (HPV), Epstein–Barr virus (EBV), cytomegalovirus (CMV), parvovirus B-19 and human immunodeficiency virus (HIV)
- Testicular trauma
- High maternal oestrogen levels
- Carcinoma in situ (intratubular germ cell neoplasia)
- Prior history of testis cancer or extragonadal germ cell tumour

SIGNS AND SYMPTOMS:

- Unilateral lump or painless swelling in the testicle. Sometimes there may be dull pain.
- Symptoms of metastases, e.g. anorexia, malaise, weight loss.

- Pulmonary metastasis—cough or shortness of breath.
- Lymphatic metastasis—cervical or supraclavicular lymphadenopathy, central or peripheral nervous system symptoms from the cerebrum, spinal cord or peripheral nerve root involvement.

INVESTIGATIONS:

- Serum tumour markers (AFP, alpha-fetoprotein; beta-hCG, subunit of human chorionic gonadotropin; LDH, lactate dehydrogenase)
- Imaging—CT (chest, abdomen and pelvis) for staging, USS

Staging Testicular Germ Cell Tumours

Criteria Based on AJCC			
Stage	**Criteria**		
Stage I	IA—disease limited to testis and epididymis		
	IB—disease limited to testis and epididymis, with tumour invasion into spermatic cord or scrotum with or without vascular or lymphatic involvement		
Stage II	IIA—involvement of lymph nodes with a mass ≤2 cm		
	IIB—involvement of lymph nodes with a mass >2 cm but <5 cm		
	IIC—involvement of lymph nodes with a mass >5 cm		
Criteria Based on IGCCCG			
Stage	**Risk**	**Seminoma**	**Non-seminoma**
Stage III	Good risk	Any primary site No non-pulmonary visceral sites Normal AFP, any β-hCG or LDH	Testicular or retroperitoneal primary tumour No pulmonary or visceral metastases Postorchiectomy values— AFP <1,000 ng/mL, β-hCG <5,000 IU/L, LDH <1.5× normal
Distant metastasis	Intermediate risk	Any primary site with non-pulmonary visceral metastasis Normal AFP, any β-hCG or LDH	Testicular or retroperitoneal primary tumour Non-pulmonary or visceral metastases Postorchiectomy values (any)—AFP 1,000–10,000 ng/mL, β-hCG 5,000–50,000 IU/L, LDH 1.5–10× normal
	High risk	No patients classified as poor risk	Mediastinal primary tumour or non-pulmonary visceral metastases Postorchiectomy markers (any)—AFP >10,000 ng/mL, β-hCG >50,000 IU/L, LDH >10× ULN

Abbreviations: AFP: alpha-fetoprotein; AJCC: American Joint Committee on Cancer; êžµ-hCG: beta-human chorionic gonadotropin; IGCCCG: International Germ Cell Cancer Collaborative Group; LDH: lactic dehydrogenase; ULN: upper limit of normal.

MANAGEMENT:

The International Germ Cell Cancer Collaborative Group (IGCCCG)-based clinical staging is used to tailor management strategies in patients with testicular malignancies. It is an MDT approach and treatment strategies involve surgery (orchidectomy), chemotherapy and radiotherapy.

TESTICULAR TORSION

- This is a time-dependent urological emergency. Testicular viability significantly decreases 6 hours after the onset of symptoms. Most cases occur in younger patients and are usually due to a congenital abnormality of the processus vaginalis.
- As the testicle twists, venous blood flow is compromised. The result is venous congestion and ischaemia of the testicle.

SYMPTOMS

- Short history of pain (few hours).
- Sudden onset—maximal immediately, may have occurred when inactive, e.g. sitting, or woke patient up from sleep.
- Most likely differential—epididymo-orchitis.
- If suspicious clinically, needs urgent surgical exploration, (i.e. immediately to theatre). Average rates of positive diagnosis in theatre are 25%, rest are torted hydatid, epididymo-orchitis or normal testicle.

In addition to these symptoms, the testicular workup for ischaemia and suspected torsion (TWIST) score is a clinical decision tool that may be used where torsion is suspected.
It comprises the following criteria:

- Hard testis—2
- Swelling—2
- Nausea/vomiting—1
- Absent cremasteric re ex—1
- High-riding testis—1

The higher the score, the greater the likelihood that the patient has torsion.
Ultimately, it is a clinical diagnosis, and prompt urological intervention is required for surgical exploration in theatre.

SCROTAL EXPLORATION:

1. Normal testicle/epididymo-orchitis—leave it as is.
2. Twisted and viable—untwist, three-point fixation, then fix the other side.
3. Twisted and ischaemic/compromised—untwist, warm moist compress; if shows signs of viability, three-point fixation bilaterally.
4. Twisted and ischaemic with no response to untwist and warm compress—orchidectomy.

PENILE CANCER

This is an uncommon cancer of the penis. 95% of cases are SCC. Other cell types include BCC, melanoma, sarcomas and adenosquamous carcinoma. The exact cause is unclear, but it is associated with some risk factors such as phimosis, balanitis, lichen planus and sexually trans-mitted diseases particularly HIV and HPV.

SIGNS AND SYMPTOMS:

- Lesion affecting the glans (and tend to affect the glans prior to invading the penile shaft)
- Lesions vary in appearance—some may be flat, other raised, discoloured and ulcerated.
- Bleeding or persistent discharge from behind the foreskin
- Patients may have presented to their GP with this lesion before and there may be a history of the lesion being persistent or worsening in appearance.
- Inguinal lymphadenopathy

INVESTIGATIONS:

- Bloods: FBC, U&Es, LFTs, Ca2+, CRP, ALP (if bone pain) viral serology
- Biopsy of lesion
- Radiology—CT, MRI, inguinal USS +/− biopsy, CXR

MANAGEMENT:

Depends on the stage of penile cancer, the degree of spread and treatment intent. All cases are discussed at MDT.

Surgery is the mainstay of treatment the aim of which is to remove the tumour whilst also bearing in mind cosmesis and penile function. Surgical options include glansectomy +/− cre-ation of a neoglans using split skin grafts or partial amputation with reconstructive split skin grafts. These cases are often referred to and performed in specialist centres.

Radiotherapy may also be offered in cases where surgery is contraindicated. Strategies may be as follows:

- T1N0 (tumour limited to the glans or prepuce)—local electron beam irradiation.
- T2N0 (tumour invading the corpora or deep invasion of the shaft)—irradiation of the whole shaft of the penis.
- T3N0 (tumour invading the urethra or prostate gland)—consider radical radiotherapy, but large volume disease may be more appropriately managed with palliative radiotherapy.
- T4/inoperable nodal disease—consider palliative radiotherapy.

Radiotherapy +/− chemotherapy may be considered for advanced and inoperable disease.

With regard to lymph nodes, aspiration cytology confirms the diagnosis of metastasis. Patient may undergo bilateral lymph node dissection. Post-operative radiotherapy to iliac nodes may be considered. Patients are counselled carefully given the significant morbidity associated with lymph node dissection.

PENILE FRACTURE

Uncommon but severe injury, which is a time critical urological emergency. The commonest cause is trauma during sexual intercourse, resulting in rupture of the tunica albuginea.

SIGNS AND SYMPTOMS:

- Pain in the genitals
- Hearing a pop

- Ecchymosis to the penis/genital area
- Angulated / flaccid penis
- Blood around the urethral meatus and haematuria—may indicate concomitant urethral injury

INVESTIGATIONS:

- Bloods—FBC, U&Es, CRP
- Radiology—USS, CT, MRI

MANAGEMENT:

Prompt surgical management to repair the rupture of the tunica albuginea +/– repair of urethral injury.

Delay >8 hours is associated with increased risk of erectile dysfunction.

COMPLICATIONS:

- Erectile dysfunction
- Curvature of the penis
- Mild chordee
- Urethral injury-related complications

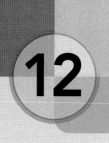

Orthopaedics

12

FRACTURES

There are many different types of fractures, and they may be defined:

- By location
- As open (compound) or closed
- As intra- or extra-articular
- As displaced or not displaced
- By type, i.e.
  - *Complex*—comminuted, segmental
  - *Non-complex*—transverse, oblique, spiral, avulsion, etc.
  - *Specific*—e.g. Greenstick
- By disease involvement, e.g. osteoporosis

Fractures must be further assessed using X-ray (most commonly two views, lateral and AP, but in the case of hand fractures, three views) and a description of impaction, angulation and translocation must be reported.

There are many complications associated with fractures that are outlined herein.

General Complications of Fractures

Complication	Comments
General	Haemorrhage
	Shock
	Infection
	Fat embolus (most commonly from long bone fractures) resulting in pulmonary embolism and respiratory distress syndrome
	Rhabdomyolysis
Associated with prolonged bedrest	DVT and PE
	Pressure sores
	Muscle wasting
	Infection

(Continued)

DOI: 10.1201/9781003292005-15

General Complications of Fractures   (Continued)

Complication	Comments
Associated with plaster casts	Remember as "**SPAN**" **S**—Stiffness **P**—Pressure **A**—Allergy **N**—Nerve and circulatory disturbance
Associated with anaesthesia	Anaphylaxis Aspiration

Specific Complications of Fractures

Complication	Comments
Immediate	Haemorrhage Neurovascular complications
Early	Infection Compartment syndrome: • Fractures cause swelling, which increases pressure within the compartment. This results in decreased capillary blood flow. Ischaemia develops when capillary pressure is less than that of the compartment pressure. Irreversible changes result after 6 hours. • Symptoms include pain which is out of proportion with the presenting injury. This pain is present/worsened on passive stretching, with paraesthesia and tightness.
Late	Malunion • Two different forms: 1. *Hypertrophic*—plenty of new bone growth, but these fail to unite. 2. *Atrophic*—lack of new bone growth. Osteopenic in appearance. • Avascular necrosis • Complex regional pain syndrome • Two different forms: 1. No underlying nerve problem 2. Underlying, demonstrable nerve problem • *Myositis ossificans*—calcification of the soft tissues which occurs after surgery or injury • *Growth disturbance*—occurs after damage to the growth plate. This is described using the **Salt**er–**Harris** **C**lassification. Remember as **SALT C** **S**—**S**eparate (fracture occurs through the growth plate) **A**—**A**bove (above the growth plate, most common type) **L**—**L**ower (below the growth plate) **T**—**T**hrough (both upper and lower, commonest cause of premature growth arrest) **C**—**C**rushed physis (worst injury)

PRINCIPLES OF FRACTURE MANAGEMENT

In the context of trauma, the primary concern is patient assessment and resuscitation in line with up-to-date Advanced Trauma Life Support (ATLS) guidelines. This is beyond the scope of this book.

With regard to fractures, it is important to follow the 3 R's:

1. *Reduce*—restoration of anatomical bone alignment by correcting deforming forces on the limb.
   Fracture reduction may be performed via open or closed techniques depending on the nature of the injury.
2. *Retain*—immobilisation of the fracture once reduced. This is typically achieved using plaster casts or splints.
3. *Rehabilitate*—physiotherapy. This period of physiotherapy helps to facilitate recovery and improve clinical/functional outcomes.

NECK PATHOLOGY

CERVICAL SPONDYLOSIS

Degenerative arthritis of the cervical vertebrae. It can affect all components of the cervical spine including the intervertebral discs, facet joints and laminae. There is increased risk with age.

CAUSES:

- Osteoarthritis (if bony spurs present, this may result in cervical radiculopathy or myelopathy). This is associated with age-related degeneration. Such degenerative change may compress the spinal cord and vasculature. Thus patients may present with myelopathy and radiculopathy.
- Trauma

SYMPTOMS:

- May be asymptomatic
- Reduced range of movement
- Pain (axial neck pain)
- Paraesthesia following a dermatomal distribution

INVESTIGATIONS:

- Thorough physical examination
- Radiology—CT/MRI scan

TREATMENT:

- *Conservative*—physiotherapy
- *Medicinal*—NSAIDs, codeine, etc.; follow the WHO analgesic ladder
- *Surgical*—anterior cervical discectomy, cervical laminectomy, posterior approaches e.g. partial discectomy, laminoplasty, laminectomy and laminotomy-foraminotomy

COMPLICATIONS:

- Vertebrobasilar insufficiency

CERVICAL SPONDYLOLISTHESIS

This is when a superiorly located cervical vertebra is displaced anteriorly relative to the vertebra below. This may narrow the vertebral canal and results in deformity.

CAUSES:

- *Congenital*—failure of ondontoid process fusion
- *Trauma*—resulting in instability
- Softening of the transverse ligament due to inflammation

SYMPTOMS:

- *Pain*—may be radicular or may radiate between the shoulder blades and to the back of the head

INVESTIGATIONS:

- Thorough physical examination
- *Radiology*—CT/MRI scan
- *Meyerding's grading system*—describes percentage slippage

TREATMENT:

- *Conservative*—physiotherapy
- *Medicinal*—NSAIDs, codeine, etc.; follow the WHO analgesic ladder; consider corticosteroid injections
- *Surgical*—microdiscectomy, hemilaminectomy, anterior cervical discectomy +/− fusion

CERVICAL DISC PROLAPSE

This occurs when the nucleus pulposus herniates through a tear in the annulus fibrosus. Typically affects C5/6 and C6/7 since these are the most mobile segments. Prolapses may be central or lateral.

SYMPTOMS:

- Brachialgia with associated radiculopathy
- Pain, paraesthesia, weakness

INVESTIGATIONS:

- Bloods: FBC, CRP (query infection/malignancy)
- Thorough physical examination. Special tests include; Hoffman test (for spinal cord compression/myelopathy), Spurling test (for acute radiculopathy) and Lhermitte sign (for spinal cord compression/myelopathy)
- *Radiology*—MRI scan, x-rays (for overall spine alignment and fractures), CT (best for bone assessment - loss, destruction), EMG (if nerve symptoms)

TREATMENT:

Depends on the extent of the prolapse and the presence or absence of neurological symptoms.

- *Mild*—no neurological symptoms. Physiotherapy and analgesia may suffice.
- *Moderate*—only radicular symptoms. Surgery may be required, e.g. discectomy or laminectomy.
- *Severe*—urgent surgical decompression.

SHOULDER PATHOLOGY

SHOULDER DISLOCATION

This is when there is a loss of congruity between the head of the humerus and the glenoid fossa. There are two types—anterior and posterior.

CAUSES:

- *Anterior*—commonest. Trauma. Increased risk in those with connective tissue disorders or those with prior shoulder dislocations.
- *Posterior*—rare. Present in seizures (although anterior dislocations are still more common in this patient group) and electrocution.

SYMPTOMS:

- Pain
- Decreased range of movement
- *Anterior*—humeral head is prominent and held in an abducted, externally rotated position

INVESTIGATIONS:

- *Radiology*—X-ray (lateral, AP and scapula Y views). Lightbulb sign is positive for posterior dislocation.

TREATMENT:

- Closed reduction and sling immobilisation
- Adequate analgesia

COMPLICATIONS:

- Axillary nerve or artery damage
- Damage to the brachial plexus
- Increased risk of recurrent dislocations
- Specific lesions
  - *Bankhart's lesion*—avulsion of antero-inferior glenoid labrum
  - *Hill–Sachs lesion*—indentation fracture of the postero-lateral humeral head

ROTATOR CUFF TEARS

WHAT ARE ROTATOR CUFF TEARS?

- The rotator cuff comprises four tendons and muscles that provide stability to the highly mobile shoulder joint.
- The four muscles (remembered as "**SITS**") are the **S**upraspinatus (most commonly torn), **I**nfraspinatus, **T**eres minor and **S**ubscapularis. Further important anatomical details about these muscles are provided in the table below.

Anatomical Details of the Rotator Cuff

Muscle	Action	Innervation	Specific test
Supraspinatus	Abducts humerus	Suprascapular nerve (C5)	Empty beer can test (eliminates deltoid)
Infraspinatus	Externally rotates humerus	Suprascapular nerve (C5–6)	Resisted external rotation
Teres minor	Externally rotates humerus	Axillary nerve (C5)	-
Subscapularis	Internally rotates humerus	Upper and lower subscapular nerve (C5–6)	Lift-off test

CAUSES:

- Degeneration
- Trauma

SYMPTOMS:

- Partial tears result in a painful arc syndrome.
- Complete tears limit shoulder abduction +/– rotation.
- Pain to a variable degree depending on the significance of the tear.
- Shoulder tenderness on palpation.
- Weakness.

INVESTIGATIONS:

- Thorough examination with specific tests, as outlined in the table above
- *Radiology*—X-ray, MRI

TREATMENT:

- *Conservative*—rest and physiotherapy
- *Medicinal*—adequate pain relief
- *Surgical*—arthroscopy +/– repair if indicated, can also be done open

COMPLICATIONS:

- Decreased range of movement that may inhibit daily activities such as reaching high shelves.
- Complications associated with surgery include general risks from anaesthesia and infection to specific risks such as damage to the axillary nerve.

ADHESIVE CAPSULITIS

Adhesive capsulitis is also known as frozen shoulder. It may be classified as primary or secondary. Primary adhesive capsulitis is idiopathic in nature but may be associated with other factors such as diabetes and thyroid disease. Secondary adhesive capsulitis is usually a result of trauma. Typically, the pathology encompasses three phases:

1. Pain with freezing
2. Thawing
3. *Resolution*—may take up to and possibly more than 2 years

CAUSES:

- The exact aetiology of this condition is not known, but it is linked to trauma and past shoulder surgery. Such trauma is likely to stimulate reactive inflammation and scar tissue development.

RISK FACTORS:

- Increased age
- Female
- Diabetes mellitus
- Rheumatoid arthritis

SYMPTOMS:

- *Pain*—on active and passive movement.
- *Restricted range of movement*—actively and passively. External rotation is often affected first.
- Often no movement at the glenohumeral joint.
- Difficulty sleeping on the affected side.

INVESTIGATIONS:

- Thorough physical examination
- *Radiology*—USS and MRI

TREATMENT:

- *Conservative*—physiotherapy
- *Medicinal*—adequate analgesia, steroid injections
- *Interventional radiology*—hydrodilatation
- *Surgery*—only performed in severe cases, e.g. capsular release via arthroscopy

COMPLICATIONS:

- Stiffness
- Loss of function

ARTHRITIS

RHEUMATOID ARTHRITIS (RA)

This is a chronic autoimmune type III hypersensitivity reaction that principally affects the joints but may also affect other organs. Joint involvement is characterised by symmetrical deformation with early morning stiffness that lasts >30 minutes. RA commonly presents in the hands and feet initially with red, hot, swollen joints. This condition is associated with HLA DR4 and HLA DR1.

CAUSES:

The exact cause RA is unknown, but it is thought to involve a type III hypersensitivity reaction.

SIGNS AND SYMPTOMS:

- *Hands*—Z deformity, Boutonnière deformity, swan neck deformity, ulnar deviation, subluxation of the fingers, Raynaud's association
- *Wrist*—carpal tunnel syndrome
- *Feet*—subluxation of the toes, hammer toe deformity
- *Skin*—rheumatoid nodule, vasculitis
- *Cardiovascular*—atherosclerosis is increased in RA
- *Respiratory*—pulmonary fibrosis
- *Bones*—osteoporosis
- Pain and stiffness

INVESTIGATIONS:

- *Blood tests*
  - 80% test positive for rheumatoid factor
  - ESR and CRP raised
  - Cyclic citrullinated peptide (CCP)
- *Radiology*—radiological signs of RA are visualised on plain film
  - Bony erosion
  - Subluxation
  - Carpal instability
  - Joint involvement of MCPJ and MTPJ
  - Periarticular osteoporosis

TREATMENT:

- *Conservative*—patient education. Encourage exercise. Refer to physiotherapy who will assess activities of daily living (ADL).
- *Medicinal*—glucocorticoids, disease-modifying antirheumatic drugs (DMARDs), e.g. methotrexate, sulfasalazine. Anti-cytokine therapies may be considered in patients intolerant to methotrexate.
- *Surgery*—excision arthroplasty or replacement may be considered in severely affected joints.

COMPLICATIONS:

- Carpal tunnel syndrome
- Pericarditis
- Cervical myopathy
- Tendon rupture

OSTEOARTHRITIS (OA)

This is a degenerative arthritis affecting synovial joints and is characterised by cartilage degeneration, associated response of the periarticular tissue and pain that is typically worse at the end of the day.

CAUSES:

Damage to the joints and general wear and tear of the joint over time is thought to be the primary cause of OA. There are certain factors that increase the risk of OA such as:

- Increased age
- Obesity
- Trauma to the joint
- Conditions such as haemochromatosis and Ehlers–Danlos syndrome

SIGNS AND SYMPTOMS:

- Pain and stiffness
- Swelling around joint involved
- Crepitus
- Heberden's nodes (DIP)
- Bouchard's nodes (PIP)

INVESTIGATIONS:

- *Blood tests*—not usually diagnostic but may be relevant when OA is related to another condition such as haemochromatosis.
- *Radiology*—radiological signs: "**LOSS**"

    L—**L**oss of joint space
    O—**O**steophytes
    S—**S**ubchondral cysts
    S—**S**clerosis

TREATMENT:

- *Conservative*—patient education. Encourage exercise and weight loss.
- *Medicinal*—analgesia, e.g. paracetamol or NSAIDs. Gels such as capsaicin may be useful. Steroid injections.
- *Surgical*—arthroplasty, (concerning OA of the hand one might consider joint fusion or other procedures like trapeziectomy depending on the location of disease)..

COMPLICATIONS:

- Increased risk of gout
- Chondrocalcinosis

ELBOW PATHOLOGY

TENNIS ELBOW

Tennis elbow is also known as lateral epicondylitis and is the most common elbow overuse injury.

CAUSES:

Tennis elbow is a form of repetitive strain injury, e.g. playing sports such as tennis and squash or undertaking other activities such as gardening and painting. This results in microruptures/microtears and eccentric overload at the origin of the common extensor tendon leading to tendinosis and inflammation of the extensor carpi radialis brevis (ECRB).

SYMPTOMS:

- Aching elbow pain, typically over the lateral epicondyle, which worsens with activity
- Typically affects the dominant arm
- Worse during simple daily tasks utilising extensors such as lifting a cup of coffee
- Decreased power grip in affected arm

INVESTIGATIONS:

- No specific tests or imaging required
- Clinical diagnosis
- Mills' test and Cozen's test

TREATMENT:

- *Conservative*—usually a self-limiting condition, stop/decrease triggering activity tennis elbow, ice elbow, utilise an elbow strap, physiotherapy may be required
- *Medicinal*—painkillers, e.g. paracetamol and NSAIDs, local steroid injections if severe and other methods have failed
- *Surgery*—only considered if above methods have failed, and even if pain lasts >4 months, surgery is very unlikely

COMPLICATIONS:

- Loss of function
- Chronic pain

GOLFER'S ELBOW

Golfer's elbow is also known as medial epicondylitis and is a type of elbow overuse injury.

CAUSES:

Golfer's elbow is an overuse tendinopathy due to chronic repetitive concentric or eccentric loading of the wrist flexors and pronator teres, resulting in microruptures/microtears, angiofibroblastic changes, tendinosis and inflammation.

SYMPTOMS:

- Aching elbow pain, typically over the medial epicondyle, which worsens with activity
- Typically affects the dominant arm
- Worse during simple daily tasks utilising flexors
- Decreased grip power in affected arm

INVESTIGATIONS:

- No specific tests or imaging required
- Clinical diagnosis
- Golfer's elbow test

TREATMENT:

- *Conservative*—usually a self-limiting condition, stop/decrease activity which triggered golfer's elbow, ice elbow, utilise an elbow strap, physiotherapy may be required
- *Medicinal*—painkillers, e.g. paracetamol and NSAIDs, local steroid injections if severe and other methods have failed
- *Surgery*—only considered if above methods have failed, and even if pain >4 months, surgery is very unlikely

COMPLICATIONS:

- Loss of function
- Chronic pain
- Associated ulnar neuropathy

HAND PATHOLOGY

DUPUYTREN'S CONTRACTURE

Dupuytren's contracture is a proliferative fibroplasia of the palmar and digital fascia. Over time, this leads to formation of nodules, cords and finger flexion contractures. Genetic mutations affecting chromosome 16q and subsequent downregulation in collagen breakdown have been implicated in the development of the disease. It affects men more than women. The ring finger is most commonly affected.

CAUSES:

The exact cause of this pathology is unknown. It is known that it is more common in males than females as well as those with a positive family history. It is associated with the following:

- Diabetes mellitus
- Hepatic cirrhosis
- Certain drugs, e.g. phenytoin
- Trauma

The aggressive form of the disease is called Dupuytren's diathesis and is associated with Peyronie's disease (penile fibromatosis) and Ledderhose's disease (plantar fascia fibromatosis).

SYMPTOMS:

- Flexion contracture of the fingers. The Tubiana classification may be used to aid evaluation of the contractures at each joint.

- Nodular thickening of palmar fascia and cord development. There are different types of named cord. For example, pretendinous cords (which are estimated to contributed to more than 80% of MCPJ contracture and 40% PIPJ contracture), retrovascular cords and spiral cords (which may contribute to up to 20% PIPJ contracture).

INVESTIGATIONS:

- No specific test, but can test for underlying associations
- Perform Heuston tabletop test

TREATMENT:

- *Surgical*—only perform fasciotomy, fasciectomy or dermofascietomy if contracture is causing functional problems. Physiotherapy and splinting required after treatment. A full-thickness skin graft is sometimes considered in severe cases of Dupuytren's contracture with skin shortage or radical dermofasciectomy.

COMPLICATIONS:

- Loss of function
- Complications associated with surgery, e.g. haematoma formation, infection, nerve injury and recurrence. There is also a risk of devascularising the digit during surgery.

DE QUERVAIN'S SYNDROME

De Quervain's syndrome, also known as washerwoman's sprain, is a stenosing tenosynovitis of the extensor pollicis brevis and the abductor pollicis tendons. The extensor pollicis brevis and abductor pollicis are found in the first extensor compartment.

CAUSES:

- The exact cause of this condition is unknown, but it is associated with overuse/repetitive tasks.

SYMPTOMS:

- Wrist pain (radial side), which is worse on movement

INVESTIGATIONS:

- *Finkelstein's test*—pain on passive ulnar deviation (fist formed over thumb)
- *Radiology*—X-ray to rule out other conditions such as osteoarthritis

TREATMENT:

- *Conservative*—rest and avoidance of precipitating factors
- *Medicinal*—analgesia, steroid injections
- *Surgery*—last resort for severe cases, release of first extensor compartment

COMPLICATIONS:

- Decreased range of movement of the wrist

STENOSING TENOSYNOVITIS

This is also known as trigger finger.

- It occurs, often from repetitive movements.
- This leads to inflammation of the tendon and sheath.
- Localised nodal formation on the tendon, distal to the pulley. The ring and middle finger are the most commonly affected.

CAUSES:

- Typically trauma
- Associated with diabetes mellitus, rheumatoid arthritis and gout

SYMPTOMS:

- Trapped flexor tendon, usually related to the A1 pulley
- Digit locked in flexion and must be passively released

INVESTIGATIONS:

- Clinical diagnosis

TREATMENT:

- *Conservative*—immobilisation
- *Medicinal*—analgesia, steroid injections
- *Surgery*—intractable cases may require surgical A1 pulley release

COMPLICATIONS:

- Related to surgery, e.g. infection, nerve injury, tendon bowstringing

CARPAL TUNNEL SYNDROME

Carpal tunnel syndrome may be defined as compression of the median nerve as it passes through the carpal tunnel, beneath the flexor retinaculum. It is more common in females than males.

CAUSES:

- Remember as "**MEDIAN TRAP**"

  M—**M**yxoedema
  E—o**E**dema
  D—**D**iabetes mellitus
  I—**I**diopathic
  A—**A**cromegaly
  N—**N**eoplasm
  T—**T**rauma
  R—**R**heumatoid arthritis
  A—**A**myloidosis
  P—**P**regnancy

SYMPTOMS:

Remember as "**3 P's**":

- *Pain*—in the median nerve distribution, worse at night.
- *Paraesthesia*—in the median nerve distribution, relieved by shaking hands.
- *Patch*—on thenar eminence is preserved since the superficial branch of the median nerve supplies this area. Thenar muscle may atrophy in advanced disease.

INVESTIGATIONS:

- Usually a clinical diagnosis after examination including thorough physical examination with specific Tinel's and Phalen's tests
- *Nerve conduction studies*—to differentiate from cervical spondylosis (C6/7)

TREATMENT:

- *Conservative*—splinting
- *Medicinal*—steroid injection
- *Surgical*—carpal tunnel release

SCAPHOID FRACTURE

The scaphoid is the most commonly fractured carpal bone. The reason this fracture is so important to assess fundamentally rests in the blood supply to this bone. The blood supply enters the distal part of the scaphoid bone and runs proximally. This means that there is a risk of proximal avascular necrosis if fractured.

CAUSES:

- *Trauma usually due to a fall on an outstretched hand.*

SYMPTOMS:

- Pain over the scaphoid bone, i.e. on palpation of the anatomical snuff box

INVESTIGATIONS:

- *Radiology*—X-ray. Fracture may not be seen initially. If not seen but suspected clinically, immobilise in a scaphoid splint and repeat the X-ray in 10 days to 2 weeks. If clinical suspicion persists in the absence of radiographic findings a CT/MRI may be warranted.

TREATMENT:

- Scaphoid plaster Surgery may be indicated in the following circumstances; fracture displacement >1mm, intrascaphoid angle >35 degrees, radiolunate angle > 15 degrees, comminuted fractures, avascular necrosis cases.

COMPLICATIONS:

- Avascular necrosis (proximal third)
- Osteoarthritis
- Malunion/nonunion

SPINAL PATHOLOGY

SCOLIOSIS

This is a lateral curvature of the spine that is >10° (Cobb angle). It may be structural or non-structural, and broadly speaking, there are five different types. Remember as "**PONDS**":

P—**P**ostural, non-structural compensatory scoliosis.
O—**O**steopathic, structural abnormality. Mostly congenital but some cases may be associated with bone disease.
N—**N**euromuscular, associated with cerebral palsy, Friedreich's ataxia, etc.
D—**D**egenerative, associated with facet joint failure.
S—**S**tructural idiopathic, may be subdivided into five types:

1. *Thoracolumbar*—usually curves to the right
2. *Lumbar*—usually curves to the left
3. *Infantile thoracic*—usually curves to the left
4. *Adolescent thoracic*—usually curves to the right
5. *Double major*—two curves, one in each direction

CAUSES:

See above. Remember to ask about family history and pregnancy.

SYMPTOMS:

- Cosmetic deformity.
- Aching, but not severe pain. If very severe, it is important to exclude spinal tumours/osteoid osteomas.

INVESTIGATIONS:

- Thorough spinal examination
- *Radiology*—X-ray (AP and lateral views) and Cobb angle measurement
- Investigations concerning an underlying cause if suspected

TREATMENT:

- *Conservative*—physiotherapy, exercise particularly swimming, brace (Boston or Milwaukee)
- *Medicinal*—adequate analgesia
- *Surgery*—only in severe cases

COMPLICATIONS:

- Psychological implications, e.g. depression
- Restrictive lung disease
- Cardiac complications
- Nerve compression

KYPHOSIS

This is an exaggerated anterior curvature of the thoracic spine. Kyphosis may be classified as fixed, as in ankylosing spondylitis, or mobile, as in postural kyphosis. It may also be defined related to shape, i.e. regular or angular (gibbus).

There are many different types of kyphosis. Remember as "**PONDS**":

P—Postural, more common in adolescent girls
O—Osteoporotic
N—Neuromuscular
D—Degenerative
S—Scheuermann's disease, also known as spinal osteochondrosis, defined as kyphosis >40° and wedging of individual vertebra of 5° (since the vertebra grows more thickly posteriorly than anteriorly)

CAUSES:

- *Infection*—TB, polio
- Malignancy
- *Bone disease*—osteoporosis, Paget's disease
- Ankylosing spondylitis
- Calve's disease

SYMPTOMS:

- Cosmetic deformity.
- Aching, but not severe pain. If very severe it is important to exclude spinal tumours/ osteoid osteomas.
- Symptoms of underlying condition.

INVESTIGATIONS:

- Thorough spinal examination
- *Radiology*—X-ray (AP and lateral views) and Cobb angle measurement
- Investigations concerning an underlying cause if suspected

TREATMENT:

- *Conservative*—physiotherapy, exercise particularly swimming
- *Medicinal*—adequate analgesia
- *Surgery*—only in severe cases

COMPLICATIONS:

- Psychological implications, e.g. depression
- Restrictive lung disease
- Cardiac complications
- Cord compression
- Paraplegia

ANKYLOSING SPONDYLITIS

This is a chronic inflammatory disease of the spine and sacroiliac joints. There is predominance in young males and the condition is associated with HLA B27 (positive in 95%).

CAUSES:

- The exact cause and pathophysiology of this condition are not known. However, it is thought to be associated with HLA B27.

SIGNS AND SYMPTOMS:

- Symptoms improve with exercise
  - Question mark posture
  - Pain and stiffness—this is progressive
- Extra-articular features
  - Iritis
  - Aortitis
  - Apical pulmonary fibrosis
  - Amyloidosis (secondary)
  - Irritable bowel disease (IBD)
  - Cardiac conduction defects
  - Specific spinal symptoms
  - *Bamboo spine*—due to calcification of ligaments (seen on x-ray)
  - Low back pain and stiffness—this pathology is characterised by involvement of the sacroiliac joints (as well as peripheral joint stiffness)
  - Loss of lumbar lordosis
  - Compensatory fixed kyphosis

INVESTIGATIONS:

- *Wall test*—diminished spine extension means that the patients occiput, scapula, buttocks and heels cannot contact the wall simultaneously.
- *Blood tests*—seronegative for rheumatoid factor.
- *Radiology*—chest X-ray and MRI scan assess changes in the spine.

TREATMENT:

- *Conservative*—patient education, refer to physiotherapy
- *Medicinal*—analgesia (NSAIDs) and DMARDs, e.g. sulfasalazine (first line)
- *Surgery*—corrective spinal surgery

COMPLICATIONS:

- Osteoporosis
- Spinal fractures
- Increased risk of cardiovascular disease, e.g. stroke and MI

SPINAL STENOSIS

This is a narrowing of the spinal canal, which results in compression of the spinal cord and corresponding nerves. The level at which the spine is affected will produce different symptoms.

CAUSES:

The cause of spinal stenosis may be congenital or acquired. These are outlined below.

- *Congenital causes*: osteopetrosis, achondroplasia, shortened pedicles, Morquio syndrome (mucopolysaccharidosis type IV).
- *Aquired causes*: trauma, degenerative arthritis, space occupying lesion.

SYMPTOMS:

- In the cervical spine: nerve root compression resulting in radicular symptoms or spinal cord compression resulting in myelopathy.
- In the lumbar spine: unilateral or bilateral leg symptoms including neurogenic claudication, myelopathy, radiculopathy as well as altered reflexes.
- Unilateral or bilateral leg pain +/– back pain, which is usually of gradual onset.
- Numbness and weakness that worsens with walking.
- Pain relieved by sitting and leaning forwards.

INVESTIGATIONS:

- Thorough physical examination.
- *Radiology*—MRI is the gold standard investigation. Other investigations include CT (or CT myelogram if patient has an MRI incompatible pacemaker).

TREATMENT:

- *Conservative*—physiotherapy
- *Medicinal*—effective analgesia
- *Surgical*—laminectomy, surgical decompression +/– fusion

COMPLICATIONS:

- Paralysis
- Incontinence
- Difficulty balancing

HIP PATHOLOGY

NECK-OF-FEMUR FRACTURE

- Fractures may be defined as a discontinuity of bone and, where the proximal femur is concerned, it usually occurs in the elderly and is more common in women.
- Neck of femur fractures may be defined as extra-capsular or intra-capsular. Intra-capsular fractures are further subdivided into subcapital, transcervical or basicervical types, whereas extra-capsular fractures may be categorised as inter-trochanteric and

sub-trochanteric. There is a high risk of avascular necrosis with intra-capsular fractures due to the anatomy of the blood supply. The blood supply of the head of femur is from:

1. The medial femoral circumflex artery
2. The lateral femoral circumflex artery
3. The artery of the ligamentum teres

CAUSES:

- Osteoporosis
- Trauma

SYMPTOMS:

- Pain
- Shortening of the affected leg
- External rotation of the affected leg

INVESTIGATIONS:

- Routine pre-op blood tests
- *Radiology*—X-ray
- Garden classification is used to describe femoral neck fractures:
  - *Type I*—undisplaced and incomplete fracture
  - *Type II*—undisplaced but complete fracture
  - *Type III*—displaced fracture but still bony contact
  - *Type IV*—completely displaced

TREATMENT:

- Extra-capsular fractures
- Dynamic hip screw
- Intra-capsular fractures
  - *Undisplaced*—internal fixation or hemiarthroplasty
  - *Displaced*—hemiarthroplasty or total hip replacement

COMPLICATIONS:

- Avascular necrosis
- Thromboembolism

SLIPPED UPPER FEMORAL EPIPHYSIS (SUFE)

This is a rare condition in which the upper femoral epiphysis slips postero-inferiorly from the femoral neck. It may occur bilaterally in 20% of cases. It is very difficult to diagnose.

CAUSES:

- Cartilaginous physis failure
- Risk factors include
  - Obesity
  - Male sex
  - Endocrine imbalances, e.g. hypothyroidism, decreased sex hormones

SYMPTOMS:

- *Pain*—tends to be localised to the knee and thigh. This is often coupled with the inability to weight bear.
- Decreased leg abduction, increased adduction, slight leg shortening and external rotation
- Loss of internal rotation

INVESTIGATIONS:

- *Radiology*—X-ray
- Severity assessed using the Southwick angle

TREATMENT:

- External in situ pinning or open reduction and pinning

COMPLICATIONS:

- Chondrolysis
- Deformity
- Osteoarthritis
- *Avascular necrosis*—high risk from reduction of SUFE

DEVELOPMENTAL DYSPLASIA OF THE HIP (DDH)

This ranges from mild dysplasia to irreducible dislocation due to a developmental deformation of the hip joint. Females are affected more than males. The condition may be bilateral.

CAUSES:

The exact cause of this condition is unknown, but several risk factors have been identified such as:

- Female sex
- First-born child
- Breech delivery
- Oligohydramnios
- Positive family history
- *Ethnicity*—Caucasian and North American Indians
- Twins

DDH IS ASSOCIATED WITH:

- Congenital talipes equinovarus
- Torticollis
- Metatarsus adductus

SYMPTOMS:

- Asymptomatic
- Asymmetric gluteal skin folds
- Reduced abduction (difficult to put nappy on)
- Clicking/clunking hips
- Limp

INVESTIGATIONS:

- DDH screening.
- Ortolani's and Barlow's tests. These are screening tests. They are done at birth and 6-week checks for all UK infants. If suspicion of DDH, referral to orthopaedics and USS to confirm.
- *Radiology*—USS.

TREATMENT:

Depends on age of diagnosis.

- *Closed reduction*—Pavlik harness/hip spica to immobilise—not necessarily involving a reduction. If dislocated, reduce and immobilise.
- *Open reduction*—derotation varus osteotomy, Salter osteotomy.

COMPLICATIONS:

- Gait abnormalities
- Limb shortening
- External rotation of the foot

PERTHES DISEASE

This is also known as Legg–Calve–Perthes disease and is osteonecrosis of the femoral head resulting in deformation of the epiphysis (fragmentation and flattening). There are three phases in the disease process:

1. *Initial*—crescent-shaped femoral head
2. *Resorption*—rarefaction (Gage's sign on X-ray)
3. *Reparative*

CAUSES:

- Unknown. Some risk factors associated with the condition include; positive family history, HIV infection (AVN of the hip), thrombophilias, inherited coagulopathies (e.g. Factor V Leiden), low birth weight.

SYMPTOMS:

- Child with a limp (boys affected more than girls)
- Hip pain which may radiate to the knee and groin
- Decreased range of hip movement. Patients often have reduced internal rotation and abduction of the hip and there may be a leg length discrepancy

INVESTIGATIONS:

- *Radiology*—X-ray. May show several features, for example:
  A—Abnormal physeal growth
  B—Bone density increased at epiphysis
  C—Calcification lateral to epiphysis, **C**rescent sign (subchondral fracture)

TREATMENT:

- *Conservative*—physiotherapy, brace, traction
- *Medicinal*—adequate analgesia
- *Surgical*—femoral +/– pelvic osteotomy

COMPLICATIONS:

- Gait abnormalities
- Arthritis
- Age range usually affected by pathologies:
  - *DDH*—infants
  - *Perthes*—3–10 years
  - *SUFE*—adolescents

KNEE PATHOLOGY

Knee Pathology

Pathology	Cause	Symptoms	Investigations	Treatment	Complications
Anterior cruciate ligament (ACL) tear	The function of the ACL is to: 1. Prevent backwards displacement of the femur on the tibia 2. Prevent rotation 3. Prevent hyperextension Any type of trauma that involves twisting of a slightly flexed knee, e.g. football injuries, or over-extension of the knee can damage the ACL Females (post-puberty) are more likely to damage their ACL than males. The reason for this is debated but is potentially due to: • Hormones—which cause laxity of ligaments • A narrower intercondylar notch • A larger Q angle in women	Pain Knee swelling Hearing or feeling a "pop"	Anterior draw test positive/ Lachman test positive Pivot shift test Radiology: • *X-ray*—rule out fracture • *MRI*—confirms diagnosis	Conservative—employ "**RICE**" techniques: **R**—Rest **I**—Ice **C**—Compression **E**—Elevation physiotherapy, knee brace Medical—analgesia Surgical—ACL reconstruction	Knee instability Osteoarthritis Complications relating to surgery such as the general complications of anaesthesia, infection, DVT, damage to surrounding structures Other complications include missed concomitant injuries, tunnel malposition, patellar fracture and complications related to graft harvest

Pathology	Cause	Symptoms	Investigations	Treatment	Complications
Posterior cruciate ligament (PCL) tear	The function of the PCL is to prevent forwards displacement of the femur on the tibia Injury to the PCL is very rare. It tends to occur in road traffic accident dashboard injuries	Pain Knee swelling	Positive posterior draw test Radiology: • X-ray—rule out fracture • MRI— confirm diagnosis	Conservative—employ "**RICE**" techniques: **R**—**R**est **I**—**I**ce **C**—**C**ompression **E**—**E**levation physiotherapy, knee brace Medical—analgesia Surgical—PCL reconstruction	Knee instability Osteoarthritis Complications relating to surgery such as the general complications of anaesthesia, infection, DVT, damage to surrounding structures Other complications related to PCL reconstruction include neurovascular injury, compartment syndrome, posterior laxity, osteonecrosis and heterotopic ossification
Meniscal tears	The medial meniscus is torn more frequently than the lateral meniscus. The reason for this rests in anatomical differences. The medial meniscus is firmly attached to both the medial collateral ligament and the joint capsule. The lateral meniscus is still "C"-shaped, but more circular. It is also thinner Trauma as a result of twisting is the common mechanism of injury. Tears may be categorised as complete or incomplete The combination of a medial meniscus tear, medial collateral ligament tear and a torn ACL is known as O'Donoghue's unhappy triad	Knee locking Giving way of the knee Pain Swelling Decreased range of movement	Positive McMurray test Radiology: • X-ray—rule out fracture • MRI— confirms diagnosis Arthroscopy can also confirm	Conservative—employ "**RICE**" techniques: **R**—**R**est **I**—**I**ce **C**—**C**ompression **E**—**E**levation physiotherapy, knee brace Medical—analgesia Surgical—depends on the location and the extent of the tear. If located in the outer third of the meniscus, also known as the "red zone", the tear will heal on its own since this is a region of copious blood supply. However, if located in the inner two-thirds, the "white zone", patients may require surgical intervention	Knee instability Osteoarthritis
Osgood–Schlatter disease	This is a tibial tuberosity apophysitis that typically affects athletic males aged 10–15 years The exact cause is not known but overuse is thought to play a role	Pain, swelling and tenderness of the tibial tuberosity Difficulty jumping/kneeling	Usually a clinical diagnosis Radiology— X-ray may show signs of tuberosity enlargement	Conservative—rest, physiotherapy, knee brace Medical—analgesia	Unlikely to cause serious complications, but pain may persist

(Continued)

Knee Pathology   (Continued)

Pathology	Cause	Symptoms	Investigations	Treatment	Complications
Osteochondritis dissecans	This is a partial or complete detachment of either bone or articular cartilage caused by avascular necrosis of the subchondral bone. It results in microfracture without remodelling. Other causes include: • Genetics • Repetitive minor trauma • Drugs, e.g. steroids	Pain—worsens with exercise Swelling Locking and giving way	Radiology: • X-ray to rule out fracture • MRI confirms diagnosis Anderson staging criteria are employed	Conservative—watchful waiting, rest Medical—analgesia Surgical—arthroscopy, osteochondral autograft transplantation	Osteoarthritis
Patellar subluxation syndrome	Exact cause is unknown, but some factors have been suggested such as • Gait abnormalities • Shallow patellar groove • Wide pelvis More common in women	Knee that gives way or locks during movement Sliding and highly mobile patella Pain—when sitting and worsens with movement Swelling	Radiology—X-ray, MRI	Conservative—physiotherapy, braces, orthotics Medical—analgesia Surgical—medial patellofemoral ligament reconstruction. This ligament may tear when the patella dislocates outwards	Knee instability Recurrent subluxation or dislocation

Notes: The knee is susceptible to both primary and secondary osteoarthritis, but the stability of the knee rests upon intra- and extra-articular ligaments and menisci, which are susceptible to injury.

FOOT PATHOLOGY

Foot Pathology

Pathology	Cause	Symptoms	Investigations	Treatment	Complications
Hallux valgus (bunion)	The exact cause is unknown, but it is associated with: • Female sex • Positive family history • Increased age • Wearing heels	The hallux deviates laterally at the MTP joint Pain Erythematous, irritated skin overlying the bunion	Thorough physical examination including an assessment of gait Radiology—X-ray will visualise the deformity	Conservative—appropriate footwear Medical—analgesia Surgery—only indicated if there is severe pain or if the deformity significantly impacts on walking/quality of life. There are different types of operative techniques. Examples include the scarf osteotomy and the Chevron osteotomy	Osteoarthritis Complications relating to surgery such as infection, DVT, damage to surrounding structures, overcorrection and undercorrection

Pathology	Cause	Symptoms	Investigations	Treatment	Complications
Pes planus	Collapse of the medial longitudinal arch	Asymptomatic Pain—over the tibialis posterior tendon Progressed disease—inability to raise heel Forefoot— abducted Hindfoot—valgus	Paediatrics—foot proforma Thorough physical examination including an assessment of gait Radiology—X-ray may help evaluate the extent of the deformity	Most are asymptomatic and do not require treatment Conservative— orthotics, physiotherapy, e.g. Achilles tendon stretching Surgery—in severe cases and aims to realign the foot • Example operations include Achilles tendon lengthening, tibialis posterior tendon reconstruction and reconstructive osteotomies	Tibialis posterior tendon dysfunction May contribute to other foot conditions such as hallux valgus and plantar fasciitis
Pes cavus	The exact cause of the accentuated longitudinal arch in this condition is unknown but is associated with conditions such as: • Cerebral palsy • Spina bifida • Muscular dystrophy • Charcot–Marie– Tooth disease	Pain on walking Claw toes Ankle instability	Thorough physical examination including an assessment of gait Radiology—X-ray may help evaluate the extent of the deformity	Conservative— orthotics, physiotherapy Surgery—plantar fascia release, Jones procedure, extensor shift procedure, Girdlestone–Taylor transfer, peroneus longus to peroneus brevis tenodesis	Complications relating to surgery such as infection, DVT, damage to surrounding structures, malunion Other complications include incomplete healing of the bone, recurrence of deformity and incomplete correction of the deformity
Stress fracture	Fractures tend to affect the shaft of the second or third metatarsal since these are less robust than the other metatarsal bones.	Pain on walking and over the metatarsal	Radiology—X-ray	Conservative—rest, plaster cast may be required Medical—analgesia Surgery — fracture fixation may be required depending on the fracture pattern	Complications of fracture e.g. non-union Osteoarthritis
Talipes equinovarus (club foot)	The exact cause of this condition is unknown, but it is associated with: • A positive family history • DDH • Oligohydramnios • Spina bifida	Inverted and supinated foot Adducted forefoot Inwardly rotated heel held in plantarflexion	USS during pregnancy Diagnosis based on typical appearance Investigate underlying cause	Ponseti method May require surgery later if Ponseti method fails	Gait abnormality Arthritis Smaller shoe size of affected foot

ORTHOPAEDIC INFECTIONS

SEPTIC ARTHRITIS

This is infection of any joint by a micro-organism. It is a surgical emergency.

CAUSES:

The exact mechanism by which the organism invades the joint is unknown. Spread may be systemic, from a penetrating wound or from prior osteomyelitis.

Causative organisms include:

- *S. aureus* (commonest)
- *Neisseria gonorrhoeae*
- *Haemophilus influenzae*
- *Pneumococcus*
- Group B streptococci
- *E. coli*
- *Pseudomonas*
- *Proteus*
- Fungi

SEPTIC ARTHRITIS IS ASSOCIATED WITH:

- Diabetes mellitus
- IV drug abuse
- Trauma
- Joint replacement surgery
- Extremes of age, i.e. the very young/old

SYMPTOMS:

- The characteristic patient presents with a red-hot, swollen, immobile joint.
- General features of infection—spiking pyrexia, malaise.
- Decreased range of movement of affected joint.
- Inflammation and pain of affected joint.

INVESTIGATIONS:

- *Blood tests*—FBC, WCC, U&Es, CRP, blood cultures, uric acid to exclude gout
- *Specific tests*—joint aspiration and culture
- *Radiology*
  - X-ray of joint (and chest if TB suspected).
  - USS—allows diagnostic joint aspiration. Most joints may be aspirated without USS, except the hip, which needs to be done in theatre with X-ray present to confirm needle placement. If the joint is prosthetic, aspiration must be done in a sterile environment, i.e. theatre.

TREATMENT:

This must be done without delay since septic arthritis is an emergency.

SURGERY:

Joint aspiration and surgical washout followed by antibiotics sensitive to causative organism.

COMPLICATIONS:

- Joint destruction
- Secondary osteoarthritis
- Fibrous ankylosis
- *In children*—growth disruption

OSTEOMYELITIS

This is a bacterial infection of the bone, which may be spread to the bone haematogenously, traumatically or from infection of soft tissue. It may have an acute or chronic presentation. Osteomyelitis of long bones may be classified by the Cierny-Mader classification. The Cierny-Mader classification is based on anatomic, clinical, and radiologic features. Anatomical stages are as follows; Stage 1: Disease confined to the medullary region of the bone, Stage 2: Superficial disease, Stage 3: Localised spread and Stage 4: Diffuse disease.

Clinical aspects of the classification system define host health into the following categories:

A: Normal host, B1 (systemic): Host with systemic compromising factors, B2 (local): Host with local compromising factors,

B3 (systemic and local): Host with both local and systemic compromising factors and C: Host for whom treatment of osteomyelitis is worse than the disease itself.

Examples of systemic compromising factors are malnutrition, renal and hepatic failure and diabetes mellitus. Examples of host local compromising factors are chronic lymphoedema, venous stasis, peripheral neuropathy, and smoking.

CAUSES:

Causative organisms include:

- *S. aureus* (commonest)—adhesin permits attachment of *S. aureus* to bone cartilage
- *H. influenzae* (more common in children)
- *Salmonella* (more common in patients with sickle cell disease)

OSTEOMYELITIS IS ASSOCIATED WITH:

- Diabetes mellitus
- IV drug abuse
- Extremes of age, i.e. the very young/old
- Sickle cell disease
- Immunocompromise
- *Chronic osteomyelitis*—smoking, steroid use and vascular disease

SYMPTOMS:

- *General features of infection*—pyrexia, malaise
- Decreased range of movement of affect joint
- Inflammation and pain of affected joint

INVESTIGATIONS:

- *Blood tests*—FBC, WCC, U&Es, CRP, ESR, blood cultures, uric acid to exclude gout
- *Specific tests*—joint aspiration and culture. Histopathology in acute osteomyelitis shows microorganisms, neutrophils and congested blood vessels. In chronic osteomyelitis histology findings include mononuclear cells, fibrous tissue and sinus tract formation.
- *Radiology*
  - X-ray of joint (no abnormal features in the first 10–14 days)
  - USS—allows diagnostic joint aspiration
  - CT—may be used to guide needle aspiration
  - MRI

TREATMENT:

- *Conservative*—splintage, rehabilitation and physiotherapy
- *Medicinal*—IV antibiotics (in all cases) Follow local hospital microbiology advice but usually parenteral targeted antibiotic therapy is required for at least 6 weeks

SURGERY:

- Guided aspiration and surgical evacuation
- Amputation

COMPLICATIONS:

- Joint destruction
- Chronic osteoarthritis
- Septic arthritis
- Pathological fracture
- *In children*—growth disruption from growth plate damage

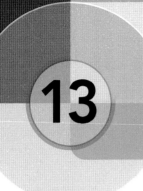

Paediatric Surgery

The best indicator of shock in paediatric patients is tachycardia.

DIFFERENTIALS FOR NON-BILIOUS VOMITING IN CHILDREN

PYLORIC STENOSIS

Presents between weeks 3 and 6 of life, projectile vomiting, palpable olive-shaped mass in the abdomen, dehydrated, characteristic metabolic disturbance is hypochloraemic, hypokalaemic, metabolic alkalosis and a paradoxical aciduria. The exact cause of pyloric stenosis is unknown. There is hypertrophy as well as hyperplasia of the pyloric circular and longitudinal muscle layers. Eventually symptoms of gastric outlet obstruction result. It has been associated with exposure to macrolide antibiotics in the postnatal period. Other factors that are associated with increased risk include preterm birth, bottle feeding and c-section delivery.

- USS—pylorus >4 mm thick and >14 mm long. One may see a "target sign" and the absence of gastric emptying.

MANAGEMENT:

This is a medical emergency and as such, the first step is resuscitation in line with local guidance and correction of any metabolic disturbance. Surgical management is pyloromyotomy.

TRACHEOOESOPHAGEAL FISTULA

Tracheooesophageal fistulas are a common congenital abnormality. Infants may present with feeding difficulties or with respiratory distress. The exact cause of the condition is unknown, although defects in the sonic hedgehog gene have been implicated. It has been postulated that during development there is an abnormality in mesenchymal proliferation that results in a fistula to form between the respiratory and digestive tracts. Five different types. Type A and type C are the most tested in the exam setting.

- Type C is the commonest. Upper portion of oesophagus ends in a blind pouch. Lower end is connected to the trachea via fistula.
- Type A is the only type without a tracheal–oesophageal fistula.

DOI: 10.1201/9781003292005-16

INVESTIGATIONS:

- Abdominal X-ray.
- Type C—there will be gas present with a distended stomach. This will not be the case in type A.
- Associated with VACTERL i.e. Vertebral defects, Anorectal anomalies, Cardiac defects, Tracheo-oesphageal fistula/oesophageal atresia, Renal anomalies and Limb hypoplasia.

TREATMENT:

Resuscitation, double-lumen tube to suck out saliva and keep oesophagus patent.

SURGERY:

Open surgical repair of TOF involves a right postero-lateral thoracotomy, fistula ligation and the creation of a primary oesophageal anastomosis.

COMPLICATIONS OF REPAIR:

Stricture, fistula, GORD, leak.

INTUSSUSCEPTION

When part of the bowel telescopes into itself.

CAUSE:

Often unknown. It can occur post viral illness, with inflammation of a Peyer's patch acting as the pathological lead point. Associated with cystic fibrosis, leukaemia, Meckel's diverticulum and intestinal polyps.

SYMPTOMS:

The main signs are bilious or non-bilious vomiting and abdominal pain. Others include redcurrant jelly stools and small-bowel obstruction.

INVESTIGATIONS:

USS (target sign).

MANAGEMENT:

Initial resuscitation, then either enema reduction, or laparoscopic reduction.

DIFFERENTIALS FOR BILIOUS VOMITING IN CHILDREN

MALROTATION +/– MIDGUT VOLVULUS

This occurs due to the failure of normal 270° rotation during intestinal development and Ladd's bands. Usually occurs during the first year of life. It is associated with congenital diaphragmatic hernias. (For details regarding diaphragmatic hernias, please refer to the Anatomy section and further details later in this chapter). The exact cause of malrotation remains unclear however, the BCL6 gene plays an important role in directing intestinal rotation during development. Thus, defects in this gene may be implicated in the development of this pathology.

MANAGEMENT:

- *Ladd's procedure*—the steps are:
  - Laparoscopy or laparotomy to gain access
  - Untwist volvulus anti-clockwise
  - Divide Ladd's bands
  - Straighten duodenum
  - Caecum fixation in LUQ

DUODENAL ATRESIA

This is the commonest cause of duodenal obstruction in neonates. Neonates may present with bilious or non-bilious vomiting in the first few days of life. Diagnosis is sometimes made during antenatal scans and is associated with polyhydramnios.

CAUSE:

- Failure of recanalisation. Duodenal recanalisation typically occurs during week 8 – 10 of embryological development. Associated with polyhydramnios, cardiac, GI anomalies and Down's syndrome.

INVESTIGATIONS:

- *AXR*—double bubble sign

MANAGEMENT:

- Resuscitation, duodenoduodenostomy.

MECONIUM ILEUS

No meconium passes in the first 24 hours. Associated with cystic fibrosis (diagnosed via sweat chloride test or Guthrie heelprick test) and Hirschsprung's disease.

MANAGEMENT:

Resuscitation, gastrograffin enema, N-acetylcysteine enema.

HIRSCHSPRUNG'S DISEASE

Congenital disorder characterised by the absence of ganglion cells at the Meissner's plexus (submucosa) and Auerbach's plexus (muscularis) of the terminal rectum that extends proximally to a variable distance. *Often starts with non-bilious vomiting progressing to bilious (as with any low intestinal obstruction in paediatrics).* The exact cause is unknown, but there is an association with proto-oncogene RET mutations. It is more common in males and histopathologic examination of an aganglionic rectal biopsy confirms the diagnosis.

MANAGEMENT:

Resect the aganglionic colon +/– ostomy +/– anastomosis.

CYSTIC FIBROSIS

This is an autosomal recessive condition that occurs in 1 in 2,500 live births and has a carrier rate of 1 in 25. It occurs due to a deletion in phenylalanine, meaning that an abnormal cystic fibrosis transmembrane conductance regulator (CFTR) protein is then created. This, in turn, decreases Cl^- ion transport, resulting in thickened dehydrated secretions.

CAUSES:

It is caused by a deletion in phenylalanine, most commonly at position 508 on chromosome 7.

SYMPTOMS:

Symptomology can vary with age.

- *Neonate*—meconium ileus. Most are diagnosed via Guthrie heelprick test. Genetic testing is available for prospective parents where one has CF.
- *Young child*
  - Failure to thrive
  - Frequent chest infection
  - Steatorrhoea
  - Signs of clubbing commence
- *Older child*
  - Frequent chest infections
  - Asthma
  - Allergic bronchopulmonary aspergillosis
  - Steatorrhoea
- *Adulthood*
  - As per older child
  - Bronchiectasis
  - Infertility
  - Diabetes
  - Cor pulmonale
  - Depression
  - Cirrhosis

INVESTIGATIONS:

Depend on age of patient and when the disease presents.

- Specific tests—Guthrie heelprick
- All babies—immunoreactive trypsinogen (IRT)
- Sweat test
  - Cl^- >50 mmol/L
  - Na^+ >60 mmol/L

- Blood tests with every acute exacerbation—FBC, U&E, LFT
- Sputum and blood cultures
- Identify cause of infection using sputum analysis. Common organisms include *Staphylococcus aureus*, *Haemophilus influenzae* and *Pseudomonas aeruginosa*
- *Radiology*—chest X-ray
- *Bronchiectasis*—"tram tracks"
- Consolidation
- Fibrosis

TREATMENT:

- *Conservative*
  - Parent education, e.g. keep children with CF separate to avoid cross-infection
  - Continual monitoring with MDT involvement
  - Up-to-date immunisations
  - Physiotherapy sputum clearance techniques, with or without adjuncts such as PEP (positive expiratory pressure) devices
- *Medicinal*—treat infections according to cultural sensitivities. Consult microbiology and hospital guidelines. Some examples are given below:
  - Piperacillin in combination with tazobactam
  - Tobramycin
  - Meropenem
  - Imipenem
  - Pancreatic enzyme supplements, e.g. Creon
  - Fat-soluble vitamins

COMPLICATIONS:

- Increased frequency of respiratory tract infections
- Bronchiectasis
- Respiratory failure
- Infertility
- Diabetes
- Gallstones
- Cor pulmonale
- Malnutrition
- Nasal polyps
- Depression

DIFFERENTIALS FOR BLOODY STOOLS

1. *Intussusception*—redcurrant jelly stools.
2. *Necrotising enterocolitis*—usually premature babies, septic, abdominal distension.
   - *AXR*—pneumatosis, free air, portal venous gas, look for perforation.
   - *Management*—resuscitation, septic six, stop enteral feeding, TPN, surgical resection +/− exteriorisation of bowel surgery if free air and peritonitis/deteriorating clinical.

3. *Meckel's diverticulum*—incomplete obliteration of the vitelline (omphalomesenteric) duct.
   a. The "rule of two's":
      - It is the most common congenital GI anomaly which occurs in about **2%** of infants.
      - It usually measures **two** inches long.
      - It is located in the ileum approximately **two** feet from the ileocecal valve.
      - It is **twice** as common in males.
      - It can contain **two** types of tissue (gastric or pancreatic. Gastric tissue is more likely to bleed since it produces acid which irritates bowel mucosa).
   b. *Management*—may need resuscitation, surgical excision.

ABDOMINAL WALL DEFECTS

The two main types to be aware of are omphalocele and gastroschisis. The differences between the two are summarised herein.

OMPHALOCELE

This is a protrusion of the abdominal contents covered with peritoneum through the base of the umbilical cord.

CAUSE:

Defect in abdominal wall development. The bowel herniates at the normal gestational time but does not return to the abdominal cavity. The bowel usually herniates at week 6 gestation and returns at week 12 gestation.

ASSOCIATIONS:

About 50% of these infants also have a chromosomal disorder. Some associations include Beckwith–Wiedemann syndrome and trisomies 13, 18 and 21.

GASTROSCHISIS

The intestinal protrusion is usually to the right of the midline, and there is no involvement of the umbilical cord.

CAUSE:

- The exact cause is unknown although it is thought to be due to in utero rupture of the umbilical vein or compromise to the omphalomesenteric artery. This in turn results in ischaemia to and therefore, weakness of the abdominal wall. It may be diagnosed during antenatal scans and is associated with an elevated serum AFP. Some other risk factors associated with the development of gastroschisis include; nitrosamine exposure, aspirin exposure, tobacco exposure, young maternal age (<20 y) and Hispanic ethnicity.
- Characterised by free-floating bowel loops without peritoneal cover.

The following table summarises the differences between omphalocele and gastroschisis.

Differences between Omphalocele and Gastroschisis

Characteristic	Omphalocele	Gastroschisis
Position	Central	Right
Hernia sac	Present	Absent
Present with other hernia	Yes	Rarely
Associated with other anomalies	Yes	Rarely
Present with intestinal problems	Infrequently	More frequently

HAEMOLYTIC URAEMIC SYNDROME (HUS)

This is a syndrome that predominantly affects children.

CAUSES:

Usually *E. coli* O157:H7 or *Shigella enteritis*. These organisms enter the body via contaminated food or water. Then, they express viratoxins, which cause damage by binding to glomerular endothelial cells resulting in renal insufficiency, destruction of red blood cells leading to anaemia and platelet damage.

SYMPTOMS:

Symptoms comprise a triad. Remember as "**MAT**":

M—**M**icroangiopathic haemolytic anaemia
A—**A**cute kidney injury
T—**T**hrombocytopaenia

OTHER SYMPTOMS INCLUDE:

- Nausea
- Vomiting
- Bloody diarrhoea
- Abdominal pain
- NO FEVER

INVESTIGATIONS:

- Stool culture
- Urinalysis and eGFR
- *Blood tests*—FBC, U&E, LFT, Cr:BUN, LDH
- *Peripheral blood smear*—schistocytes

TREATMENT:

- *Conservative*
  - Involve the nephrologists and haematologists.
  - HUS is a notifiable disease in the UK.
  - Patient and parent education.
  - Monitor BP.

- *Medicinal*
  - Treatment is generally supportive.
  - Hydrate patient with IV fluids.
  - If hypertension is present, then consider calcium channel blockers.
  - Consider dialysis and RBC transfusion if needed.

COMPLICATIONS:

- Remember as "**ABCS**":

  A—**A**cute kidney injury
  B—increased **B**lood pressure
  C—**C**hronic kidney injury
  C—**C**ardiac complications, e.g. heart failure
  C—**C**oma
  S—**S**troke

HENOCH–SCHÖNLEIN PURPURA (HSP)

This is a systemic vasculitis that presents with a classic cluster of symptoms/signs.

CAUSES:

HSP is caused by IgA complex deposition in the capillaries, arterioles and venules in organs such as the skin and the kidneys. This deposition causes symptoms via the activation of complement.

SYMPTOMS:

It is comprised of a triad. Remember as **RAP**:

R—**R**enal manifestations:

- *Haematuria*—microscopic/macroscopic.
- ANCA negative glomerulonephritis.
- Nephrotic syndrome (rare).

A—**A**rthralgia and abdominal pain.

P—**P**urpura:

- This typically affects the buttocks and the lower limbs. However, it may affect the arms.

INVESTIGATIONS:

- Urinalysis and eGFR
- *Blood* tests—FBC, U&E, LFT, Cr:BUN, LDH, CRP, ESR
- IgA levels
- Skin biopsy if indicated or if there is diagnostic uncertainty:
  - Immunofluorescence shows IgA deposits and C3

TREATMENT:

- *Conservative*
  - Patient and parent education.

- *Medicinal*
  - Treatment is generally supportive due to high rates of spontaneous remission.
  - Analgesia.
  - Steroids may sometimes be used in severe cases.

COMPLICATIONS:

Remember as **ABC**:

A—**A**cute kidney injury
B—**B**owel obstruction, intussusception
C—**C**hronic kidney injury

CHILDHOOD CANCERS

Commonly Tested Childhood Cancers

Disease	Cause	Symptoms	Investigations	Treatment	Complications
Acute lymphoblastic leukaemia (ALL)	A rare neoplasm of the blood/bone marrow. The exact cause is unknown, but it is likely due to a genetic susceptibility coupled with an environmental trigger. It is the commonest cancer in children. Associated with Down's syndrome.	Bone marrow failure Bruising Shortness of breath Purpura Malaise Weight loss Night sweats	Blood tests—FBC, WCC, platelets, U&Es, LFT, ESR, CRP Bone marrow biopsy, lymph node biopsy Radiology—X-ray, ultrasound scan, CT scan, MRI ALL is classified using the French–American–British (FAB) classification	To induce remission: • Dexamethasone • Vincristine • Anthracycline antibiotics • Cyclophosphamide Maintenance: • Methotrexate • Mercaptopurine • Cytarabine • Hydrocortisone	Death Often spreads to the central nervous system Increased risk of infection Haemorrhage Depression Complications of chemotherapy
Neuroblastoma	This is a neuroendocrine tumour arising from neuroblast cells within the sympathetic nervous system. Neuroblastomas mostly originate in the adrenal glands but may develop anywhere along the sympathetic nervous system. It is the most common extracranial solid tumour of infancy. The exact cause of neuroblastoma is unknown, but *ALK* mutations have been identified in familial cases. About 50–60% present with metastases.	Symptoms differ depending on the location of the lesion. General symptoms: • Weight loss • Anorexia • Emesis Abdomen: • Abdominal pain • Swelling Chest: • Respiratory difficulty Bone/bone marrow: • Bone pain • Limpness Paraspinal cord ganglia results in neurological symptoms such as: • Weakness • Paralysis • Bladder dysfunction • Bowel dysfunction Rare symptoms: • Hypertension (renal artery compression) • Chronic diarrhoea (vasoactive intestinal peptide secretion)	Blood tests: FBC, WCC, platelets, U&Es, LFTs, TFTs, ESR, CRP, calcium, magnesium, phosphorus, uric acid, LDH, IgG levels Increased levels of urine catecholamines (or their metabolites e.g. homovanillic acid/ vanillylmandelic acid) Radiology—CT scan, meta-iodobenzylguanidine scan Histology—Homer Wright rosettes Neuroblastomas are classified using the International Neuroblastoma Staging System (INSS)	Treatment depends on the stage of the tumour and is delivered by a multidisciplinary team Medicine—common combinations include: • Vincristine, cyclophosphamide and doxorubicin • Cisplatin and etoposide • Carboplatin and etoposide • Ifosfamide and etoposide • Cyclophosphamide and topotecan Surgery: • Surgical resection in localised disease is curative • Surgery post-chemotherapy may be seen as a debulking procedure	Relapse and recurrent disease Metastasis Paraneoplastic syndromes, e.g. opsoclonus myoclonus syndrome Complications of chemotherapy

(Continued)

Commonly Tested Childhood Cancers   (Continued)

Disease	Cause	Symptoms	Investigations	Treatment	Complications
Wilms tumour	AKA nephrobastoma, is a form of renal cancer that occurs in children. It is associated with aniridia. Nephroblastomas are mostly unilateral. It is associated with WT1 gene mutations (chromosome 11p13) in 20% cases. Syndromes associated with Wilms tumours: • Denys–Drash syndrome • Frasier syndrome • Sporadic aniridia • Li–Fraumeni syndrome	Abdominal swelling Abdominal pain Haematuria Nausea Vomiting	Blood tests—FBC, WCC, platelets, U&Es, LFTs, ESR, CRP, BUN Urinalysis Radiology—abdominal USS, abdominal X-ray, chest X-ray, CT abdomen, MRI scan, IV pyelogram	Treatment depends on the stage and size of the tumour as well as histopathological and molecular tumour features Some standard therapy regimes are: Chemotherapy: • Vincristine and dactinomycin • Vincristine, dactinomycin and doxorubicin • Vincristine, doxorubicin, cyclophosphamide and etoposide Radiotherapy Surgery: • Nephrectomy	Metastasis Hypertension, particularly if bilateral renal involvement
Ewing's sarcoma	This is a rare, malignant, small round blue cell tumour affecting the bone/soft tissue. It typically affects teenagers and young adults. Usually a result of t(11; 22) translocations resulting in a *EWSR1/FLI1* fusion gene The most common regions affected are: • Pelvis • Femur • Humerus • Ribs • Clavicle	Pain in the location of the tumour, which worsens over time A swelling in the location of the tumour Swelling and decreased range of movement of the affected joint Fever of unknown origin Unprovoked bone fracture General symptoms such as lethargy and weight loss	Blood tests—FBC, WCC, platelets, U&Es, LFTs, TFTs, ESR, CRP Radiology—X-rays (show "moth-eaten" radiolucency) CT scan, MRI scan, PET scan, bone scintigraphy Histology—small blue round cell tumour. Clear cytoplasm with H&E staining.	Treatment depends on the stage and size of the tumour as well as histopathological features Some therapy regimes are: Chemotherapy: • Ifosfamide and etoposide • Vincristine, doxorubicin and cyclophosphamide Radiotherapy Surgery: • Limb amputation	Metastasis Limb amputation

Ear, Nose and Throat

HEARING LOSS

Hearing loss may be defined as conductive or sensorineural. Each has congenital and acquired causes.

Causes of conductive hearing loss:

- *Congenital:* atresia, abnormality of the ossicles
- *Acquired:* impacted wax, otitis externa, glue ear, perforated drum

Causes of sensorineural hearing loss:

- *Congenital:* infection e.g. rubella, genetics e.g. Alport's syndrome
- *Acquired:* presbycusis, infection e.g. meningitis, trauma e.g. noise injury, tumour e.g. acoustic neuroma, ototoxic drugs e.g. gentamicin, Ménière's disease

GLUE EAR

Glue ear, also known as otitis media with effusion, is a collection of fluid within the middle ear. This fluid is thought to occur due to dysfunctional Eustachian tubes, which create negative pressure. It occurs in males more than females and is more common in children. When present in adults, symptoms are more likely to be unilateral. The commonest complication is persistent otorrhea.

CAUSE:

Exact cause is unknown. It often occurs secondary to a viral upper respiratory tract infection or following repeated episodes of acute bacterial otitis media.

- Risk factors—remember as "**EARS**"

  E—**E**ustachian tube abnormalities, e.g. in Down's syndrome
  A—**A**denoids (enlarged) The thought is that enlarged adenoids obstruct the Eustachian tube. Such obstruction would enable bacterial proliferation and subsequent inflammation.
  R—**R**espiratory infections
  S—**S**moking (usually parents), **S**eason (winter)

DOI: 10.1201/9781003292005-17

CLINICAL FEATURES:

May vary depending on age of child/adult. Bulging drum of varying colour. A fluid level may be present. Often presents as behavioural/developmental issues in young children, which on investigation are found to be due to hearing difficulties. There is opacification of thee tympanic membrane and an absent light reflex.

INVESTIGATIONS:

Audiograms (conductive defects), impedance audiometry.

TREATMENT:

- *Conservative*
  - Often self-limiting
  - Hearing aids only if bilateral symptoms
- *Medicinal*
  - NICE does not recommend antibiotics
- *Surgery*
  - Myringotomy
  - Grommets +/− adenoidectomy

MÉNIÈRE'S DISEASE

Ménière's disease, also known as endolymphatic hydrops, is a cause of sensorineural hearing loss. It is more common in females than males and presents most commonly in middle aged adults.

CAUSES:

It is thought to be caused by dilatation and excessive fluid collection within the endolymphatic spaces.

SYMPTOMS:

Presents with a characteristic triad:

1. Vertigo
2. Low pitch tinnitus
3. Sensorineural hearing loss

Other features include aural fullness, a positive Romberg test and nystagmus.

INVESTIGATIONS:

Clinical diagnosis, but also perform cranial MRI to rule out space-occupying lesions.

- Complete physical examination including neurological examination
- Rinne and Weber tests to show sensorineural hearing loss
- Audiometric evaluation
- Cranial MRI to rule out space-occupying lesion

TREATMENT:

Conservative: Patient education

- *Medicinal*
  - *Acute attacks*—cyclizine or prochlorperazine
  - *Long-term treatment*—betahistine or thiazide diuretics
  - Treat symptoms, e.g. vomiting with buccastem
- *Surgical*
  - Endolymphatic shunts
  - Ototoxic drugs

OTOSCLEROSIS

This is an autosomal dominant condition that typically affects females aged 20–40 years. There are two subtypes; fenestral/stapedial (80%) and retrofenestral/cochlear (20%). The former and more common of the two typically presents with conductive hearing loss whereas the latter may present with sensorineural hearing loss.

CAUSES:

Normal ossicle bone is replaced by vascular bone, which is spongy. The exact cause of this condition is unknown by some aetiologies have been postulated:

- Positive family history in up to 50% of patients
- Persistent embryologic cartilage
- Possible role of oestrogens proposed, which may be why it is more common in females
- Post viral infection

SYMPTOMS:

Conductive hearing loss, tinnitus, flamingo-tinge appearance to the tympanic membrane (Schwart's sign).

INVESTIGATIONS:

- *Audiometry*
  - Rinne and Weber tests—conductive hearing loss (Weber test will lateralise to the affected ear)
  - Audiometry and tympanometry
  - Histology—blue mantles of manasse (new bone formation stains blue on haematoxylin and eosinophil staining).
  - CT scan of the temporal bones
  - The Symons and Fanning CT grading system may be use to further clarify otosclerosis

TREATMENT:

- *Conservative*—patient education
- *Medicinal*—sodium fluoride (efficacy controversial)
- *Surgical*—stapedectomy +/– prosthesis

BENIGN PAROXYSMAL POSITIONAL VERTIGO (BPPV)

This pathology of the inner ear results in the sudden onset of nausea, vertigo and nystagmus upon certain movements of the head.

CAUSES:

- BPPV is thought to be caused by the displacement of otoconia (small calcium carbonate crystals) from the utricle into the semicircular canals. Movement of these crystals along the canal in question stimulates the sensation of rotation.
- There are many factors that contribute to the displacement of otoconia. The commonest is head injury, but others include infection and degeneration attributed to old age.

SYMPTOMS:

- Vertigo
- Nausea
- Light-headedness
- Imbalance
- Nystagmus

The above symptoms are nearly always precipitated by a sudden change in head position such as lying down.

INVESTIGATIONS:

A diagnosis is made depending on symptoms, patient history and examination.

- Dix–Hallpike test—a positive test stimulates bursts of nystagmus
- Undertake vestibular and auditory tests

TREATMENT:

- *Conservative*
  - *Patient education*—said to be a self-limiting condition than may resolve ~2 months after onset.
  - *Epley manoeuvre*—attempts to reposition the displaced otoconia.
- *Medicinal*
  - Anti-emetics for nausea if severe.
- *Surgery*
  - Very rarely performed and should not be considered unless the above methods have failed. Examples include posterior canal plugging.

COMPLICATIONS:

- Dizziness, therefore increased risk of falls.

EPISTAXIS

Epistaxis is the term used for nosebleed. It is very common and there are two major types:

1. *Anterior epistaxis*—most common. Often presents as unilateral nasal bleeding and occurs from the Kiesselbach's plexus (also known as Little's area). Please refer to the Anatomy section.

2. *Posterior epistaxis*—less common but more difficult to manage. Presents with bilateral nasal bleeding and postnasal bleeding into the oropharynx.

CAUSES:

There are many different causes of nosebleeds ranging from the idiopathic to foreign bodies and tumours. Some causes are listed below. Remember as "**EPISTAXIS**":

E—**E**pistaxis past history, e.g. anatomical deformities or hereditary haemorrhagic telangiectasia

P—**P**unch to the face/trauma

I—**I**nflammatory reactions, e.g. recent upper respiratory tract infection

S—**S**ystemic factors, e.g. hypertension

T—**T**hrombocytopenia

A—**A**lcohol, causes vasodilation

X—Factor **X** deficiency

I—**I**ntranasal tumours

S—**S**prays, e.g. prolonged use of nasal steroids

RISK FACTORS:

- Trauma
- Anticoagulation medication
- Hypertension
- Recent upper respiratory tract infection
- History of epistaxis
- Drugs—cocaine use

SYMPTOMS:

- Haemorrhage of varying severity from one or both nostrils
- Presence of blood in the oropharynx

INVESTIGATIONS:

It is essential in all cases to examine both nostrils with a nasal speculum and a pen torch to identify whether bleeding is unilateral or bilateral as well as to identify the source of the bleed. It is also vital to assess whether postnasal bleeding has compromised breathing.

In most acute cases, specific tests are unnecessary. However, recurrent cases require:

- *Blood tests*—FBC, coagulation studies
- *Radiology*—CT scan (if malignancy suspected)
- *Other*—nasopharyngoscopy (if malignancy suspected).

TREATMENT:
- *Conservative*
  - ABCDE—emergency care.
  - Pinch fleshy parts of the nose together and tilt head forwards. Place an ice pack on the bridge of the nose or the back of the neck. Do this for 20–30 minutes.

- *Medicinal*
  - Anterior epistaxis:
    - Adrenaline solution to clean the nose and cause vasoconstriction. Reassess to identify bleed.
    - Silver nitrate sticks—used for nasal cautery if bleeding point is clearly identified. Apply to this point and a small area around it.
      - *Caution*—do not use bilaterally since there is a risk of nasal perforation. Always prescribe Naseptin cream after cautery. This consists of neomycin and chloramphenicol.
      - *Contraindications*—peanut allergy.
    - If bleeding still perfuse after cautery, then consider nasal packing with either (1) rapid rhino, (2) Merocel or (3) BIPP gauze.
  - Posterior epistaxis
    - ENT team required to posteriorly package the nasal cavity with a foley catheter. Anterior packing is applied as well.
- *Surgery*
  - Refer to ENT team for sphenopalatine artery ablation.

COMPLICATIONS:

- Compromise to airway
- Anaemia

NASOPHARYNGEAL CANCER

Nasopharyngeal cancer is typically a squamous cell carcinoma (85%). Other cell types include adenocarcinoma, lymphoma and melanoma. It is more common in Asian populations and in males.

CAUSES:

The exact cause of nasopharyngeal tumours is unknown, but risk factors include:

- *Genetics*—Family clusters (15% of patients have a first-degree relative with the disease). HLA-A, B, C and D haplotypes confer increase risk
- *Infection*—EBV
- *Diet*—nitrosamines and vitamin C deficiency

SYMPTOMS:

Remember as "**NOSE**":

N—**N**eck lump (usually high level V and level II)
O—**O**talgia, nasal, **O**bstruction, Otitis media with effusion
S—**S**ymptoms of spread, e.g. nerve palsies—mandibular nerve, Horner's syndrome.
The most commonly affected cranial nerves are CN V, VI, IX, X and XII
E—**E**pistaxis

INVESTIGATIONS:

- *Blood tests*—FBC, WCC, U&Es, LFTs, ESR, EBV and viral capsid antigen
- *Specific tests*—audiogram, tympanogram and visual fields
- *Radiology*—CT, MRI with TNM classification. Angiography for angiofibroma

TNM Staging for Nasopharyngeal Carcinoma

Category	Description
T1	Tumour confined to nasopharynx, oropharynx or nasal fossa
T2	Tumour extends to parapharyngeal space
T3	Tumour invades bony structures of skull base or paranasal sinuses
T4	Tumour with intracranial extension or involvement of cranial nerves, masticator space, orbit or hypopharynx
N	Regional lymph nodes
N1	Retropharyngeal lymph node, either unilateral or bilateral
N2	Unilateral metastasis in lymph nodes, ≤ 6 cm in greatest dimension, above supraclavicular fossa
N3	Bilateral metastasis in lymph nodes, ≤ 6 cm in greatest dimension, above supraclavicular fossa
N4	Metastasis in lymph nodes, > 6 cm in dimension or in the supraclavicular fossa
M	Distant metastasis
M0	No distant metastasis
M1	Distant metastasis

TREATMENT:

- *Conservative*—patient education, McMillan nurse referral
- *Medicinal*—chemotherapy and radiotherapy
- *Surgical*—for angiofibroma/resection as appropriate post-MDT discussions

Definitive management depends on the stage of the disease and also the nature of treatment intent e.g. curative or palliative. Potential treatment options include the following:

- *Stage I–II*: radiation alone
- *Stage III–IV*: chemotherapy and radiotherapy
- *For persistent disease*: salvage surgery
- *For recurrent disease*: salvage surgery or reirradiation

Contraindications to surgery in nasopharyngeal cancer surgery include: clival erosion and carotid artery encasement.

COMPLICATIONS:

- Metastasis
- Invasion of local structures
- Death
- *Early side effects of radiation*: xerostomia, sinusitis and mucositis
- *Late side effects of radiation*: CN VIII palsy, CN XII palsy and trismus
- *Complications of reirradiation*: temporal lobe necrosis, trismus, transverse myelitis, palatal dysfunction, cranial nerve palsies

OROPHARYNGEAL CANCER

Most oropharyngeal cancers are squamous cell carcinomas (85%). There are two subtypes of SCC to consider. The first is the traditional subtype. This is negative for HPV and mediated by tobacco and alcohol. The spindle cell variant is particularly aggressive and the verrucous subtype tends to be relatively radioresistant. The second subtype is HPV-mediated SCC. HPV 16 is the commonest and this variation tends to affect younger patients. Other cell types of oropharyngeal cancer include; lymphoma (the palatine tonsil is the commonest extranodal site of non-Hodgkin lymphoma), sarcomas (which are rare) and salivary gland neoplasms such as adenoid cystic carcinoma (commonest) or mucoepidermoid carcinoma.

CAUSES:

The exact cause of oropharyngeal tumours is unknown, but risk factors include:

- Smoking/tobacco chewing
- Alcohol
- HPV infection (types 8 and 16)
- Ionising radiation

SYMPTOMS:

- Odynophagia
- Otalgia
- Neck lump
- Trismus
- Sore throat
- Leucoplakia

INVESTIGATIONS:

- *Blood tests*—FBC, WCC, U&Es, LFTs, ESR HPV testing
- *Specific tests*—FNAC of nodes, panendoscopy
- *Radiology*—CT, MRI with TNM classification. USS liver (for metastases). USS +/– fine needle aspiration of primary site and/or lymph node(s)

AJCC (8th Edition) TNM Categories and Definitions for HPV-Associated (p16+) OPSCC

T category*	Criteria
T0	No primary tumour identified
T1	Tumour size ≤ 2 cm in greatest dimension
T2	Tumour size > 2 cm but ≤ 4 cm in greatest dimension
T3	Tumour size > 4 cm in greatest dimension or extension to lingual surface of epiglottis
T4	Moderately advanced tumour invading larynx, extrinsic tongue muscles, medial pterygoid, hard palate, or mandible or beyond
Clinical N category	**Criteria**
Nx	Regional nodes cannot be assessed
N0	No regional nodal metastasis
N1	Metastasis to one or more ipsilateral nodes, ≤ 6 cm
N2	Metastasis to contralateral or bilateral lymph nodes, ≤ 6 cm
N3	Metastasis in any cervical lymph node >6 cm
Pathologic N category	**Criteria**
Nx	Regional nodes cannot be assessed
pN0	No regional nodal metastasis identified
pN1	Metastasis to four or fewer lymph nodes
pN2	Metastasis to five or more lymph nodes
M category	**Criteria**
M0	Absence of distant metastasis
M1	Presence of distant metastasis

* Clinical and pathologic T classification schemes are similar.

Abbreviations: AJCC = American Joint Committee on Cancer; HPV = human papillomavirus; OPSCC = oropharyngeal squamous cell carcinoma.

TREATMENT:

Treatment depends on the cell type and the TNM grading.

- SCC—radiotherapy and surgery There are many different types of surgical approaches depending on the stage of disease, anatomical location of the tumour, structures involved and treatment intent. These are beyond the scope of the MRCS examination but some approaches include; 1. transoral techniques e.g. transoral robotic surgery and 2. open techniques e.g. transhyoid pharyngotomy, lip split with mandibulotomy.
- Carcinoma of the soft palate:
  - *T1/T2*—radiotherapy
  - *T3/T4*—resection
- Posterior pharyngeal wall carcinoma:
  - *T1/2*—radical radiotherapy, resection
- Tonsil carcinoma:
  - *T1/2*—radical radiotherapy, trans-oral surgery
  - *T3/4*—resection +/– dissection and reconstruction
- Post-operative radiotherapy required for nodal involvement.

COMPLICATIONS:

- Metastasis
- Invasion of local structures
- Death

LARYNGEAL CANCER

Laryngeal tumours may be benign or malignant. Tumours may affect different sites of the larynx; the supraglottis (subdivided into the epiglottis, aryepiglottic folds, arytenoids and false vocal folds), the glottis (subdivided into the true vocal folds, anterior commissure, posterior commissure and the ventricle) and the subglottis. Laryngeal cancers tend to spread via the following routes; the paraglottic space, the preepiglottic space and Broyle's tendon (the vocalis tendon insertion into the thyroid cartilage).

MALIGNANT:

Squamous cell carcinomas, adenocarcinomas, sarcoma, verrucous carcinoma, undifferentiated.

BENIGN:

Papillomas, chondromas, lipomas.

CAUSES:

The exact cause of laryngeal tumours is unknown, but risk factors include:

- Age
- Male gender
- Smoking
- Alcohol

SYMPTOMS:

- Cough
- Hoarse voice—recurrent laryngeal nerve involvement
- Lymphadenopathy
- Stridor
- Cough
- Difficulty swallowing
- Referred otalgia
- Nodal/fixed masses in the neck
- Thyroid cartilage tenderness—may indicate tumour extension
- Tenderness superior to the thyroid notch—may indicate pre-epiglottic space invasion

INVESTIGATIONS:

- *Blood tests*—FBC, WCC, U&Es, LFTs, ESR
- *Specific tests*—laryngoscopy, fibreoptic endoscopy, EUA and biopsy
- *Radiology*—CXR, CT, MRI

Tumour Staging for Laryngeal Cancer

Supraglottis	
T1	Tumour limited to one subsite of supraglottis with normal vocal cord ability
T2	Tumour invades mucosa of more than one adjacent subsite of supraglottis, glottis or region outside the supraglottis (e.g. mucosa of base of tongue, vallecula, medial wall or pyriform sinus) without fixation of the larynx
T3	Tumour limited to larynx with vocal cord fixation or invades any of the following: postcricoid area, pre-epiglottic tissues, paraglottic space or minor thyroid cartilage erosion (e.g. inner cortex)
T4a	Tumour invades through the thyroid cartilage or invades tissues beyond the larynx (e.g. trachea, soft tissues of neck including deep extrinsic muscle of the tongue, strap muscles, thyroid or oesophagus)
T4b	Tumour invades prevertebral space, encases carotid artery or invades mediastinal structures
Glottis	
T1	Tumour limited to the vocal cord(s) (may involve anterior or posterior commissure) with normal mobility
T1a	Tumour limited to one vocal cord
T1b	Tumour involves both vocal cords
T2	Tumour extends to supraglottis or subglottis, or with impaired vocal cord mobility
T3	Tumour limited to the larynx with vocal cord fixation or invades paraglottic space, or minor thyroid cartilage erosion (e.g. inner cortex)
T4a	Tumour invades through the thyroid cartilage or invades tissues beyond the larynx (e.g. trachea, soft tissues of neck including deep extrinsic muscle of the tongue, strap muscles, thyroid or oesophagus)
T4b	Tumour invades prevertebral space, encases carotid artery or invades mediastinal structures

TREATMENT:

- *Conservative*—patient education, McMillan nurse referral
- *Medicinal*—radiotherapy and chemotherapy
- *Surgery*—endoscopic laser resection +/– diathermy/argon, laryngectomy, neck dissection. Indications for total laryngectomy include: T3/4 tumours with cartilage destruction, subglottic extension with cricoid cartilage involvement, circumferential submucosal disease and radiation necrosis of the larynx

COMPLICATIONS:

- Metastasis
- Invasion of local structures
- Death
- Vocal cord paralysis.
- Early complications from total laryngectomy include: haematoma, infection, pharyngocutaneous fistula, hypoglossal nerve injury.
- Late complications from total laryngectomy include: pharyngoesophageal stenosis, pharyngoesophageal stricture, stomal stensois, hypothyroidism.

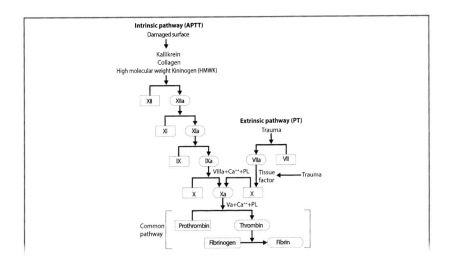

Key points about factors within the coagulation cascade:
- Factor VII has the shortest half-life.
- Factors V and VIII are the most labile factors. Their activity is lost in stored blood but not in FFP.
- Factor VIII is the only factor that is not synthesised by the liver. It is made by endothelium.
- Factors II, VII, IX and X are vitamin K dependent (along with proteins C and S).
- Factor X is the common point of both pathways.
- Factor XIII helps to cross-link fibrin.

Thrombin is the key to coagulation. It converts fibrinogen to fibrin, it activates factors V and VIII and it stimulates platelets. Fibrin links platelets together. Binding of GPIIb/IIIa promotes platelet plug formation.

Coagulation measurements:
PT measures factors II, V, VII, X and fibrinogen. It is the best marker of synthetic liver function.
PTT measures most factors except VII and XIII.

Problem	PT	APTT
Platelet problem	Normal	Normal
Factor VII problem	Increased	Normal
Common pathway problem	Increased	Increased
Intrinsic pathway problem	Normal	Increased
Extrinsic pathway problem	Increased	Normal

Figure 15.1 The coagulation cascade.

DOI: 10.1201/9781003292005-18

ACQUIRED THROMBOCYTOPENIA:

This can be caused by heparin and H_2 blockers.

GLANZMANN'S THROMBOCYTOPENIA:

GP IIb/IIIa receptor deficiency of the GP IIb/IIIa receptor on platelets. This means that they can no longer bind to each other.

BERNARD–SOULIER SYNDROME:

This is a rare inherited disorder of coagulation characterised by unusually large platelets, thrombocytopenia and prolonged bleeding time. It is caused by GPIb receptor deficiency. Treatment is platelet transfusion.

URAEMIA:

This inhibits platelet function.

HEPARIN-INDUCED THROMBOCYTOPENIA (HIT):

This thrombocytopenia is due to antiplatelet antibodies (IgG PF4Ab). It can result in platelet aggregation and subsequent thrombosis (HITT). Treatment is to stop heparin, start argatroban (a direct thrombin inhibitor) for anticoagulation.

DISSEMINATED INTRAVASCULAR COAGULATION (DIC):

This is an acquired syndrome characterised by the activation of coagulation pathways, resulting in the formation of intravascular thrombi and the depletion of platelets and coagulation factors. Therefore, in this condition, there is uncontrollable bleeding as well as clot formation. It is characterised by thrombocytopenia, low fibrinogen levels, increased fibrin degradation products, increased D-dimer levels and increased PT and aPTT.

VON WILLEBRAND'S DISEASE:

- This is an inherited disorder resulting from the complete absence or the dysfunction of von Willebrand factor. There are three major types of VWD: types 1, 2 and 3. Type 1 is the commonest. Type 2 is subdivided into 2A, 2B, 2M, 2N. The pathophysiology of each type depends on the defects in von Willebrand factor.
- von Willebrand factor is a glycoprotein present in plasma. It is made in Weibel–Palade bodies (in the endothelium), α-granules of platelets and by sub-endothelial connective tissue.

HAEMOPHILIA A:

This is sex-linked recessive deficiency in factor VIII.

HAEMOPHILIA B:

This is a sex-linked recessive deficiency in factor IX.

WARFARIN-INDUCED SKIN NECROSIS:

Always question whether there is an underlying protein C deficiency. It is a result of the shorter half-life of proteins C and S compared with that of the other vitamin K-dependent factors. This results in a hypercoagulable state just after starting warfarin.

INDICATIONS FOR SPLENECTOMY:

Include unstable trauma (grade III/IV) and haematological disorders, e.g. spherocytosis, splenic abscess, symptomatic splenic cysts, malignancy.

WANDERING SPLEEN:

This is due to the failure of the dorsal mesogastrium to fuse, meaning that the splenic ligaments do not form. There is a risk of infarction and splenic torsion. May result in the need for splenectomy or splenopexy.

HEREDITARY SPHEROCYTOSIS:

This can be autosomal dominant or autosomal recessive. Occurs due to a defect in genes related to membrane proteins, e.g. spectrin or ankyrin. This means that the red blood cells are less deformable thereby resulting in haemolysis. Children often need a splenectomy, and cholecystectomy is also considered due the risk of gallstones from the haemolysis.

PYRUVATE KINASE DEFICIENCY:

This is the most common hereditary non-anatomical cause of elective splenectomy that is not related to a structural issue. It is a congenital abnormality related to impaired glucose metabolism.

ANGIOSARCOMA:

This is a primary malignant tumour of the spleen associated with vinyl chloride exposure.

SPLENIC ARTERY ANEURYSM:

This is the commonest visceral artery aneurysm. It is more common in females and can be fatal, particularly in pregnant women. It is associated with the double rupture sign whereupon the patient initially presents with abdominal pain but then transiently improves. This is because the splenic artery bleed is tamponaded by the lesser sac. The lesser sac eventually overflows into the peritoneal cavity, and the patient becomes haemodynamically unstable.

OPSI:

The spleen is vital in the formation of IgM and IgG. Equally, it makes proteins like tufscin, which is important in the opsonisation of encapsulated organisms. The fenestrations of the spleen filter encapsulated organisms. Some examples of encapsulated organisms are *Streptococcus pneumoniae, N. meningitidis* and *H. influenzae*. It is important that patients receive their vaccines in line with hospital/national guidance as well as an annual flu jab. They should have a medi-alert bracelet and may require lifelong/long-term prophylaxis with penicillin.

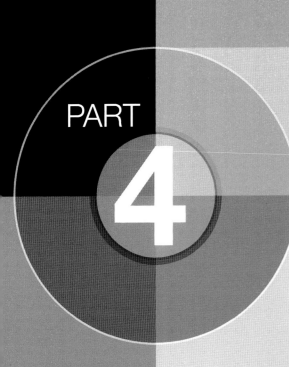

PART 4

PHARMACOLOGY

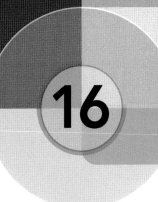

A–Z of Core Topics

16

There are currently eight questions pertaining to pharmacology centred around the safe prescribing of common drugs as applied to surgical practice. Commonly encountered agents include analgesics, antibiotics, cardiovascular drugs and anticoagulants as well as drugs used for the management of endocrine disorders (including diabetes) and local anaesthetics. This section of the book aims to provide high-yield information pertaining to these drugs in a way to aid memory recall. An A–Z pharmacology table provides a list of uses, mechanisms of action and side effects of commonly used drugs that are highly testable.

KEY TERMS AND TOPICS:

- *Zero-order kinetics*—this is the constant amount of drug eliminated regardless of dose.
- *First-order kinetics*—drug is eliminated in proportion to the dose.
- *Bioavailability*—amount of unchanged drug reaching the systemic circulation. Assumed to be 100% for IV drugs.
- *ED_{50}*—level of drug at which the desired effect occurs in 50% of the population.
- *LD_{50}*—level of drug at which death occurs in 50% of the population.
- *Tachyphylaxis*—tolerance after x doses.
- *Potency*—dose of drug required to reach effect.
- *Minimal alveolar concentration (MAC)*—the smallest concentration of inhalational agent at which 50% of patients will not move with incision/painful stimulus.

ANTIBIOTICS:

A summary of mechanisms of actions of commonly used antibiotics:

- *Inhibit cell wall synthesis*—penicillin, cephalosporins, carbapenems, vancomycin
- *Inhibit 30s ribosomes*—gentamicin, linezolid, tetracyclines
- *Inhibit 50s ribosomes*—erythromycin, clindamycin
- *Inhibit DNA gyrase*—quinolones
- *Inhibit dihydrofolate reductase*—trimethoprim
- *Inhibit purine synthesis*—sulphonamides
- *Stimulate oxygen free radicals that subsequently break up DNA*—metronidazole

COMMONLY ASKED ABOUT ANTIBIOTIC SIDE EFFECTS:

- *Piperacillin*—inhibits platelet function
- *Third generation cephalosporins*—cholestatic jaundice
- *Quinolones*—tendon rupture
- *Gentamicin*—ototoxicity, nephrotoxicity
- *Erythromycin*—cholestasis (IV administration), prokinetic for bowel
- *Vancomycin*—ototoxicity, nephrotoxicity, red man syndrome (histamine release)
- *Metronidazole*—peripheral neuropathy, disulfiram-like reaction
- *Tetracycline*—tooth discolouration in children, photosensitivity

ANTI-FUNGAL AGENTS:

The mechanisms of action and side effects of commonly used anti-fungal drugs are as follows:

- **Amphotericin**
  - Binds to sterol in fungal wall thus altering the permeability of the membrane.
  - *Side effects*—nephrotoxicity, hyperkalaemia, hypotension, anaemia
- **Voriconazole/itraconazole**
  - Inhibits ergosterol synthesis

ANTI-TUBERCULOSIS DRUGS:

The mechanism of action and side effects of commonly used anti-tuberculosis drugs are as follows:

- **Rifampicin**
  - Inhibits RNA polymerase
  - *Side effects*—hepatotoxicity
- **Isoniazid**
  - Inhibits mycolic acids
  - *Side effects*—hepatotoxicity, Vit B_6 deficiency, peripheral neuropathy, seborrheic dermatitis, seizures; give with pyridoxine
- **Pyrazinamide**
  - Activated to pyrazinoic acid, which interferes with fatty acid synthesis
  - *Side effects*—hepatotoxicity
- **Ethambutol**
  - Inhibits arabinosyl transferase
  - *Side effects*—retrobulbar neuritis

HAEMATOLOGY:

Heparin
- Binds to and potentiates the action of antithrombin III (ATIII)
- Reversed with protamine
- *Side effects*—bleeding, can cause osteoporosis and alopecia with long-term use
- Does not cross the placenta

Streptokinase
- Plasminogen activator, results in thrombolysis.
- Aminocaproic acid is the treatment for thrombolytic overdose.

Clopidogrel
- ADP receptor antagonist.

Warfarin
- Vitamin K antagonist, therefore stops the action of clotting factors II, VII, IX and X as well as protein C and S.
- Reversal of warfarin—vitamin K takes 6 hours to work. Prothrombin complex reverses it immediately.

Low Molecular Weight Heparin (LMWH)
- Neutralises factor Xa

ANTI-EMETICS:
Ondansetron
- Inhibits $5HT_3$ receptor
- *Side effects*—headache, dizziness, tiredness, constipation, chest tightness, convulsions

Metoclopramide
- Inhibits dopamine receptors
- *Side effects*—prokinetic, increased gastric motility, gut motility, dystonic reactions (more likely in children and young adults <30 years)

GOUT DRUGS:
Colchicine
- Binds tubulin and inhibits WBC migration
- *Side effects*—abdominal pain, nausea, vomiting, diarrhoea

Allopurinol
- Xanthine oxidase inhibitor
- *Side effects*—nausea, vomiting, deranged liver function, gout flare

CARDIAC DRUGS:
Digoxin
- Inhibits Na^+/K^+ ATPase and increases myocardial Ca^{2+}
- Slows AV conduction and is an inotrope
- *Side effects*—fatigue, arrythmias, yellow vision, skin rashes
- Hypokalaemia increases heart sensitivity to digoxin and may precipitate arrythmias

Statins
- Inhibit HMG-CoA reductase
- *Side effects*—deranged liver function, myalgia, rhabdomyolysis

Amiodarone
- A class III anti-arrhythmic, blocks K^+ rectifier currents
- *Side effects*—arrhythmias, pulmonary fibrosis, thyroid dysfunction, hepatic disorders, skin reactions/photosensitivity, corneal deposits, sleep disorders, altered taste

ACE inhibitors, e.g. ramipril
- Inhibit angiotensin-converting enzyme (ACE) thereby preventing the formation of angiotensin II. The result is vasodilation and reduced blood pressure.
- *Side effects*—dry cough, arrythmias, GI tract discomfort, may precipitate renal failure (particularly in patients with renal artery stenosis), rhinitis, tinnitus, vertigo, eosinophilia, hepatitis, neutropenia.

Atropine
- Antimuscarinic, acetylcholine antagonist, therefore increases heart rate
- *Side effects*—dry mouth, constipation, palpitations, anxiety, dizziness, dyspepsia, vision disorders

GI DRUGS:

Cholestyramine
- Binds bile in the GI tract and decreases level of cholesterol
- Can also bind vitamin K, resulting in bleeding
- *Side effects*—abdominal pain, diarrhoea, constipation, skin irritation

Proton pump inhibitors
- Inhibit the H^+/K^+ ATPase pump, therefore lowering acid levels in the stomach
- *Side effects*—abdominal pain, constipation, diarrhoea, dry mouth, bone fractures, arthralgia, myalgia, peripheral oedema, agranulocytosis, alopecia, gynaecomastia, hepatic disorders, *C. difficile*, low magnesium

Octreotide
- Somatostatin analogue, reduces GI secretions, used to treat carcinoid symptoms, VIPomas and glucagonomas as well as the initial treatment in acromegaly prior to operative management
- *Side effects*—alopecia, cholecystitis, cholelithiasis (with long-term use), hyperglycaemia/impaired glucose tolerance, hypoglycaemia, sinus bradycardia, arrhythmias, thyroid disorders

Biologic Agents

Agent	Mechanism of action
Infliximab	Inhibits TNF-α
Bevacizumab	Anti-VEGF
Trastuzumab	HER receptor blocker
Imatinib	Inhibits tyrosine kinase
Basiliximab	Targets IL-2 binding site
Cetuximab	Inhibits ECF

LOCAL ANAESTHETIC AGENTS

Most local anaesthetics are weak bases. They have a pH 5–6 without adrenaline and pH 2–3 with adrenaline, which is why the latter group sting more when injected. They block Na^+ channels, thereby preventing membrane depolarisation. They work faster in smaller unmyelinated nerves, e.g. C fibres. Adrenaline counteracts the vasodilatory effects of most local anaesthetics, resulting in a longer duration of action as well as faster onset of action.

Local anaesthetics fall into two groups—amides and esters. Amides are agents such as lidocaine, bupivacaine and prilocaine. They are degraded by the liver. Esters are agents such as cocaine and procaine. They are hydrolysed in plasma by pseudocholinesterase to para-aminobenzoic acid (PABA), and PABA can trigger antibody formation as well as lymphocyte stimulation. Amides are the more commonly used local anaesthetic.

Properties of Amides and Esters

	Esters	Amides
Stability	Less heat stable	Heat stable (can be autoclaved)
Shelf life	Short	Approximately 2 years
Metabolism	Plasma cholinesterase	Slow, hepatic
Allergy	Metabolism produces para-aminobenzoate (higher risk of allergic reactions)	Rare

CLINICAL CHARACTERISTICS OF LOCAL ANAESTHETIC AGENTS

Local anaesthetic	Type	Onset of action	Duration of action	Uses	Recommended maximum dose
Lidocaine	Amide	Fast (2–4 minutes)	Moderate (30–60 minutes)	Infiltration Nerve blocks Topical	3 mg/kg without adrenaline 7 mg/kg with adrenaline
Prilocaine	Amide	Fast (2–4 minutes)	Moderate (30–90 minutes)	Infiltration Dentistry Intravenous regional anaesthesia Can induce methemoglobinemia at high doses	6 mg/kg
Lidocaine and prilocaine cream	Amide	Slow (needs at least an hour to work)	EMLA® (eutectic mixture containing lidocaine 2.5% and prilocaine 2.5%). Tubes contain 5 g or 30 g	Before cannulation Skin graft harvest site	-
Bupivacaine	Amide	Moderate (6–10 minutes)	Long (120–140 minutes)	Infiltration Nerve block Epidural Subarachnoid block Ophthalmology Can last 180–420 minutes with adrenaline	2 mg/kg
Levobupivacaine	Amide	Moderate	Long	Infiltration Nerve blocks Spinal Epidural	2 mg/kg
Ropivacaine	Amide	Moderate	Long (120–360 minutes)	Infiltration Nerve blocks Epidural For continuous infusion	3 mg/kg
Cocaine	Ester			ENT All cocaine mixtures are controlled drugs	-

SIDE EFFECTS OF LOCAL ANAESTHETICS

- Pain at injection site.
- Pain if needle directly hits a nerve.

- Allergy (true allergy is rare but if it does occur it is more common with esters).
- Methemoglobinemia. This most commonly happens with prilocaine or benzocaine and occurs due to the oxidation of ferric iron to ferrous iron. It results in cyanosis and is treated with methylene blue.
- Adrenaline toxicity, e.g. hypertension, tachycardia and arrhythmias.
- Local anaesthetic toxicity—this can be subdivided into the effects on the central nervous system, and those on the cardiovascular system. These are summarised in the table below.

CLINICAL MANIFESTATIONS OF LOCAL ANAESTHETIC TOXICITY*

Central nervous system effects	Cardiovascular system effects
Dizziness	Myocardial depression
Tinnitus	Cardiac arrhythmias (ventricular re-entrant)
Perioral numbness	Ventricular arrest
Tremor	
Confusion	
Seizures	
Respiratory depression	

* Classically, central nervous system effects precede cardiovascular effects.

Anaesthetic Agents

Agent	Mechanism of action	Notes
Propofol	• Modulation of the inhibitory function of the neurotransmitter gamma-aminobutyric acid (GABA) through GABA-A receptors	• Rapid onset anaesthesia • Antiemetic action • Rapidly metabolised
Sodium thiopental	• Binds at a binding site associated with a Cl⁻ ionophore at the $GABA_A$ receptor. This increases the duration of time for which the Cl⁻ ionophore is open	• Rapid onset • Rapid induction • Marked myocardial depression
Ketamine	• Activation of the N-Methyl-D-Aspartate (NMDA) receptor	• Little myocardial depression • Associated with nightmares • Good in presence of haemodynamic instability
Etomidate	• Activates the $GABA_A$ receptor	• Good cardiac safety profile • May result in adrenal suppression • Post-operative vomiting is common

Antidiabetic Agents

Class of antidiabetic agent	Example	Mechanism of action	Uses	Side effects	Contraindications	Drug interactions
Biguanides	Metformin	↑ Peripheral insulin sensitivity ↑ Glucose uptake into and use by skeletal muscle ↓ Hepatic gluconeogenesis ↓ Intestinal glucose absorption	Type 2 DM (first choice in overweight patients) Polycystic ovarian syndrome	Gastrointestinal tract (GIT) disturbance, e.g. diarrhoea Nausea Vomiting Lactic acidosis	Renal failure Cardiac failure Respiratory failure Hepatic failure (The above increase the risk of developing lactic acidosis)	Contrast agents Angiotensin-converting enzyme (ACE) inhibitors Alcohol Non-steroidal anti-inflammatory drugs (NSAIDs) Steroids
Sulphonylureas	Glipizide	Block potassium channels on the pancreatic beta cells, thus stimulating insulin release	Type 2 DM	GIT disturbance Hypoglycaemia Weight gain	Renal failure Hepatic failure Porphyria Pregnancy Breastfeeding	ACE inhibitors Alcohol NSAIDs Steroids
Meglitinides (glinides)	Repaglinide	Block potassium channels on the pancreatic beta cells, thus stimulating insulin release	Type 2 DM	Weight gain Hypoglycaemia	Hepatic failure Pregnancy Breastfeeding	Ciclosporin Trimethoprim Clarithromycin
Thiazolidinediones (glitazones)	Pioglitazone	Activates nuclear peroxisome proliferator-activated receptor (PPAR)	Type 2 DM	Weight gain Hypoglycaemia Hepatotoxicity Fracture risk	Type 1 DM Hepatic disease Heart failure Bladder cancer	Rifampicin Paclitaxel
Incretins	Exenatide	Analogue of glucagon-like peptide (GLP)-1	Type 2 DM	GIT disturbance, e.g. diarrhoea Acute pancreatitis	Thyroid cancer Multiple endocrine neoplasia (MEN) 2 syndrome	Bexarotene
	Saxagliptin	Inhibits dipeptidyl peptidase	Type 2 DM	GIT disturbance, e.g. diarrhoea Infection of the respiratory and urinary tract Hepatotoxicity Peripheral oedema	History of serious hypersensitivity reaction	Thiazolidinedione
Alpha-glucosidase inhibitors	Acarbose	Inhibits alpha-glucosidase	Type 2 DM	GIT disturbance, e.g. diarrhoea	Inflammatory bowel disease (IBD) Intestinal obstruction Hepatic cirrhosis	Orlistat Pancreatin
Amylin analogues	Pramlintide	Analogue of amylin	Type 1 DM Type 2 DM	Severe hypoglycaemia	Gastroparesis Hypersensitivity to pramlintide	Acarbose
Sodium-glucose co-transporter-2 (SGLT2) inhibitors	Canagliflozin, dapagliflozin and empagliflozin	Inhibit SGLT2	Type 2 DM	Genital mycotic infections Urinary tract infections Increased urination Dizziness Dyslipidaemia Hypoglycaemia (Very rarely angioedema and Fournier's gangrene)	Type 1 DM (high risk of diabetic ketoacidosis)	Dapagliflozin

(Continued)

Antidiabetic Agents (Continued)

Class of antidiabetic agent	Example	Mechanism of action	Uses	Side effects	Contraindications	Drug interactions
Insulin therapy	Rapid-acting, e.g. insulin lispro Short-acting, e.g. soluble insulin Intermediate-acting, e.g. isophane insulin Long-acting, e.g. insulin glargine Biphasic, e.g. biphasic isophane insulin	Replaces insulin Insulin binds to tyrosine kinase receptors, where it initiates two pathways by phosphorylation: 1. *The MAPK signalling pathway*—this is responsible for cell growth and proliferation. 2. *The PI3K signalling pathway*—this is responsible for the transport of GLUT4 receptors to the cell surface membrane; GLUT4 transports glucose into the cell. This pathway is also responsible for protein, lipid and glycogen synthesis.	Type 1 DM Type 2 DM	Weight gain Hypoglycaemia Localised lipoatrophy Hypokalaemia	Hypersensitivity to any of the therapy ingredients Hypoglycaemia	Repaglinide increases risk of myocardial infarction (MI) and hypoglycaemia Monoamine oxidase inhibitors may increase insulin secretion Corticosteroids decrease the effect of insulin Levothyroxine decreases the effect of insulin Thiazide diuretics decrease the effects of insulin

Anticonvulsant Drugs

Anticonvulsant agent	Mechanism of action	Uses	Side effects	Contraindications	Drug interactions
Carbamazepine	Blocks voltage-dependent Na⁺ channels	All seizures except absence seizures Neuropathic pain, e.g. trigeminal neuralgia Manic-depressive illness	Rash Sedation Drowsiness Hyponatraemia Dry mouth Blurring of vision Neutropenia Hallucinations	Pregnancy (it is teratogenic) Past history of bone marrow depression Acute porphyria	Alters metabolism of oral contraceptive pills Alters metabolism of warfarin Alters metabolism of corticosteroids

Anticonvulsant agent	Mechanism of action	Uses	Side effects	Contraindications	Drug interactions
Phenytoin	Blocks voltage-dependent Na$^+$ channels	All seizures except pure absence seizures Seizure prevention post-neurosurgery Trigeminal neuralgia Arrhythmia Digoxin toxicity	Rash Hypersensitivity reactions Ataxia Megaloblastic anaemia Hirsutism Gum hypertrophy Purple glove syndrome	Pregnancy (it is teratogenic) Sinus bradycardia Stokes–Adams syndrome Sinoatrial block Second-degree heart block Third-degree heart block	Sodium valproate alters (increases or decreases) phenytoin concentration Phenytoin increases metabolism of drugs like anticoagulants by enzyme induction Phenytoin reduces concentration of mirtazapine This drug has a narrow therapeutic index
Sodium valproate	Blocks voltage-dependent Na$^+$ channels Weakly inhibits gamma-amino butyric acid (GABA) transaminase	All seizures Anxiety disorders Anorexia nervosa Manic-depressive illness	Nausea Vomiting Weight gain Hair loss • Thinning of hair • Curling of hair Hepatotoxicity Tremor Parkinsonism Thrombocytopenia Encephalopathy	Pregnancy (it is teratogenic) Hepatic failure History of mitochondrial disease	Aspirin increases levels of sodium valproate Sodium valproate may enhance effects of anticoagulant coumarins Carbamazepine decreases levels of sodium valproate
Ethosuximide	Inhibits T-type Ca^{2+} channels	Absence seizures (used more frequently in children)	Nausea Vomiting Anorexia Hypersensitivity reactions Blood dyscrasias Ataxia	Pregnancy (it is teratogenic) Hepatic failure Affective disorders Systemic lupus erythematosus	Metabolism is inhibited by isoniazid Sodium valproate increases the level of ethosuximide Phenytoin and carbamazepine decrease the level of ethosuximide
Phenobarbital	Acts on GABA$_A$ receptors, enhancing synaptic inhibition	All seizures except absence seizures Status epilepticus (third line) Anaesthesia Neonatal seizures Cyclical vomiting syndrome Crigler–Najjar syndrome Gilbert syndrome	Rash Sedation Depression Ataxia Amelogenesis imperfecta	Pregnancy (it is teratogenic) History of porphyria	Phenobarbital increases metabolism of coumarins Carbamazepine increases concentration of phenobarbital Phenobarbital decreases levels of itraconazole

(Continued)

Anticonvulsant Drugs   (Continued)

Anticonvulsant agent	Mechanism of action	Uses	Side effects	Contraindications	Drug interactions
Benzodiazepines	Allosterically modifies $GABA_A$ receptor, thereby increasing Cl^- conductance	Lorazepam used to treat status epilepticus (first line) Anxiety disorders Insomnia Seizures Alcohol withdrawal	Sedation Withdrawal syndrome Respiratory depression	Chronic obstructive pulmonary disease Sleep apnoea Myasthenia gravis Severe depression (increased suicidal tendencies)	Use cautiously with other central nervous system depressants, e.g. opioids and barbiturates Increasing sedative effect when used with antihistamines Increasing sedative effect when used with antipsychotics
Vigabatrin	Inhibits GABA transaminase	All seizures Seizures in patients who are resistant to other anticonvulsant medication	Sedation Headache Peripheral visual field defect Depression Psychosis Hallucinations	Hypersensitivity	Vigabatrin increases the clearance of carbamazepine Vigabatrin decreases levels of phenytoin
Lamotrigine	Blocks voltage-dependent Na^+ channels Inhibits L-, N- and P-type Ca^{2+} channels	All seizures Manic-depressive illness Severe depression Neuropathic pain, e.g. trigeminal neuralgia	Stevens–Johnson syndrome Toxic epidermal necrolysis (Lyell's syndrome) Rashes Nausea Ataxia	Hypersensitivity Hepatic failure	The oral contraceptive pill decreases levels of lamotrigine Carbamazepine decreases lamotrigine levels Rifampicin decreases levels of lamotrigine Valproate increases levels of lamotrigine
Gabapentin and pregabalin	Gabapentin is a GABA analogue Pregabalin is an analogue of gabapentin	All seizures Neuropathic pain Manic-depressive illness	Sedation Ataxia	Hypersensitivity	When used with propoxyphene, patients are more at risk of side effects such as dizziness and confusion Bioavailability of gabapentin increased by morphine

Key Drugs A–Z

Drug	Uses	Mechanism of action	Side effects
Acetylcysteine (N-acetylcysteine or NAC)	Paracetamol overdose	Replenishes stores of glutathione	Anaphylactoid reactions
Adenosine	SVT	Adenosine receptor agonist and activation of G protein coupled receptors Reduces automaticity and increases atrioventricular node refractoriness	Bradycardia Feeling of impending doom Breathlessness

Drug	Uses	Mechanism of action	Side effects
Adrenaline	Cardiac arrest Anaphylaxis Mixed with local anaesthetic to prolong local anaesthetic action	Agonist of α_1, α_2, β_1 and β_2 receptors	Adrenaline-induced hypertension Headache Tremor Palpitations In those with pre-existing heart disease it may cause angina, myocardial infarction and arrhythmia
Aldosterone antagonists, e.g. spironolactone	Hypertension Hyperaldosteronism Diuretic in liver cirrhosis Heart failure	Competitively binds to aldosterone receptors	Hyperkalaemia Gynaecomastia Hepatic impairment
Allopurinol	Gout Renal stones caused by uric acid Tumour lysis syndrome	Xanthine oxidase inhibitor	Skin rash Stevens–Johnson syndrome May worsen acute gout episode
Alpha blockers, e.g. tamsulosin	Benign prostatic hypertrophy	Usually selective blocking of β_1 receptors	Postural hypotension Syncope Dizziness
Aminoglycosides, e.g. gentamicin	Infections—typically good antibiotics against Gram-negative organisms	Irreversibly bind to 30s ribosomes, thereby inhibiting protein synthesis	Ototoxicity Nephrotoxicity
Aminosalicylates, e.g. mesalazine	Ulcerative colitis	Releases 5-aminosalicylic acid	Headache Renal impairment Leukopaenia Thrombocytopenia Oligospermia
Amiodarone	Tachyarrhythmias (various)	Blocks sodium, calcium and potassium channels Antagonist of α and β receptors	Hypotension Bradycardia Pneumonitis Hepatitis Thyroid abnormalities Photosensitivity
ACE inhibitors, e.g. ramipril	Hypertension Heart failure Ischaemic heart disease	Inhibits angiotensin-converting enzyme thereby stopping the formation of angiotensin II	Dry cough Hypotension Hyperkalaemia Renal impairment
Angiotensin receptor blockers, e.g. losartan	Hypertension Heart failure Ischaemic heart disease	Blocks the action of angiotensin II at the AT_1 receptor	Hypotension Hyperkalaemia Renal impairment
Anti-emetics (1) dopamine antagonists, e.g. metoclopramide	Nausea and vomiting	Antagonist to the D_2 receptor in the chemoreceptor trigger zone	Diarrhoea Oculogyric crisis (particularly in young women)
Anti-emetics (2) histamine antagonists, e.g. cyclizine	Nausea and vomiting	Antagonist to the H_1 receptor and to the acetylcholine receptor in the vomiting centre and vestibular system	Dry mouth Drowsiness Palpitations

(Continued)

Key Drugs A–Z   (Continued)

Drug	Uses	Mechanism of action	Side effects
Anti-emetics (3) **phenothiazines, e.g.** **prochlorperazine**	Nausea and vomiting Schizophrenia	Antagonist to the D_2 receptor in the chemoreceptor trigger zone also, antagonist to the H_1 receptor and to the acetylcholine receptor in the vomiting centre and vestibular system	Drowsiness Palpitations Postural hypotension Extrapyramidal side effects, e.g. oculogyric crisis Prolonged QT interval
Anti-emetics (4) **serotonin receptor antagonists,** **e.g. ondansetron**	Nausea and vomiting	Antagonist to the serotonin $(5\text{-}HT_3)$ receptor in the chemoreceptor trigger zone	Bowel disturbance— constipation or diarrhoea Headache
Anti-fungals e.g. nystatin	Fungal infections	Nystatin is a polyene anti-fungal. It binds to ergosterol in the fungal membrane creating a pore Imidazoles and triazoles fluconazole inhibit the synthesis of ergosterol	Nystatin and clotrimazole have very few side effects since they are topical and may cause local irritation Fluconazole—bowel disturbance, headache, hepatitis, prolonged QT interval and very rarely hypersensitivity reactions including anaphylaxis
Antihistamines, e.g. **fexofenadine**	Allergic reactions	Antagonist to the H_1 receptor	Drowsiness
Aspirin	Coronary syndromes Stroke Peripheral vascular disease Pain	Irreversibly inhibits cyclooxygenase (COX), thereby affecting arachidonic acid metabolism and reducing the amount of thromboxane produced and thus reducing platelet aggregation	Bleeding Gastric irritation including the formation of gastric ulcers Bronchospasm
Beta₂-agonists, e.g. salbutamol	Asthma COPD Acute management of hyperkalaemia	Agonist to β_2 receptors	Tachycardia Palpitations Tremor Anxiety
Beta-blockers, e.g. bisoprolol	Ischaemic heart disease Heart failure Atrial fibrillation Hypertension	Blocking β_1 receptors results in reduced force of myocardial contraction as well as reduced speed of conduction	Headache Fatigue Cold extremities Impotence in men
Bisphosphonates, e.g. **alendronic acid**	Osteoporosis Myeloma Paget's disease	Inhibits the action of osteoclasts thus decreasing bone turnover	Oesophagitis Low phosphate Osteonecrosis of the jaw Atypical fractures
Calcium channel blockers, e.g. **amlodipine**	Hypertension Angina	Blocks calcium channels, thereby reducing calcium entry into cardiac and vascular cells. The resultant effect is relaxation and vasodilation of arterial smooth muscle	Headache Flushing Palpitations Ankle swelling Bradycardia Heart block

Drug	Uses	Mechanism of action	Side effects
Clopidogrel	Acute coronary syndromes Ischaemic heart disease Atrial fibrillation	Irreversibly inhibits adenosine diphosphate (ADP) receptors (the $P2Y_{12}$ subtype). These are present on the surface on platelets	Bleeding Gastrointestinal upset Thrombocytopaenia
Corticosteroids, e.g. prednisolone	Allergic reactions Autoimmune diseases Adrenal insufficiency Tumour-related swelling	The exact mechanism is unknown. The immune response is modified and anti-inflammatory genes are upregulated	Immunosuppression Osteoporosis Bruising Skin thinning Hypertension Hypokalaemia Oedema
Digoxin	Atrial fibrillation Heart failure	Inhibits the Na^+/K^+ ATPase pump on the cardiac myocytes. It is negatively chronotropic and positively inotropic	Yellow vision Bradycardia Rash Dizziness Arrhythmias Digoxin toxicity increases with hypokalaemia
Diuretics (1) loop, e.g. furosemide	Hypertension Oedema Chronic heart failure Pulmonary oedema	Inhibits $Na^+/K^+/2Cl^-$ co-transporter in the ascending loop of Henle	Hypotension Hyponatraemia Hypokalaemia Hypochloraemia Hypocalcaemia Hypomagnesaemia Metabolic alkalosis Tinnitus/hearing loss
Diuretics (2) potassium sparing, e.g. amiloride	Hypertension Hyperkalaemia	Inhibits the reabsorption of sodium and therefore water via epithelial sodium channels in the distal convoluted tubule	Hypotension Gastrointestinal upset Hyperkalaemia Hyponatraemia
Diuretics (3) thiazides, e.g. bendroflumethiazide	Hypertension	Inhibits the Na^+/Cl^- co-transporter in the distal convoluted tubule of the nephron	Hypotension Hyponatraemia Hypokalaemia Impotence in men
Fibrinolytic drugs, e.g. streptokinase	Stroke Acute coronary syndromes Pulmonary embolism	Promotes the cleavage of the Arg/Val bond in plasminogen to form the proteolytic enzyme plasmin, which then dissolves clots	Bruising Bleeding Allergic reactions
H_2 antagonists	Peptic ulcer disease GORD	Antagonist to H_2 receptors present on parietal cells	Diarrhoea Constipation Headache Dizziness
Heparins, e.g. enoxaparin	Prophylactic against clots Treatment of deep vein thrombosis and pulmonary embolism Acute coronary syndromes Acute limb embolism	LMWHs, e.g. enoxaparin, inhibit factor Xa Fondaparinux inhibits Xa only Unfractionated heparin activates antithrombin, which then inactivates thrombin and factor Xa	Bleeding Heparin-induced thrombocytopaenia Injection site reactions

(Continued)

299

Key Drugs A–Z (Continued)

Drug	Uses	Mechanism of action	Side effects
Laxatives (1), e.g. bulk-forming like ispaghula husk	Constipation and faecal impaction	Hydrophilic substances within the laxative cause movement of water into the stool resulting in an increase in stool bulk. An increase in stool bulk stimulates bowel peristalsis	Flatulence Abdominal cramping Diarrhoea Rarely, bowel obstruction
Laxatives (2), e.g. osmotic laxatives like lactulose	Constipation Faecal impaction Hepatic encephalopathy	Osmotically active substances remain within the bowel lumen therefore retain water within the stool and increases stool bulk. An increase in stool bulk stimulates bowel peristalsis In cases of hepatic encephalopathy, lactulose inhibits ammonia absorption	Flatulence Abdominal cramping Diarrhoea
Laxatives (3), e.g. stimulant laxatives like senna	Constipation Faecal impaction	Increase electrolyte and water secretion from the mucosa of the colon, resulting in an increase in stool bulk. An increase in stool bulk stimulates bowel peristalsis	Flatulence Abdominal cramping Diarrhoea Melanosis coli
Lidocaine	Local anaesthetic	Blocks voltage-gated sodium channels	Pain on local administration Neurological symptoms, e.g. perioral anaesthesia, drowsiness, tremor, seizures Cardiovascular symptoms, e.g. hypotension, arrhythmias.
Macrolides, e.g. clarithromycin	Covers atypical organisms that cause pneumonia (*Legionella pneumophilia*, *Mycoplasma pneumoniae*) Penicillin alternative in certain skin/ soft tissue infections and respiratory tract infections. *H. pylori* eradication therapy	Inhibits bacterial protein synthesis by binding to the 50s ribosomal subunit. It is bacteriostatic	Nausea Vomiting Diarrhoea Cholestatic jaundice Ototoxic at high doses Prolongation of the QT interval
Metformin	Type 2 diabetes mellitus	A biguanide that increases peripheral sensitivity to insulin	Gastrointestinal upset Lactic acidosis
Methotrexate	A disease-modifying drug for conditions such as rheumatoid arthritis or psoriasis Chemotherapy	Inhibitor of dihydrofolate reductase. This enzyme coverts folic acid to tetrahydrofolate, which is needed for protein and DNA synthesis. Thus, the overall action of methotrexate is to prevent cell replication	Bone marrow suppression Sore mouth Hypersensitivity reactions Hepatic cirrhosis Pulmonary fibrosis
Metronidazole	Treatment against anaerobic bacteria, e.g. *Clostridium difficile* Treatment of protozoal infections, e.g. giardiasis	Stimulates nitroso free radicals that subsequently bind to DNA resulting in DNA degradation and cellular death	Gastrointestinal upset Hypersensitivity reactions Neurological effects at high doses, e.g. optic neuropathy, peripheral neuropathy, seizures

Drug	Uses	Mechanism of action	Side effects
Naloxone	Opiate toxicity	Competitive antagonist of μ receptors	Opioid withdrawal reaction
Nicorandil	Stable angina	Causes venous and arterial dilatation by acting as a nitrate and by activating K^+ ATP channels. K^+ efflux causes hyperpolarisation and thus inactivation of voltage-gated Ca^{2+} channels. Decreased levels of intracellular calcium mean that vasodilatation occurs	Flushing Headache Dizziness Hypotension
Nitrofurantoin	Urinary tract infections	It is metabolised by bacterial cells, creating an active metabolite that damages DNA	Gastrointestinal upset Hypersensitivity reactions Rarely it may cause pneumonitis, hepatitis and peripheral neuropathy Haemolytic anaemia in neonates
Non-steroidal anti-inflammatory drugs, e.g. naproxen	Pain Inflammation	Inhibit cyclooxygenase to prevent the formation of products of arachidonic acid metabolism	Gastrointestinal upset Gastrointestinal bleeding Renal impairment
Opioids, e.g. morphine	Acute pain Chronic pain As part of palliative symptom control in the context of end-of-life care Acute pulmonary oedema	Agonist of μ receptors	Nausea and vomiting Respiratory depression Neurological depression Constipation Pupillary constriction Dependence/tolerance
Paracetamol	Acute pain Chronic pain Anti-pyretic	Not completely understood. Weak inhibitor of cyclooxygenase-2	Hepatic failure in overdose
Penicillin, e.g. flucloxacillin	Infections, e.g. skins and soft tissue, tonsillitis, meningitis	β-lactam ring is responsible for the anti-microbial activity Penicillin antibiotics weaken enzymes that cross-link peptidoglycans in bacterial cell walls	Gastrointestinal upset Penicillin allergy Neurological effects at very high doses or in renal impairment (impaired excretion)
Proton pump inhibitors, e.g. lansoprazole	Gastro-oesophageal reflux Peptic ulcer disease *H. pylori* infection	Irreversibly inhibits H^+/K^+ ATPase in gastric parietal cells	Gastrointestinal upset Hypomagnesaemia *Clostridium difficile*
Quinolones, e.g. ciprofloxacin	Infections, e.g. lower respiratory tract, urinary tract	Inhibit DNA synthesis	*Clostridium difficile* Gastrointestinal upset Tendon rupture Hypersensitivity reactions Prolongation of the QT interval Neurological effects (by lowering the seizure threshold)

(Continued)

Key Drugs A–Z   (Continued)

Drug	Uses	Mechanism of action	Side effects
Statins	Hypercholesterolaemia Primary and secondary risk reduction in cardiovascular/peripheral vascular disease	Inhibit 3-hydroxy-3-methyl-glutaryl coenzyme A (HMG-CoA) reductase	Gastrointestinal upset Headache Myopathy Rhabdomyolysis Drug-induced hepatitis
Tetracyclines, e.g. doxycycline	Infections, e.g. lower respiratory tract, pelvic inflammatory disease, Lyme disease Acne vulgaris	Inhibits protein synthesis by binding to the 30s ribosomal subunit	Gastrointestinal upset Hypersensitivity reactions Dental discolouration in children Photosensitivity Oesophageal irritation
Trimethoprim	Urinary tract infections	Inhibits dihydrofolate reductase, folate is needed for bacterial DNA synthesis	Gastrointestinal upset Hypersensitivity reactions Skin rash Haematological disorders Hyperkalaemia
Vancomycin	Gram-positive infections or in situations of penicillin allergy	Inhibits cell wall synthesis in Gram-positive bacteria by inhibiting cross-linking of peptidoglycan chains	Gastrointestinal upset Hypersensitivity reactions Red man syndrome Thrombophlebitis Nephrotoxicity Ototoxicity Haematological disorders
Warfarin	Deep vein thrombosis Pulmonary embolism Anticoagulation in atrial fibrillation or heart valve replacement	Antagonises vitamin K and therefore inhibits the production of vitamin K-dependent coagulation factors—II, VII, IX and X as well as proteins C and S	Bleeding
Z drugs, e.g. zopiclone	Insomnia	Enhances binding of GABA to $GABA_A$ receptor	Rebound insomnia Headache Confusion Daytime sleepiness Taste disturbance Gastrointestinal upset Dependence Withdrawal symptoms

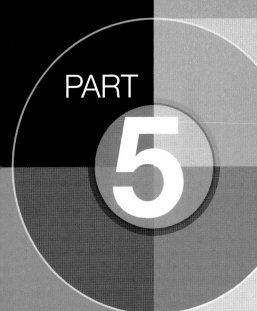

PART

5

MATHS FOR THE MRCS

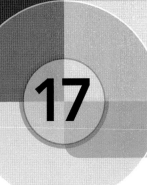

Practice Questions with Answers

17

There are at least two to four questions within the MRCS Part A examination which require candidates to perform some simple calculations. These are easy marks to gain if you know the formulae. Below I have provided frequently occurring formulae as well as some worked examples.

LIST OF KEY EQUATIONS:

- Mean arterial pressure (MAP) = Diastolic blood pressure + 0.33 (systolic blood pressure – diastolic blood pressure)

- Cerebral perfusion pressure (CPP) = MAP – Intracerebral pressure (ICP)

- Stroke volume = Cardiac output/heart rate

- Cardiac output = Stroke volume × Heart rate

- Total peripheral resistance = MAP/Cardiac output

- Cardiac output = Oxygen consumption per minute/oxygen content of blood taken from the pulmonary artery (representing venous blood) – Oxygen content of blood from a cannula in a peripheral artery

  - i.e. $VO_2/C_aO_2 - C_vO_2$

- Cardiac output = Oxygen uptake/(aortic – mixed venous oxygen content)

- Pulmonary vascular resistance (PVR) = (mean pulmonary artery pressure – pulmonary capillary wedge pressure)/cardiac output

  - i.e. PVR = (MAP – PCWP)/cardiac output

- Excretion = (filtration + secretion) – Reabsorption

- Renal clearance = (urine concentration × urine flow rate)/plasma concentration

  - i.e. $(U_x \times V)/P_x$

- MCV = Haematocrit × 1000/Red blood cells

- MCHC = Concentration of haemoglobin/haematocrit

DOI: 10.1201/9781003292005-22

- Calculation for burns—*check the latest ATLS guidelines for the most up-to-date Parkland Formula*

- In adults = 2 mL × % Body surface area burns × Weight

- In children < 14 years = 3 mL × % Body surface area burns × Weight

- Electrical injury all ages = 4 mL × % Body surface area burns × Weight

MATHS—QUESTIONS

1. A 43-year-old gentleman is a patient in the ICU after being involved in a road traffic collision. His blood pressure is currently 138/75. Your consultant asks you to calculate the mean arterial pressure (MAP).

2. A medical student is learning about MAP as part of his physiology class and wishes to calculate his own. His blood pressure (BP) is 120/80; what is his MAP?

3. A 50-year-old alcoholic woman has presented to your surgical ward with severe pancreatitis. She has now been moved to the HDU. Her BP is currently 95/75; what is her MAP?

4. A 25-year-old university student was playing rugby when he took a blow to the side of his head during a difficult tackle. He appeared to lose consciousness for 15 seconds and then continued to watch the rest of the match from the sidelines. Later that day his friend found him collapsed. He is currently in the ICU with a confirmed extradural haematoma, and his intracranial pressure (ICP) is currently 16 mmHg. His BP is 130/80. Calculate the cerebral perfusion pressure (CPP).

5. A 68-year-old man with known hypertension was walking with his family by the coast on holiday when he complained of a sudden-onset headache and collapsed. He is in the ICU with a subarachnoid haemorrhage and an ICP of 15 mmHg. His BP is 156/90. What is the CPP?

6. A 30-year-old gentleman has attended his preassessment appointment with you prior to an elective inguinal hernia repair. Apart from mild asthma he has no other medical issues and attends the gym regularly. His stroke volume at rest is 75 cm^3 and his resting heart rate is 58 bpm. What is his cardiac output?

7. If a patient has a cardiac output of 5100 cm^3/min and a heart rate of 70 bpm, what is the stroke volume?

8. A patient attends your vascular clinic and has a blood pressure of 140/80 and a cardiac output of 4 L/min. What is his total peripheral resistance?

9. A 69-year-old woman who had rheumatic fever as a child is undergoing cardiac function tests prior to an elective procedure. She has a resting heart rate of 80 bpm, which is irregular at times. Her oxygen consumption is 250 mL/min, arterial oxygen content is 20 mL/100 mL blood and pulmonary artery oxygen content is 15 mL/100 mL. What is her cardiac stroke volume?

10. A 70-year-old gentleman unfortunately suffers from an anterior myocardial infarction. Whilst undergoing percutaneous intervention, some measurements are made. He has an

oxygen uptake of 150 mL/min, a venous oxygen concentration of 5 mL oxygen/100 mL blood and an oxygen concentration in the pulmonary artery of 10 mL oxygen/100 mL blood. In the aorta, the oxygen concentration is 15 mL oxygen/100 mL blood. Calculate the cardiac output.

11. An 80-year-old gentleman is in the ICU after an elective right hemicolectomy for caecal cancer. His heart rate is 85 bpm, and measurements show that he has an arterial O_2 concentration of 0.25 mL O_2/min and a venous O_2 concentration of 0.15 mL O_2/min. His whole-body O_2 consumption is 500 mL/min. What is (a) the cardiac output and (b) the stroke volume?

12. An 80-year-old gentleman is in the ICU after an elective right hemicolectomy for caecal cancer. His heart rate is 85 bpm, and measurements show that he has an arterial O_2 concentration of 0.25 mL O_2/min and a venous O_2 concentration of 0.15 mL O_2/min. His whole-body O_2 consumption is 500 mL/min. He has a pulmonary wedge pressure of 5 mmHg, a pulmonary diastolic pressure of 8 mmHg and a pulmonary systolic pressure of 20 mmHg. What is the pulmonary vascular resistance?

13. How much oxygen is usually carried in 100 mL blood?

14. A 50-year-old asthmatic has a tidal volume of 350 mL on spirometry and a respiratory rate in clinic of 15 breaths per minute. What is his minute ventilation?

15. Substance X is filtered freely but is not secreted by the kidney. Substance X has a plasma volume of 500 mg/L, and the urine excretion rate is 15 mg/min. Insulin clearance is 100 mL/min. What is the rate of tubular reabsorption of substance X?

16. Calculate the renal clearance of substance X given the following:

- T_{max} of substance X = 200 mg/min
- GFR = 90 mL/min
- Plasma concentration of X = 100 mg/100 mL
- Urine volume = 60 mL/20 min
- Renal fraction = 20%
- Haematocrit = 50
- Urine concentration of X = 25 mg/10 mL
- Blood pressure = 120/85

17. A woman suffering with anaemia has arrived for her haematology clinic review. She has a haematocrit level of 45% and her red blood cell count is 7.2×10^6/μL. Calculate her MCV.

18. Your consultant reviews the above patient in the haematology clinic and asks you to calculate the mean corpuscular haemoglobin concentration (MCHC). Her Hb is 11.2 g/dL.

19. An 18-year-old man presents to the emergency department having set fire to himself in an attempt to take his own life. He weighs 70 kg and the burns cover 36% of his total body surface area. What volume of fluid will you prescribe to be given over the first 8 hours?

20. A 37-year-old soldier received a severe electrical burn that has affected both of his upper limbs, the anterior aspect of his torso and the perineum. He weighs 90 kg. What volume of fluids should he receive over the first 8 hours?

MATHS—ANSWERS

1. A 43-year-old gentleman is a patient in the ICU after being involved in a road traffic collision. His blood pressure is currently 138/75. Your consultant asks you to calculate the mean arterial pressure (MAP).

   Mean arterial pressure (MAP) = diastolic blood pressure + 0.33 (systolic blood pressure – diastolic blood pressure)

   MAP = 75 + 0.33 (138 – 75)
   = 75 + 0.33 (63)
   = 75 + 20.79
   = 95.79 mmHg

2. A medical student is learning about MAP as part of his physiology class and wishes to calculate his own. His blood pressure (BP) is 120/80; what is his MAP?

   Mean arterial pressure (MAP) = diastolic blood pressure + 0.33 (systolic blood pressure – diastolic blood pressure)

   MAP = 80 + 0.33 (120 – 80)
   = 80 + 0.33 (40)
   = 80 + 13.2
   = 93.2 mmHg

3. A 50-year-old alcoholic woman has presented to your surgical ward with severe pancreatitis. She has now been moved to the HDU. Her BP is currently 95/75; what is her MAP?

   Mean arterial pressure (MAP) = diastolic blood pressure + 0.33 (systolic blood pressure – diastolic blood pressure)

   MAP = 75 + 0.33 (95 – 75)
   = 75 + 0.33 (20)
   = 75 + 6.6
   = 81.6 mmHg

4. A 25-year-old university student was playing rugby when he took a blow to the side of his head during a difficult tackle. He appeared to lose consciousness for 15 seconds and then continued to watch the rest of the match from the sidelines. Later that day, his friend found him collapsed. He is currently in the ICU with a confirmed extradural haematoma, and his intracranial pressure (ICP) is currently 16 mmHg. His BP is 130/80. Calculate the cerebral perfusion pressure (CPP).

   This must be solved in two steps. First calculate the MAP, and then calculate the CPP.

   Step 1:
   Mean arterial pressure (MAP) = Diastolic blood pressure + 0.33 (systolic blood pressure – diastolic blood pressure)

   MAP = 80 + 0.33 (130 – 80)
   = 80 + 0.33 (50)
   = 80 + 16.5
   = 96.5 mmHg

Step 2:
Cerebral perfusion pressure (CPP) = MAP − Intracerebral pressure (ICP)
= 96.5 − 16
= 80.5 mmHg

5. A 68-year-old man with known hypertension was walking with his family by the coast on holiday when he complained of a sudden-onset headache and collapsed. He is in the ICU with a subarachnoid haemorrhage and an ICP of 15 mmHg. His BP is 156/90. What is the CPP?

Step 1:
Mean arterial pressure (MAP) = Diastolic blood pressure + 0.33 (systolic blood pressure − diastolic blood pressure)

MAP = 90 + 0.33 (156 − 90)
= 90 + 0.33 (66)
= 90 + 21.78
= 111.78 mmHg

Step 2:
Cerebral perfusion pressure (CPP) = MAP − Intracerebral pressure (ICP)

= 111.78 − 15
= 96.78 mmHg

6. A 30-year-old gentleman has attended his preassessment appointment with you prior to an elective inguinal hernia repair. Apart from mild asthma he has no other medical issues and attends the gym regularly. His stroke volume at rest is 75 cm^3 and his resting heart rate is 58 bpm. What is his cardiac output?

Cardiac output = Stroke volume × Heart rate
= 75 × 58
= 4350 cm^3 per minute

7. If a patient has a cardiac output of 5100 cm^3/min and a heart rate of 70 bpm, what is the stroke volume?

Stroke volume = Cardiac output/heart rate

= 5100/70
= 72.86 cm^3

8. A patient attends your vascular clinic and has a blood pressure of 140/80 and a cardiac output of 4 l/min. What is his total peripheral resistance?

Total peripheral resistance = MAP/cardiac output

Step 1:
Mean arterial pressure (MAP) = diastolic blood pressure + 0.33 (systolic blood pressure − diastolic blood pressure)

MAP = 80 + 0.33 (140 − 80)
= 80 + 0.33 (60)
= 80 + 19.8
= 99.8 mmHg

Step 2:
Total peripheral resistance = MAP/cardiac output
= 99.8/4
= 24.95 mmHg × min/L

9. A 69-year-old woman who had rheumatic fever as a child is undergoing cardiac function tests prior to an elective procedure. She has a resting heart rate of 80 bpm, which is irregular at times. Her oxygen consumption is 250 mL/min, arterial oxygen content is 20 mL/100 mL blood and pulmonary artery oxygen content is 15 mL/100 mL. What is her cardiac stroke volume?

Step 1:
O_2 consumption = Cardiac output × (arterial O_2 content – venous O_2 content)

Rearranging this equation:
250 = Cardiac output × (20 – 15)
250 = Cardiac output × 5 mL O_2/100 mL blood
Cardiac output = 5000 mL blood/min

Step 2:
Stroke volume = cardiac output/heart rate
= 5000/80
= 62.5 mL

10. A 70-year-old gentleman unfortunately suffers from an anterior myocardial infarction. Whilst undergoing percutaneous intervention, some measurements are made. He has an oxygen uptake of 150 mL/min, a venous oxygen concentration of 5 mL oxygen/100 mL blood and an oxygen concentration in the pulmonary artery of 10 mL oxygen/100 mL blood. In the aorta, the oxygen concentration is 15 mL oxygen/100 mL blood. Calculate the cardiac output.

Cardiac output = Oxygen uptake/(aortic – mixed venous oxygen content)
= 150 mL/min/(15 O_2/100 mL – 10 O_2/100 mL)
= 150 mL/min/5 O_2/100 mL
= 150/0.05
= 3000 mL/min

11. An 80-year-old gentleman is in the ICU after an elective right hemicolectomy for caecal cancer. His heart rate is 85 bpm, and measurements show that he has an arterial O_2 concentration of 0.25 mL O_2/min and a venous O_2 concentration of 0.15 mL O_2/min. His whole-body O_2 consumption is 500 mL/min. What is (a) the cardiac output and (b) the stroke volume?

a) Cardiac output = Oxygen consumption per minute/oxygen content of blood taken from the pulmonary artery (representing venous blood) – Oxygen content of blood from a cannula in a peripheral artery

i.e. Cardiac output = $VO_2/C_aO_2 – C_vO_2$
Cardiac output = 500/(0.25 – 0.15)
= 500/0.1
= 5000 mL/min
= 5 l/min

b) Stroke volume = Cardiac output/heart rate
= 5000/85
= 58.82 mL

12. An 80-year-old gentleman is in the ICU after an elective right hemicolectomy for caecal cancer. His heart rate is 85 bpm, and measurements show that he has an arterial O_2 concentration of 0.25 mL O_2/min and a venous O_2 concentration of 0.15 mL O_2/min. His whole-body O_2 consumption is 500 mL/min. He has a pulmonary wedge pressure of 5 mmHg, a pulmonary diastolic pressure of 8 mmHg and a pulmonary systolic pressure of 20 mmHg. What is the pulmonary vascular resistance?

Step 1: Calculate the cardiac output as described above and repeated below.

Cardiac output = Oxygen consumption per minute/oxygen content of blood taken from the pulmonary artery (representing venous blood) – Oxygen content of blood from a cannula in a peripheral artery

i.e. Cardiac output = $VO_2/C_aO_2 - C_vO_2$
Cardiac output = 500/(0.25 – 0.15)
= 500/0.1
= 5000 mL/min
= 5 L/min

Step 2: Calculate the mean arterial pressure of the pulmonary artery.

MAP pulmonary artery = 8 + 0.33 (20 – 8)
= 8 + 3.96
= 11.96

Step 3: Calculate the pulmonary vascular resistance.

Pulmonary vascular resistance (PVR) = (mean pulmonary artery pressure – pulmonary capillary wedge pressure)/cardiac output

PVR = (11.96 – 5)/5
= 6.96/5
= 1.39 resistance units (mmHg/L/min)

13. How much oxygen is usually carried in 100 mL blood?
The answer here is 20 mL O_2/100 mL of blood. This reason is that in 100 mL of blood, there is approximately 15 g of haemoglobin. One gram of haemoglobin binds to 1.34 mL of O_2 when fully saturated. Therefore, 15 × 1.34 = is 20 mL O_2/100 mL.

14. A 50-year-old asthmatic has a tidal volume of 350 mL on spirometry and a respiratory rate in clinic of 15 breaths per minute. What is his minute ventilation?

Minute ventilation = Respiratory rate × Tidal volume
= 15 × 350
= 5250 mL/min

15. Substance X is filtered freely but is not secreted by the kidney. Substance X has a plasma volume of 500 mg/L, and the urine excretion rate is 15 mg/min. Inulin clearance is 100 mL/min. What is the rate of tubular reabsorption of substance X?

Excretion = (filtration + secretion) − Reabsorption
15 = (100 + 0) − reabsorption

Rearrange the equation, such that . . .
Reabsorption = 100 − 15
= 85 mg/min

16. Calculate the renal clearance of substance X given the following:

   • T_{max} of substance X = 200 mg/min
   • GFR = 90 mL/min
   • Plasma concentration of X = 100 mg/100 mL
   • Urine volume = 60 mL/20 min
   • Renal fraction = 20%
   • Haematocrit = 50
   • Urine concentration of X = 25 mg/10 mL
   • Blood pressure = 120/85

   Renal clearance of X = (urine concentration × urine flow rate)/plasma concentration
   i.e. $(U_x \times V)/P_x$
   = 25 × 60/100
   = 15 mL/min

17. A woman suffering with anaemia has arrived for her haematology clinic review. She has a haematocrit level of 45%, and her red blood cell count is $7.2 \times 10^6/\mu L$. Calculate her MCV.

   MCV = (haematocrit (%)/red blood cells) × 10*
   = (45/7.2) × 10
   = 62.5 fl
   *If haematocrit is expressed in l/l, multiply by 1000 instead of 10.

18. Your consultant reviews the above patient in the haematology clinic and asks you to calculate the mean corpuscular haemoglobin concentration (MCHC). Her Hb is 11.2 g/dL.

   MCHC = (Hb/haematocrit) × 100
   = (11.2/45) × 100
   = 24.89 g/dL

19. An 18-year-old man presents to the emergency department having set fire to himself in an attempt to take his own life. He weighs 70 kg and the burns cover 36% of his total body surface area. What volume of fluid will you prescribe to be given over the first 8 hours?

   Parkland formula = 2 mL × % Body surface area burns × Weight
   = 2 × 36% × 70
   = 5040 mL/2

   (The reason why we divide by 2 is because, in accordance with ATLS guidelines, half of the fluid calculate by the Parkland formula is given within the first 8 hours of the injury. The remaining fluid is given over the subsequent 16 hours and titrated to urine output.)
   = 2520 mL

20. A 37-year-old soldier received a severe electrical burn that has affected both of his upper limbs, the anterior aspect of his torso and the perineum. He weighs 90 kg. What volume of fluids should he receive over the first 8 hours?

Total surface area for burns = 9 + 9 + 18 + 1 = 37%
Parkland formula = 4 mL × % Body surface area burns × Weight
= 4 × 37% × 90
= 13320 mL/2
(The reason why we divide by 2 is because, in accordance with ATLS guidelines, half of the fluid calculate by the Parkland formula is given within the first 8 hours of the injury. The remaining fluid is given over the subsequent 16 hours and titrated to urine output.)
= 6660 mL

Index

Note: Page numbers in *italics* indicate a figure and page numbers in **bold** indicate a table on the corresponding page. Page numbers followed by "n" with numbers refer to notes.

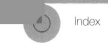

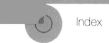

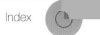

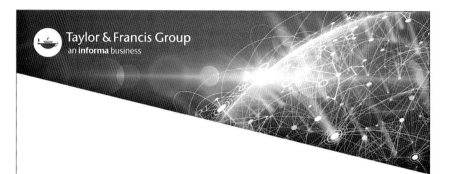